Small An Spinal Disorders

Diagnosis and Surgery

Simon J Wheeler
BVSc, PhD, MRCVS
Diplomate, European College of Veterinary Neurology
The Royal Veterinary College
University of London
UK

Nicholas J H Sharp
BVetMed, PhD, MRCVS
Diplomate, American College of Veterinary Surgeons
Diplomate, American College of Veterinary Internal Medicine (Neurology)
Diplomate, European College of Veterinary Surgeons
Department of Companion Animal and Species Medicine
College of Veterinary Medicine,
North Carolina State University
USA

Illustrations
Joseph E Trumpey
AB, MFA, CMI
Medical Illustrator, Biomedical Communications
College of Veterinary Medicine
North Carolina State University
USA

Photography
Wendy P Savage
BA
Biomedical Photographer, Biomedical Communications
College of Veterinary Medicine
North Carolina State University
USA

Mosby-Wolfe

London Baltimore Barcelona Bogotá Boston Buenos Aires Carlsbad, CA Chicago Madrid Mexico City Milan Naples, FL New York Philadelphia St. Louis Seoul Singapore Sydney Taipei Tokyo Toronto Wiesbaden

Development Editor	Gillian Harris
Cover Design	Lara Last/Rob Curran
Production	Cathy Martin
Publisher	Jill Northcott

Mosby-Wolfe

An imprint of Harcourt Publishers Limited.

Copyright © 1994 Times Mirror International Publishers Limited.
Copyright © 2000 Harcourt Publishers Limited.

Printed by Grafos S.A, Arte sobre papel, Barcelona, Spain.

Reprinted 1997
Reprinted 2000

The illustrations in this book are the copyright of North Carolina State University.

ISBN 0 7234 1897 7

All rights reserved. No part of this publication may be reproduced, stored in a retrieval system, copied or transmitted, in any form or by any means, electronic, mechanical, photocopying, recording or otherwise without written permission from the Publisher (Harcourt Publishers Limited, Robert Stevenson House, 1-3 Baxter's Place, Leitn walk, Edinburgh EH1 3AF) or in accordance with the provisions of the Copyright Act. 1988, or under the terms of any licence permiting limited copying issued by the Copyright Licensing Agency, 90 Tottenham Court Road, London, W1P OLP, UK .

Any person who does any unauthorised act in relation to this publication may be liable to criminal prosecution and civil claims for damages.

Permission to photocopy or reproduce solely for internal or personal use is permited for libraries or other users registered with the Copyright Clearance Center, and paid directly to the Copyright Clearance Center 222 Rosewood Drive, Danvers MA 01923 USA. This consent does not extend to other kinds of copying for general distribution, for advertising or promotional purposes, for creating new collected works or for resale.

A CIP catalogue record for this book is available from the British Library.

Library of Congress Cataloging-in-Publication Data has been applied for

CONTENTS

Foreword	iv
Preface	v
Acknowledgements	vi

1. FUNCTIONAL ANATOMY	**8**
Nervous tissue	8
Skeleton	12
Blood supply	18
2. PATIENT EXAMINATION	**21**
Approach to the patient	21
History	21
Physical examination	21
Neurological examination	23
Localization of lesions	29
Assessing the severity of the lesion	30
Determining the aetiology	30
3. DIAGNOSIS AND DIFFERENTIAL DIAGNOSIS	**31**
4. DIAGNOSTIC AIDS	**34**
Routine laboratory analysis	34
Cerebrospinal fluid	35
Radiography	43
Special radiographic procedures	46
Principles of spinal radiology	49
Other imaging techniques	52
Clinical electrophysiology	54
Biopsy	55
5. INSTRUMENTATION	**57**
6. PREOPERATIVE ASSESSMENT	**61**
Clinical assessment	61
Pharmacological considerations	62
Anaesthetic considerations	63
Surgical considerations	64
Client communication	66
7. CERVICAL DISC DISEASE	**68**
Clinical signs	68
Diagnosis	69
Treatment options	70
Surgery	71
Complications	82
Postoperative care	83
Prognosis	83
Cervical disc disease in cats	84
8. THORACOLUMBAR DISC DISEASE	**85**
Clinical signs	85
Diagnosis	87
Treatment	88
Surgery	89
Complications	107
Postoperative care	107
Prognosis	108
Thoracolumbar disc disease in cats	108
9. ATLANTOAXIAL SUBLUXATION	**109**
Clinical signs	110
Diagnosis	110
Treatment	111
Surgery	111
Complications	120
Postoperative care	121
Prognosis	121
Atlantoaxial subluxation in cats	121
10. LUMBOSACRAL DISEASE	**122**
Clinical signs	123
Diagnosis	124
Treatment	127
Surgery	127
Complications	134
Postoperative care	134
Prognosis	134
11. CAUDAL CERVICAL SPONDYLOMYELOPATHY	**135**
Clinical signs	135
Diagnosis	136
Presurgical evaluation	139
Treatment	140
Surgery	141
Complications	153
Prognosis	154
12. NEOPLASIA	**156**
Clinical signs	156
Diagnosis	156
Pathology	158
Treatment	159
Surgery	160
Complications	167
Postoperative care	168
Prognosis	168
Feline spinal tumours	168
13. TRAUMA	**171**
Initial assessment	171
Neurological examination	172
Radiography	172
Biomechanics	173
Treatment	178
Surgery	184
Feline spinal injuries	190
Prognosis	191
14. MISCELLANEOUS CONDITIONS	**192**
15. POSTOPERATIVE CARE	**203**
Analgesia	203
Nursing care	205
Flooring for recumbent patients	206
Physiotherapy	208
Control of urinary function	210
Postoperative complications	215
GLOSSARY OF ACRONYMS	**220**
INDEX	**221**

FOREWORD

Spinal surgery has been performed routinely in dogs and cats for only 40 years. The potential value, and complications, of laminectomy and fenestration for treatment of intervertebral disk disease were first published in the early to mid 1950s by Olsson, Hoerlein, and Vaughan, among others.[1-3] Application of these and other surgical techniques to additional spinal disorders came even later. Perhaps, not surprisingly, given spinal surgery's relatively brief history, controversy still persists among 'experts' regarding the surgical management of essentially all spinal diseases, ranging from intervertebral disk disease, to spinal fracture, to disorders affecting the caudal cervical and lumbosacral regions of large breed dogs. All who practice this rewarding, and at times frustrating, art thus remain, in a way, pioneers.

Over the past 40 years, veterinarians performing spinal surgery have been guided by two at times conflicting principles, a desire to restore complete function as soon as possible on the one hand, but with the reservation, on the other, that 'no harm be done.' In this spirit, there was initial reluctance to perform laminectomies because of the potential for iatrogenic injury. Reflecting upon this, Olsson wrote in 1951 that 'it is well known (from human medicine) that interventions into the spinal canal may cause nervous complications, however carefully the operation is performed' and that 'animal experiments had shown the same thing.[1]' Based on his own experiences and those of others, Vaughan indicated in 1958 that 'with present techniques, laminectomy is altogether too hazardous to be recommended in the treatment of a dog with disc protrusion.[3]' Veterinarians performing spinal surgery benefited from this wise counsel and took it upon themselves to refine existing techniques, and in some cases, to develop new procedures for managing spinal disorders. Improved surgical instrumentation, most notably power equipment and operating microscopes, contributed further to our progress.

As a result, veterinary surgeons are now able to routinely operate within the vertebral canal, and indeed, the dural sac itself, while in most instances, remaining true to the basic tenet of 'do no harm.' Nevertheless, all who perform spinal surgery, upon honest reflection, would admit that considerable progress is still needed. The management of many spinal disorders remains problematic, and our overall success rates, too low. In striving for additional progress, we will continue to be guided by our collective experiences, as recorded in peer-reviewed scientific papers. Summaries of this material traditionally have been presented in large multi-authored textbooks covering all aspects of small animal surgery or veterinary neurology. Technical aspects of the surgical procedures often have necessarily been short-changed. Illustrative material generally has been confined to black and white schematics and photographs of inconsistent quality. This textbook effectively brings the discussion of spinal surgery 'under one roof.' Because both authors have dual training in clinical neurology and neurosurgery, they have been able to guide readers through all steps of the neurologic evaluation, as well as the actual surgery. Material has been presented in a systematic fashion, so that both the specialist and general practitioner can benefit. Moreover, through their collaboration with Joe Trumpey and Wendy Savage, the authors have provided illustrative material of unequalled excellence. All of us involved in spinal surgery will benefit from this textbook and must commend the authors for bringing it to us.

Joe N. Kornegay DVM PhD
Professor of Neurology
Department of Companion Animal and Special Species Medicine
College of Veterinary Medicine, North Carolina State University

---

[1] Olsson S-E: On disc protrusion in dog (Endochondrosis intervertebralis). *Acta Orthoped. Scand.* (Suppl. 8): 51–62, 1951.
[2] Hoerlein BF: Further evaluation of the treatment of disc protrusion paraplegia in the dog. *J. Am. Vet. Med. Assoc.* **129**: 495–502, 1956.
[3] Vaughan LC: Studies on intervertebral disc protrusion in the dog. *Brit. Vet. J.* **105**: 458–463, 1958.

PREFACE

Spinal diseases have long been recognised as important causes of disability in animals. Early veterinary textbooks contain clearly recognizable descriptions of paralysis caused by intervertebral disc herniation.

Patients with spinal disease form a high proportion of the case load in most referral centres. In many private and academic institutions, medical neurology and neurosurgery are dealt with together. In others, neurosurgery falls under the responsibility of orthopaedic surgeons. Thus there is a diverse group of clinicians interested in spinal disease, including neurologists, surgeons, radiologists, and general practitioners. This book will help students and general practitioners to diagnose patients with spinal diseases, assess treatment options, and determine the prognosis. It should help clinicians to undertake neurosurgery, by the step by step illustrations of various surgical procedures.

Surgery and neurology residents in training will find the information valuable in learning the surgical techniques. Experienced surgeons may gain some assistance in the use of unfamiliar methods.

Clinicians unfamiliar with neurology would be best advised to read the introductory chapters on anatomy, diagnosis, and differential diagnosis. Those more familiar with the subject may wish to consult the specific chapters on disease conditions directly.

We have aimed to produce a practical guide to diagnosis and surgical treatment of spinal diseases. We have covered the most commonly used surgical procedures under the disease for which they are most likely to be used. Study of the surgical illustrations and practice on cadavers should allow the clinician to master the techniques shown. The important areas of the acute care of the spinal patient and postoperative care are covered, because these can have a significant impact on the prognosis for recovery of neurological function.

This book does not aim to be a comprehensive neurology text. There are other books that fulfil that role, and these are listed in Chapters 2 and 3. We have concentrated on the commonly encountered spinal diseases and what we believe to be the most appropriate methods of surgical treatment. There are some differences in approach throughout the world and we have found that a liberal examination of different opinions has been very instructive. As we both have had experience as neurologists and neurosurgeons in Great Britain and the USA, we have tried to embrace what we feel to be the best of these two worlds. Experienced neurosurgeons will doubtless find much to disagree with in our approach, but we hope to have provided a balanced view that should prove thought provoking.

We have aimed to use the nomenclature of the *Nomina Anatomica Veterinaria* (1983) throughout the book. Some of the anatomical terms may be unfamiliar and we have included more commonly used terms where confusion could arise.

The value of this book will be gauged by whether it meets its aims of educating clinicians in the diagnosis and surgical treatment of spinal diseases. It will be interesting to review the content in 10 years' time, to see which techniques are still in fashion and how neurosurgery in general has advanced.

Simon Wheeler
Nick Sharp

ACKNOWLEDGEMENTS

We have many people to thank for their help in producing this book.

During our time at North Carolina State University we had the opportunity to work with, and learn from, some outstanding neurologists: Drs. Joe Kornegay, Andrew Hopkins, Larry Gainsburg, Billy Thomas, Rod Bagley, Laurent Cauzinille, Steve Lane, Scott Plummer, and Christine Thomson.

W. David Fischer provided outstanding technical support during the early stages of this project, for which we are most grateful. The skills of Joe Trumpey and Wendy Savage cannot be overstated. Their contribution to this book is immense. Other members of Biomedical Communications provided expertise and assistance, including Ree Coan and Dan Tucker. Dr Kip Berry and Mr Chris Lamb were most helpful in procuring radiographs. Michelle Moore, CASS Department Secretary, has coped with many communication tasks with her usual calm authority. Dr Billy Thomas was also most helpful in chasing up various errant slides.

Peer review of the manuscript was very important and we are most grateful to the following for doing this so thoroughly and promptly: Rod Bagley, Steve Butterworth, Gary Clayton Jones, Jerry Davies, Hamish Denny, Cathy Garden, Steve Gilson, Andy Hopkins, Malcolm McKee, Russell Patterson, Ian Robertson, Geoff Skerritt, and Billy Thomas. Professor Elizabeth Stone was kind enough to review the whole manuscript and made many valuable comments. Margaret Hemingway of the Word Processing Department at NC State University edited the text with great expertise. Janet Wheeler also read the manuscript and the proofs.

Production of colour illustrations is expensive and we are grateful to two sponsors: John Lapish BVetMed, BSc, MRCVS of Veterinary Instrumentation and Mr Peter Symons of Ethicon U.K. Ltd.

Pacific Research Laboratories made the plastic vertebrae in **436**, **440**, and **450–452**.

FIGURES ACKNOWLEDGEMENTS

Several colleagues loaned illustrations and photographs for which we are indebted.
Dr C.W. Betts **169**, **276**, **411**, **445**; Mr D.G. Clayton Jones **417**; Dr J.V. Davies **65–67**, **69**, **73**, **74**, **77**, **470**; Dr A. L. Hopkins **64**, **177**, **178**; Dr J.N. Kornegay **62**; Mr Malcolm McKee **342–344**; Dr D.J. Meuten **105**; Drs R.H. Patterson and G.K. Smith **426**, **427**, **430**, **431**, **437**; Dr S.B. Plummer **40**; Dr D.C. Richardson **501**; Mr I. Robertson **182–184**; Dr. G.J. Spodnick **478**; Dr W.B. Thomas **416**, **418**.

DEDICATION

Professor Ian R. Griffiths
Glasgow University Veterinary School

For our introduction to Neurology and his continued enthusiastic support and advice, we are very grateful.

1. FUNCTIONAL ANATOMY

A knowledge of functional anatomy is important for both understanding the neurological examination and performing spinal surgery. This chapter concentrates on clinically relevant points of anatomy and physiology, including surgical landmarks. Some radiographs have been used for illustration, and the reader is also directed to the normal radiographic anatomy illustrated in Chapter 4. For more detail see 'Further Reading,' page 20.

NERVOUS TISSUE

Spinal cord
The spinal cord lies within the vertebral canal, fitting snugly in the thoracolumbar spine, but with more space in the cervical spine. The residual space is filled with epidural fat. The spinal cord extends from the caudal limit of the brain stem at the foramen magnum to the caudal lumbar vertebrae, terminating in the sixth lumbar vertebra (L_6) in most dogs, and in L_7 in cats, with some variation.

The spinal cord is divided into segments.
- Cervical 1–8.
- Thoracic 1–13.
- Lumbar 1–7.
- Sacral 1–3.
- Caudal (variable number).

It is wider at the cervical and lumbar intumescences (segments C_6–T_2 and L_4–S_3 respectively), from which the lower motor neurons (LMNs) to the thoracic and pelvic limbs arise. These segments contain the cell bodies for the LMNs, the ventral horn cells, thus the spinal cord is thicker in these areas.

The spinal cord is composed of central grey matter and peripheral white matter (**1**). A dorsal sulcus and ventral fissure, lined by pia mater, divide the spinal cord into two halves. Dorsal and ventral roots exit the spinal cord at each segment and join to form the segmental spinal nerves. There are eight cervical segments, but seven cervical vertebrae. The C_1 spinal nerves leave through the lateral foramina in C_1 vertebra. The rest of the cervical spinal nerves exit the vertebral canal cranial to the vertebrae of the same annotation, except C_8 nerves, which exit between C_7 and T_1 vertebrae.

The thoracic and lumbar spinal nerves exit behind the same-named vertebrae.

The nerve roots are partly ensheathed by meninges, which are continuous with the epineurium.

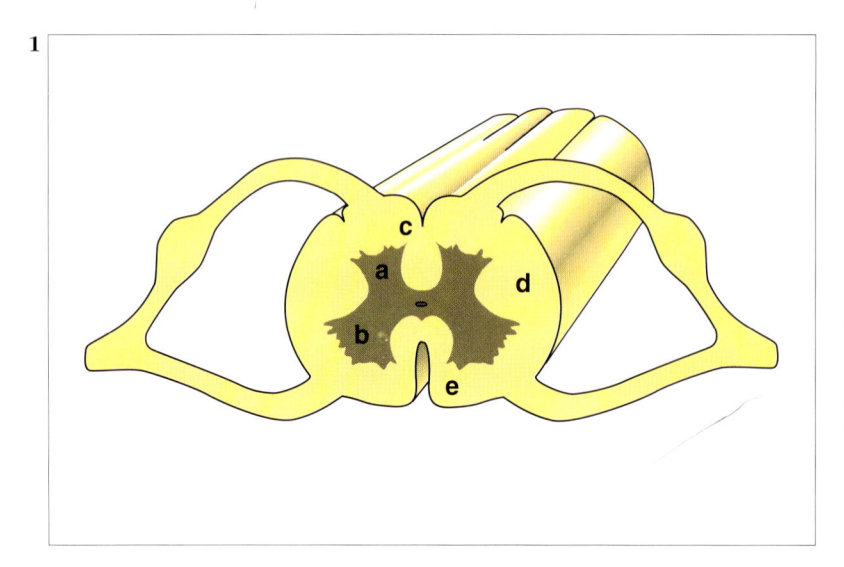

1 Spinal cord in transverse section. The grey matter forms an H shape with two dorsal horns (**a**) and two ventral horns (**b**). The white matter tracts are divided into dorsal funiculi, between the dorsal roots (**c**); lateral funiculi, between dorsal and ventral roots (**d**); and ventral funiculi, between the ventral roots (**e**).

1. FUNCTIONAL ANATOMY

Relationship of spinal cord segments to vertebrae

Some spinal cord segments lie in the vertebra of the same annotation, but others do not (**2**, **3**). Neurological lesion localization refers to spinal cord segments. It is therefore important to understand the relationship between vertebrae and spinal cord segments.

Cauda equina

The nerves of the cauda equina have a typical peripheral nerve structure and are partly ensheathed by the meninges (**4**). They tolerate deformation better than spinal cord, and there is a large epidural space in the region of the cauda equina. Thus they are usually more resistant to injury than spinal cord tissue, but if severe damage occurs, recovery is unlikely.

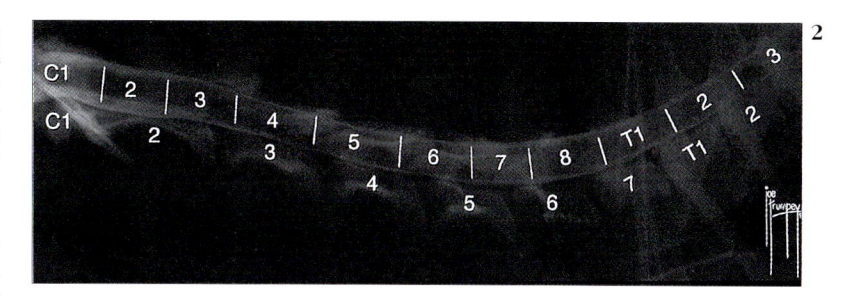

2 Position of the spinal cord segments in the cervical and cranial thoracic vertebrae. The cervical intumescence (C_6–T_2) lies within vertebrae C_4–T_2. Thus, lesions as far cranial as C_4/C_5 may cause LMN signs in the thoracic limbs.

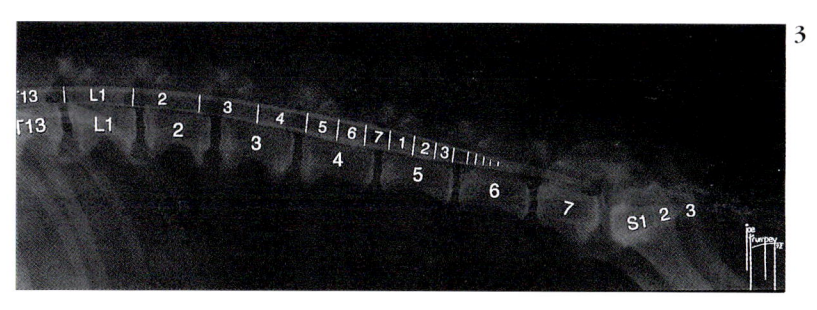

3 Position of the spinal cord segments in the lumbar vertebrae. Segments L_1 and L_2 lie in their respective vertebrae. The lumbar intumescence lies within vertebrae L_3–L_5. Thus, lesions as far cranial as L_3/L_4 intervertebral disc may cause LMN signs in the pelvic limbs. Segments L_3–L_7 lie in vertebrae L_3 and L_4. The sacral segments S_1–S_3 are in L_5 vertebrae in most dogs (This can be remembered as **5** in L_5 looks like **S** for sacral). The cord ends in L_6 in most dogs and in L_7 in cats. The cauda equina lies in the vertebral canal from L_5 vertebra into the sacrum.

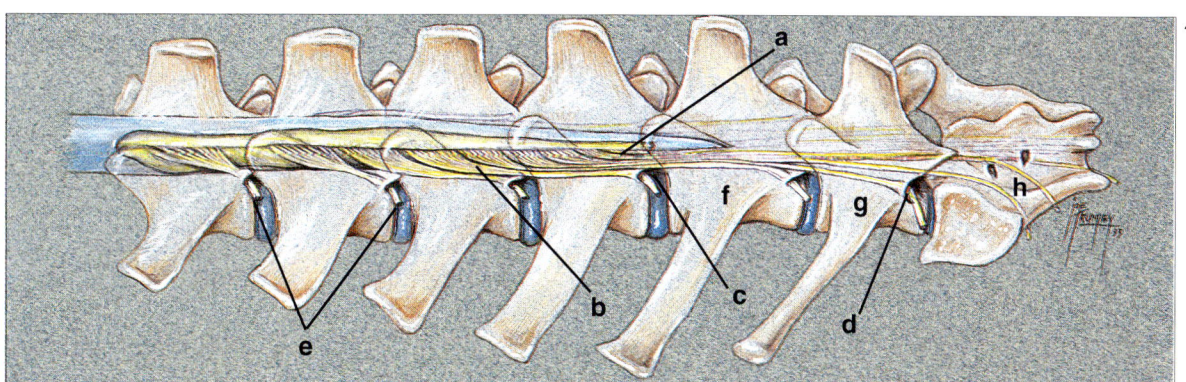

4 The terminal part of the spinal cord, comprising the sacral and caudal segments, tapers to form the conus medullaris (**a**). The nerve roots (**b**) of the caudal lumbar, sacral, and caudal spinal cord segments pass caudally and leave the vertebral canal via their respective intervertebral foraminae (**c**). The roots fuse just distal to the spinal ganglion (**d**), close to the intervertebral foramen, to form the spinal nerve (**e**). Thus, the L_7 spinal nerve roots arise from the L_7 cord segment (which lies in the vertebral canal at L_4/L_5 in dogs), and the L_7 spinal nerve leaves the vertebral canal between L_7 and the sacrum. This disparity between the location of the spinal cord segments and their respective vertebrae is a result of the differential growth of skeletal and neural structures in the embryo. The cauda equina is the collection of nerve roots descending in the vertebral canal. (Some definitions also include the conus medullaris in the cauda equina.) (**f**) L_6 vertebra; (**g**) L_7 vertebra; (**h**) sacrum.

Meninges

The meninges (**5**) surround the central nervous system (CNS). The arachnoid mater and pia mater together are termed the leptomeninges. Between the pia mater and the arachnoid mater is a space, the subarachnoid space, which is filled with the cerebrospinal fluid (CSF). The subarachnoid space is traversed by the arachnoid trabeculae, which suspend the spinal cord in the CSF. The meninges caudal to the conus medullaris form the filum terminale, which extends into the sacrocaudal vertebrae. The meningeal sac is outlined by myelography. The caudal limit to its extension varies between animals; it can terminate anywhere between L_7 and the caudal vertebrae, but usually ends in the sacrum.

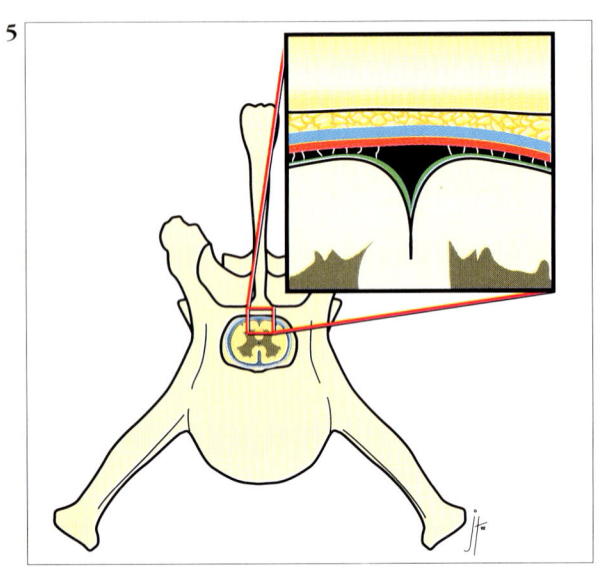

5 There are three layers of meninges. The most superficial is the dura mater, which is composed of dense connective tissue (blue). The thin arachnoid mater (red) is inside the dura mater and lies adjacent to it. These two membranes follow the larger contours of the spinal cord. The pia mater (green) is a delicate layer that lies directly on the surface of the spinal cord.

Cerebrospinal fluid

Cerebrospinal fluid is formed in the brain, mainly by the choroid plexuses, with contributions from the pia-arachnoid mater and the ependymal lining.

Cerebrospinal fluid flows mainly in a caudal direction. Most leaves the fourth ventricle of the brain through the lateral apertures into the subarachnoid space, with some entering the central canal of the spinal cord. It is absorbed through the arachnoid villi in cerebral venous sinuses, by venules in the subarachnoid space, lymphatics around the spinal nerves, and the ependymal lining.

The CSF is normally a clear, colourless fluid with a very low protein and cellular content. It suspends and protects the brain and spinal cord against shock, allows some variation in the volume of the central nervous system without altering pressure, and has some nutritional and metabolic functions.

The caudal direction of flow of CSF has some impact on clinical CSF evaluation. Fluid collected caudal to a lesion is more likely to provide diagnostic information (see Chapter 4).

Spinal cord white matter tracts

Ascending (sensory) tracts

Sensory information is gathered from the peripheral nervous system via sensory axons. The cell bodies of these axons lie in the spinal ganglia (dorsal root ganglia). Central projections of these axons ascend in the spinal cord to the brain (**6**).

Conscious proprioception is transmitted in the tracts of the dorsal funiculi. It is usually evaluated by the paw position response. From the pelvic limbs, the information is transmitted in the fasciculus gracilis, and from the thoracic limbs in the fasciculus cuneatus. These fibres project to the ipsilateral cuneate and gracile nuclei in the brain stem before the pathways cross the midline to the contralateral forebrain.

1. FUNCTIONAL ANATOMY

Unconscious proprioception is transmitted to the cerebellum in the superficial parts of the lateral funiculi. The information is carried in the dorsal and ventral spinocerebellar tracts from the pelvic limbs, and the cuneocerebellar and rostral spinocerebellar tracts from the thoracic limbs.

Temperature and superficial pain sensation are transmitted by the myelinated fibres of several tracts, including the lateral spinothalamic tract in the lateral funiculus. More severe pain (deep pain) sensation is carried by non-myelinated fibres. Both types of pain fibres cross and re-cross the midline in a multisynaptic arrangement throughout the spinal cord, thus providing a diffuse bilateral pattern of ascending pain fibres from each limb.

Information on the degree of urinary bladder filling is transmitted to the brain in the spinothalamic tract.

Descending (motor) tracts

Two systems are responsible for the transmission of motor function—the upper motor neuron (UMN) and LMN systems (7).

Function of flexor muscles is facilitated by the corticospinal and rubrospinal tracts. The fibres of the corticospinal tract arise in the cerebral cortex, and most decussate at the spinomedullary junction and descend in the lateral corticospinal tracts of the lateral funiculi. Fibres that do not decussate descend in the ventral corticospinal tracts, which lie in the ventral funiculi. The rubrospinal fibres originate in the red nucleus of the brain stem, cross the midline and descend in the rubrospinal tract of the lateral funiculus. The vestibulospinal tracts and reticulospinal tracts also influence motor function. The function of extensor muscles is facilitated by these tracts, which lie in the ventral funiculi. The

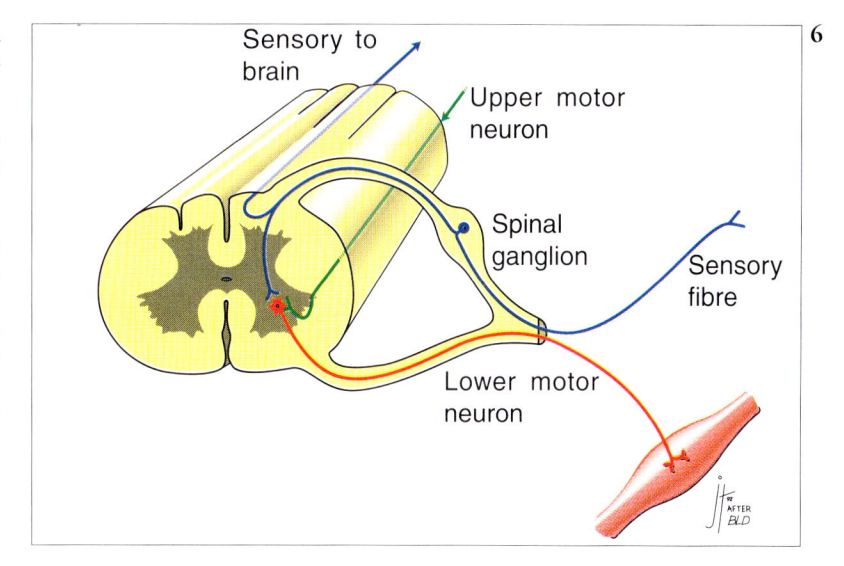

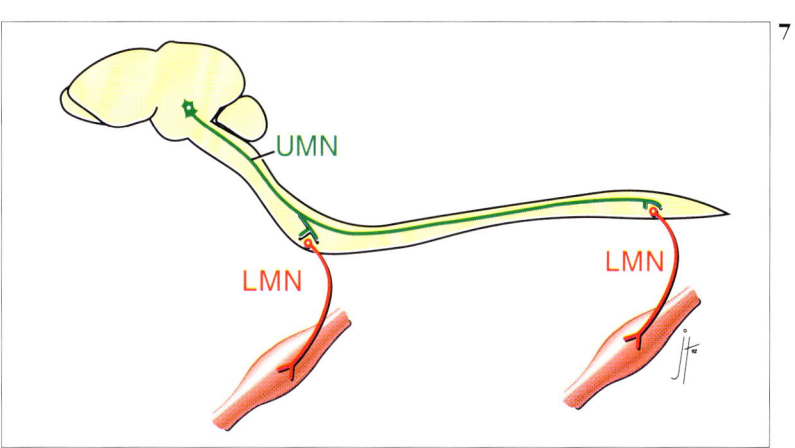

6 The LMN is the effector neuron of the reflex arc. The cell bodies are the ventral horn cells, which lie in the ventral horn grey matter of the spinal cord. The axons leave the spinal cord in the ventral roots and pass through the brachial and lumbosacral plexuses to form the periphery nerve trunks of the limbs. The sensory arm of the reflex arc is the sensory neuron. It arises in the periphery and enters the spinal cord via the dorsal root. It projects to the LMN (via an interneuron in some reflex pathways) and a branch also ascends in the spinal cord.

7 The UMN system originates in the motor cortex of the contralateral forebrain. It facilitates flexor and extensor muscles, initiating voluntary movement and maintaining muscle tone.

vestibulospinal fibres arise in the ipsilateral vestibular nuclei. They facilitate extensors and inhibit flexors on the ipsilateral side, and have the opposite effect on the muscles of the contralateral limbs.

Voluntary bladder emptying is mediated through fibres in the tectospinal and reticulospinal tracts of the ventral funiculi.

Ascending motor tract

In dogs, an ascending motor tract originates in the border cells of the dorsolateral grey matter of the lumbar spinal cord segments. Their axons pass cranially in the contralateral fasciculus proprius of the lateral funiculus and inhibit the extensor muscles of the thoracic limb.

Interference with this pathway, as seen in some severe thoracic spinal cord lesions, is manifest as the Schiff–Sherrington sign (see **40**).

Spinal cord nerve fibres and the effect of compression

The white matter tracts of the spinal cord are composed of nerve fibres of different sizes, most of which have a myelin sheath. The largest fibres are myelinated, and these are the most rapidly conducting; they transmit conscious proprioception. Motor fibres are intermediate sized myelinated fibres. Pain perception is transmitted by the smallest myelinated fibres and by nonmyelinated fibres.

Larger diameter fibres are more susceptible to damage by compression than fibres of lesser diameter; small fibres are the most resistant. The progression of clinical signs seen with increasing spinal cord compression is explained largely by this feature. Mild lesions cause loss of conscious proprioception. Increasingly severe lesions cause loss of the ability to bear weight, loss of voluntary movement and, finally, loss of deep pain sensation.

The position of the spinal cord tracts contributes to the progression of signs. The ascending conscious proprioceptive tracts (fasciculus gracilis and cuneatus) lie superficially in the dorsal funiculus and, therefore, are most susceptible to compression. In contrast, the spinothalamic tracts and ascending reticular system, which carry pain perception, are more deeply positioned, and the fibres cross the spinal cord at various levels. Thus a lesion must involve most of the diameter of the spinal cord for the patient to lose deep pain sensation. This point and the fact that pain fibres are the most resistant to pressure explains why loss of deep pain sensation is such a severe clinical sign. (See 'Assessing the severity of the lesion,' page 30).

SKELETON

The vertebral column is composed of a series of vertebrae, most of which are joined by the intervertebral discs, and synovial joints between the articular processes.

Vertebrae

The number of different types of vertebrae are as follows: cervical 7; thoracic 13; lumbar 7; sacral 3; caudal 20 (approximately). Variations are possible, particularly in the transition zones between thoracic to lumbar, and lumbar to sacral vertebrae. The most common are variations in the number of ribs, and abnormal articulations with the ilium. The importance of this is in recognizing landmarks at surgery. The sum of the thoracic and lumbar vertebrae is generally 20.

The vertebrae have various common features, but there are differences between the groups. Each vertebra has a vertebral body, which lies ventral to the spinal cord, and is joined to its neighbours by intervertebral discs. In immature animals, the vertebral bodies have cranial and caudal growth plates, which close by about 11 months of age in dogs. The centre of the vertebral body is composed of cancellous bone, which is red and relatively soft. The margins of the vertebral body are made of hard, dense, white cortical bone, which also forms the vertebral end plates adjacent to the intervertebral discs. The types of bone provide an important guide to the depth of penetration in surgical procedures (see **299**, **300**).

Each vertebra has a vertebral arch, which forms the dorsal and lateral parts of the vertebral canal enclosing the spinal cord. The arch is made up of the pedicles lateral to the vertebral canal and the lamina dorsally. The vertebral arch also has cortical and cancellous bone, although the cancellous bone may be very thin in small dogs and cats. Most vertebrae have transverse processes projecting laterally from the vertebral body, a spinous process projecting dorsally from the lamina, and cranial and caudal articular processes on the vertebral arch. Other bony processes vary with the group of vertebrae.

Between each pair of vertebrae there is an intervertebral foramen, through which pass the spinal nerves and blood vessels.

Cervical vertebrae

There are seven cervical vertebrae. The first two are distinct: the atlas (C_1) and axis (C_2) (**8**). The other cervical vertebrae each have a similar morphology (**9**). The large transverse processes of C_6 project ventrally and are important surgical landmarks; the C_5/C_6 intervertebral disc lies between the cranial edges of these transverse processes (see **151**).

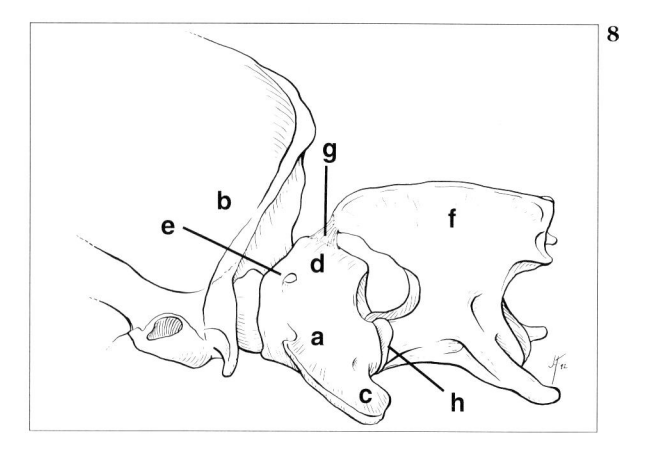

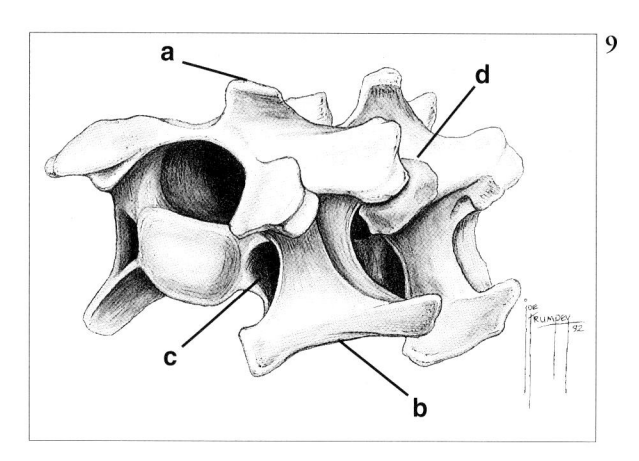

8 Atlas and axis. The atlas C_1 (**a**) articulates with the skull (**b**) via the atlanto-occipital joints. C_1 has very prominent transverse processes (**c**), which are easily palpated. There is no spinous process on the dorsal arch (**d**). The vertebral body is small, the bulk of the vertebra being composed of lateral masses. Caudally on the body there are two articular processes, which articulate with C_2. There is no intervertebral disc between C_1 and C_2. A prominent ventral tubercle lies on the caudoventral aspect of C_1. This can be palpated at surgery when the region is approached ventrally. There are lateral vertebral foraminae in the vertebral arch (**e**), through which pass the C_1 spinal nerves. Also, there are transverse foraminae in the transverse processes, through which pass the vertebral arteries (see **21**). The axis (C_2) has a large spinous process (**f**), which extends cranially over the atlas and is connected to it by the dorsal atlantoaxial ligament (**g**). The dens projects cranially from the vertebral body into the atlas and lies on the floor of the vertebral canal (see **240**). The dens originates embryologically as part of C_1. It has a growth plate at its attachment to the body of C_2, which can separate. The atlas and axis are connected by synovial joints between the articular processes, which lie ventral to the vertebral canal (**h**).

9 Cervical vertebrae. The spinous processes are small (**a**), and the transverse processes (**b**) project laterally, with the exception of C_6, where they are directed ventrally (see **68**, **151**). There are transverse foramina (**c**), through which the major blood vessels pass, except in C_7 (see **21**). The articular processes (**d**) lie in an oblique dorsal plane. The ventral tubercles can be palpated in the midline at surgery when the neck is approached ventrally. They lie caudally on the vertebral body, just cranial to the intervertebral space (see **68**).

Thoracic vertebrae
The 13 thoracic vertebrae articulate with the ribs (**10,11**).

Lumbar vertebrae
There are seven lumbar vertebrae (**12, 13**).

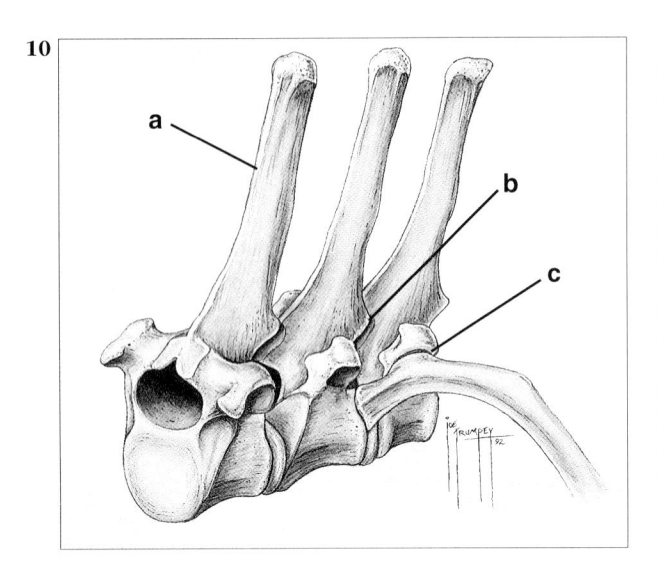

Sacral vertebrae
The three sacral vertebrae are fused into one body, which articulates with the pelvis via the sacroiliac joint. It articulates caudally with the first caudal vertebra (**13**).

10 Thoracic vertebrae. The vertebral bodies are small with large spinous processes (**a**). The spinous processes slant caudally in the cranial thoracic vertebrae (to T_{10}), and cranially in the last two thoracic vertebrae. The site of change in direction (which may vary) is termed the anticlinal vertebra (**11**). The articular processes from T_1–T_{10} are at the base of the spinous process. They are in the same oblique dorsal plane as in the cervical vertebrae, with the caudal process of the cranialmost vertebra overlying the cranial process of the caudalmost vertebra (**b**). In the caudal thoracic vertebra, the articular processes adopt a vertical orientation, as between the lumbar vertebrae. The change in orientation occurs near the anticlinal vertebra. The transverse processes are short and have a fovea (**c**) that articulates with a rib. Caudal to the mid thoracic area, caudally-projecting accessory processes are present on the pedicle.

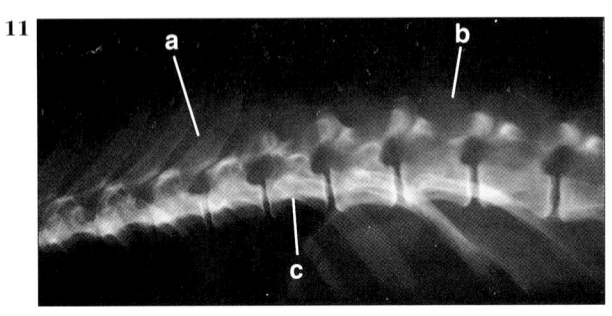

11 Radiograph of anticlinal region. Note the caudal orientation of the spinous processes in the cranial thoracic vertebrae (**a**) and the cranial orientation of the spinous processes in the caudal thoracic and lumbar vertebrae (**b**). The anticlinal vertebra is T_{11} (**c**). This can be a useful surgical landmark, but the position must be determined from the radiographs in each patient.

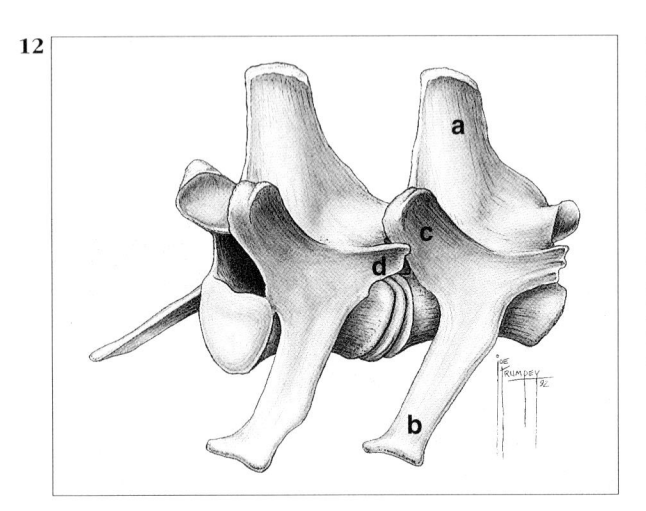

12 Lumbar vertebrae. The vertebral bodies are long (particularly in cats). The spinous processes are short and blunt, and slant cranially (**a**). The transverse processes project laterally and cranially (**b**). The L_1 transverse processes are rather small, an important feature in identifying the thoracolumbar junction at surgery. They are often difficult to palpate as they are obscured by the last rib. More caudally, the transverse processes are narrower and longer. The articular processes are vertically oriented (**c**). The caudal process of the cranialmost vertebra lies medial to the cranial process of the caudalmost vertebra. There are accessory processes on the pedicles, which project caudally (**d**). See **196**.

1. FUNCTIONAL ANATOMY

13 Lumbosacral vertebrae. L_7 differs from the other lumbar vertebrae in that the spinous process is shorter (**a**). The intervertebral foramen (**b**) between L_7 and S_1 lies cranial to the lumbosacral disc. The L_7 nerve root runs in a lateral recess in the vertebral canal of L_7 before emerging from the intervertebral foramen. The sacrum comprises the three fused sacral vertebrae (**c**), the spinous processes of which are fused and form a continuous ridge of bone (**d**). There is a marked notch in the cranial lamina of the sacrum, such that the lamina is not complete over the cauda equina at the lumbosacral junction. There are two pairs of dorsal and ventral sacral foraminae, through which pass S_1 and S_2 spinal nerves and blood vessels. The lateral wings of the sacrum (**e**) articulate laterally with the wing of the ilium.

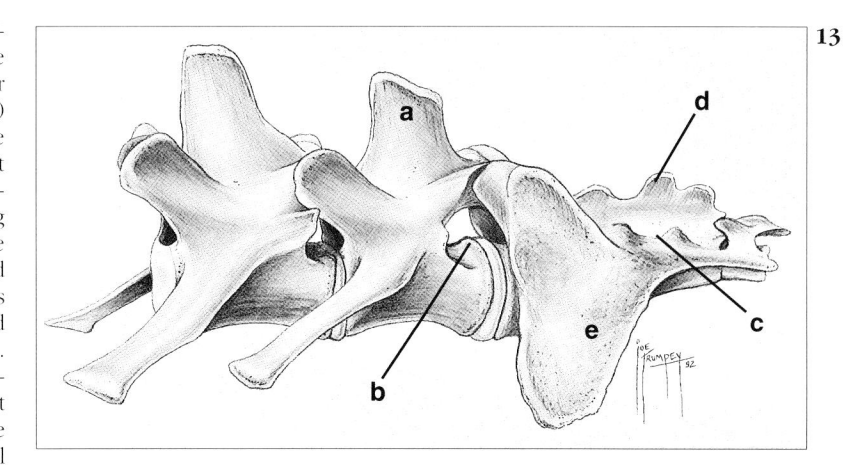

Articulations

Synovial articulations
The articular processes of the vertebral bodies have dorsal articulations, (except C_1/C_2 where the articulations are ventral, and between the fused sacral vertebrae). These joints have a joint capsule, articular cartilage and synovial fluid.

Intervertebral discs
The vertebral bodies are joined by intervertebral discs (**14**), with the exception of C_1/C_2 and the fused sacral vertebrae. The intervertebral discs provide flexibility to the vertebral column, and act as shock absorbers for the spine. The capacity to absorb shock is diminished by age changes and degeneration. They have a poor blood supply; nutrients gain access by diffusion. The anulus fibrosus has pain fibres, mainly in the outer laminae.

Intervertebral disc degeneration and disc disease
Degeneration of the intervertebral discs occurs with age and may precede disc herniation (Hansen, 1952). The two types of disc degeneration are chondroid and fibroid metamorphosis.

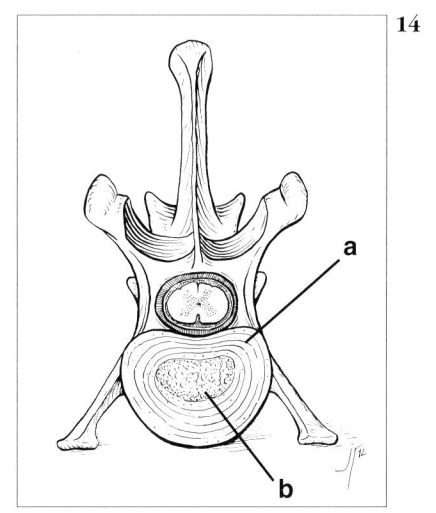

14 The divisions of the intervertebral disc. These are the outer anulus fibrosus (**a**) and the inner nucleus pulposus (**b**). The anulus fibrosus is made up of concentric fibrous laminae, the fibres of which form a strong complete structure. It is thicker ventrally and laterally than it is dorsally, and is firmly attached to the vertebral end plates by deeply penetrating fibres. The nucleus pulposus is a gelatinous structure in the young dog, but its characteristics change with age. There are a few cartilage-like cells in the normal nucleus pulposus.

- **Chondroid metamorphosis** occurs in chondrodystrophoid breeds in the first two years of life. As the disc degenerates, it dehydrates and at the same time the nucleus pulposus is invaded by hyaline cartilage. These two processes interfere with the shock absorbing capacity of the disc by reducing the hydrostatic properties of the nucleus pulposus, and by weakening the fibres of the anulus fibrosus. In most Dachshunds, by two years of age the majority of discs have undergone chondroid metamorphosis, and many nuclei have also mineralized, changing from the former jelly-like consistency to a dry, gritty substance. Normal wear and tear often causes severe weakening of the intervertebral discs, especially at the thoracolumbar junction. This explains why the peak incidence of disc disease is between three and six years of age for most chondrodystrophoid breeds of dog. Herniation of this type of disc is termed Hansen Type I herniation or *disc extrusion* (**15**).
- **Fibroid metamorphosis** occurs in nonchondrodystrophoid breeds late in life. The nucleus pulposus also dehydrates but is invaded by fibrocartilage. This process has a much later onset than chondroid metamorphosis, and the discs are usually quite normal while the dog is young and active. The nucleus pulposus does not undergo mineralization as frequently as in discs that undergo chondroid metaplasia. This occurs in older dogs and this type of herniation is termed Hansen Type II or *disc protrusion* (**16**).

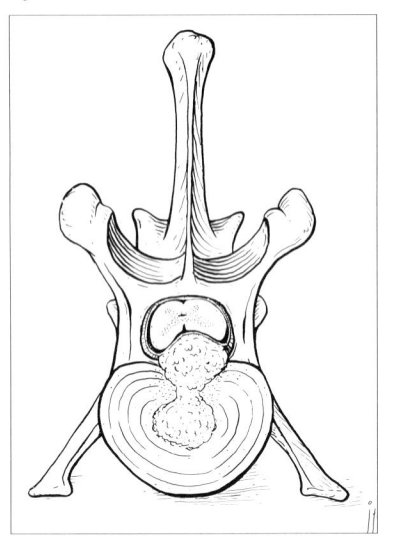

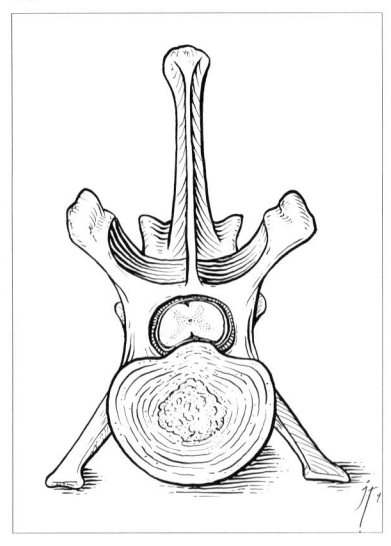

15 Hansen Type I disc extrusion. This is most common in chondrodystrophoid breeds. Following chondroid metamorphosis, the nucleus pulposus herniates into the vertebral canal through the damaged anulus fibrosus. The nucleus may take a tortuous route through the anular fibres or may explode through a large defect, when it is not unusual to find pieces of anulus fibrosus in the vertebral canal.

16 Hansen Type II disc protrusion. This occurs mainly following fibroid metamorphosis, in non-chondrodystrophoid breeds. The anulus fibrosus is damaged and there is bulging of the intervertebral disc into the vertebral canal.

1. FUNCTIONAL ANATOMY

Ligaments

The ligaments inside and outside the vertebral canal have a significant role in spinal stability and mobility (**17–20**).

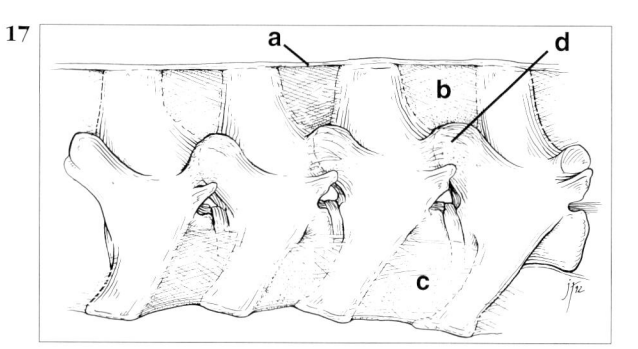

17 Ligaments and synovial articulations. The supraspinous ligament runs along the tips of the spinous processes (**a**). The lumbodorsal fascia blends with this structure in the thoracolumbar region. The interspinous ligament (**b**) is a fascial sheet that is found between the spinous processes. It is continuous with the lumbodorsal fascia in the lumbosacral region. The intertransverse ligaments (**c**) run between the transverse processes of the lumbar vertebrae. The synovial articulations between the articular processes of the vertebral arches are invested in a joint capsule (**d**).

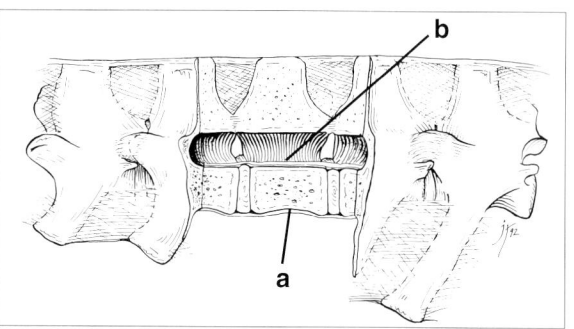

18 Cutaway diagram revealing the dorsal and ventral longitudinal ligaments. The ventral longitudinal ligament (**a**) runs along the ventral surface of the vertebral bodies; it is relatively insignificant. The dorsal longitudinal ligament (**b**) runs along the floor of the vertebral canal; it is a much more substantial structure (see **19**). The ligamentum flavum is found in the roof of the vertebral canal and in the space between adjacent vertebral laminae. It is continuous with the joint capsules of the articular processes, and may be significantly thickened in some diseases.

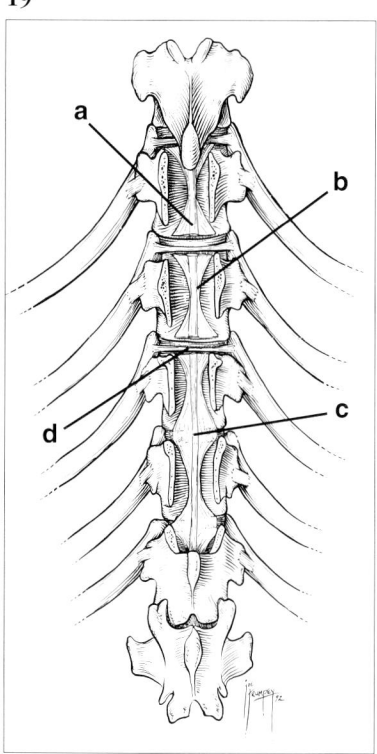

19 Ligaments. The dorsal longitudinal ligament (**a**) lies on the floor of the vertebral canal, on the dorsal surface of the vertebral bodies. The ligament is compact and narrow over the vertebral bodies (**b**). It diverges and is thus thinner over the intervertebral disc (**c**) (see also **214**). The fibres merge with those of the anulus fibrosus of the intervertebral disc. There are pain fibres in the dorsal longitudinal ligament (Forsythe and Ghoshal, 1984). Between the heads of the ribs (except T_1, T_{12}, and T_{13}) there is an intercapital ligament (**d**), which lies under the dorsal longitudinal ligament. The presence of the intercapital ligament contributes to the low incidence of intervertebral disc extrusions in the thoracic spine between T_2 and T_{11}.

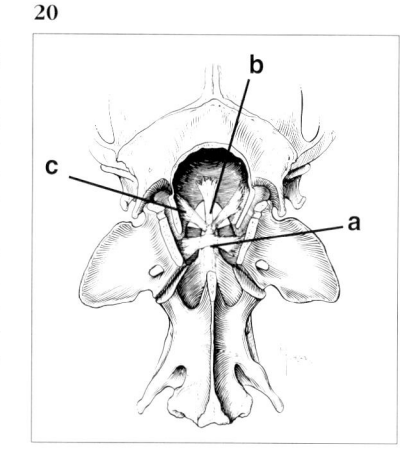

20 There are several important ligaments between C_1 and C_2. The most significant is the transverse ligament of the atlas (**a**), which runs between the sides of the atlas and over the dens. Less significant are the apical ligament of the dens (**b**) (from the dens to the foramen magnum) and the alar ligaments (**c**) (from the dens to the occipital bones). There is also a dorsal atlantoaxial ligament (see **8**) There are two ventral synovial articulations between C_1 and C_2.

The nuchal ligament extends from the dorsal arch of the axis to the spinous processes of the cranial thoracic vertebrae (see **355**). This ligament lies deep in the dorsal cervical musculature. It is a large structure but can be sectioned at surgery without impairing head and neck movement and support.

BLOOD SUPPLY

Vertebral column

The arterial supply to the vertebral column is segmental, with a spinal branch entering the vertebral canal via the intervertebral foramen, closely associated with the spinal nerve. The origin of the branches vary between the regions of the spine (**21–23**).

The venous drainage is via the internal vertebral venous plexus, which comprises two valveless veins on the floor of the vertebral canal. (These are often termed the venous sinuses.) The veins converge at midvertebral body (and sometimes join) and diverge over the intervertebral disc (see also **169**). They are thin walled and easily damaged. The venous plexus drains at the intervertebral foraminae via the intervertebral veins into the vertebral veins. The intervertebral veins may be single at each foramen, or may be paired, in which case they surround the spinal nerve. The intervertebral veins are very fragile and can bleed profusely if damaged.

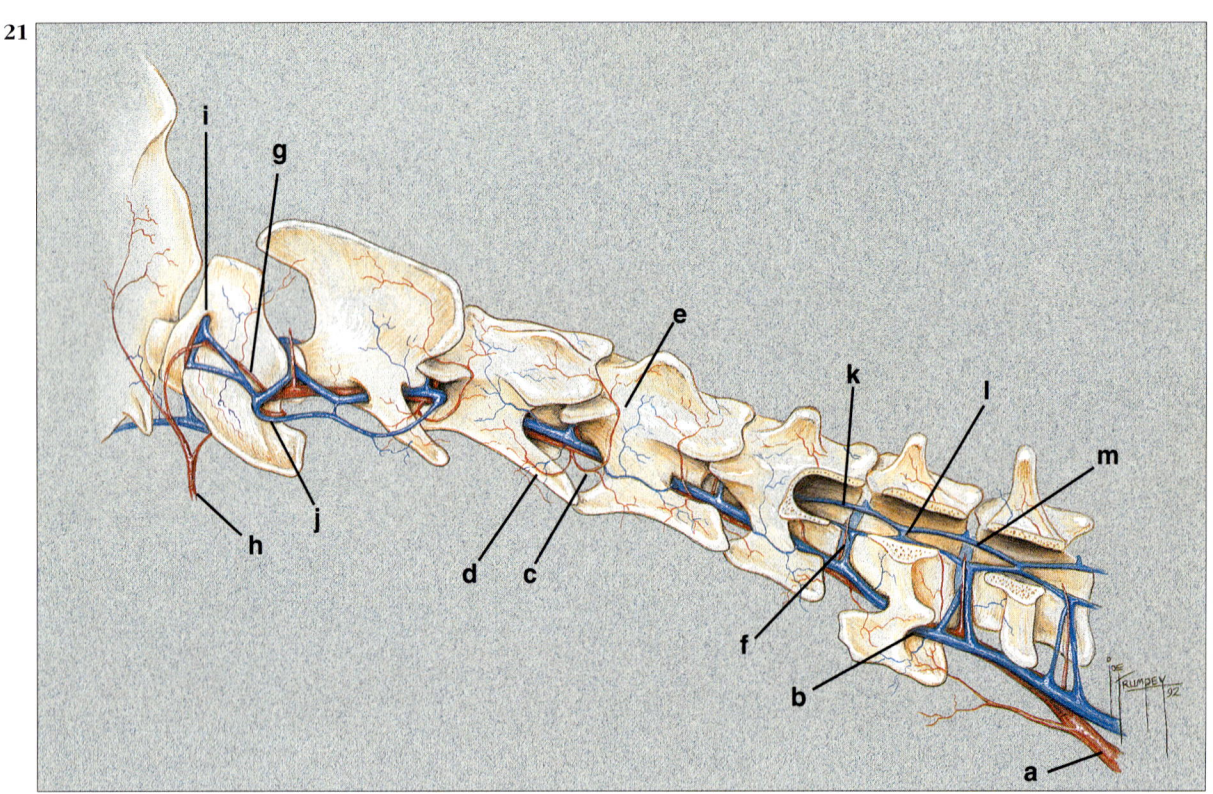

21 Blood supply to the cervical spine. The arterial supply to the cervical vertebrae is from the paired vertebral arteries (**a**), which run cranially from the subclavian arteries. The arteries run through the transverse foramina (**b**) in the transverse processes of the vertebrae (except C_7). At each segment, there are dorsal (**c**) and ventral (**d**) muscular branches. A significant vessel runs near the caudal edge of the articular processes (**e**). A spinal branch (**f**) enters the vertebral canal at each intervertebral foramen. At the atlas, the vertebral artery branches. The dorsal branch (**g**) runs over the transverse process of C_1, anastomoses with a branch of the occipital artery (**h**), and enters the vertebral canal through the lateral vertebral foramen of C_1 (**i**). The ventral branch runs under the transverse process and also anastomoses with a branch of the occipital artery (**j**). The internal vertebral venous plexus (venous sinus) (**k**) lies on the floor of the vertebral canal. The veins converge at midvertebral body (and sometimes join) (**l**), and diverge over the intervertebral disc (**m**). In the atlas and axis, the veins of the internal vertebral venous plexus are more laterally positioned.

1. FUNCTIONAL ANATOMY

22 Blood supply to the thoracic spine. This is supplied by spinal branches (**a**) from the intercostal arteries (**b**), which enter the vertebral canal via the intervertebral foramina. The internal vertebral venous plexus drains into the major veins of the dorsal thorax, mainly the azygous vein (**c**).

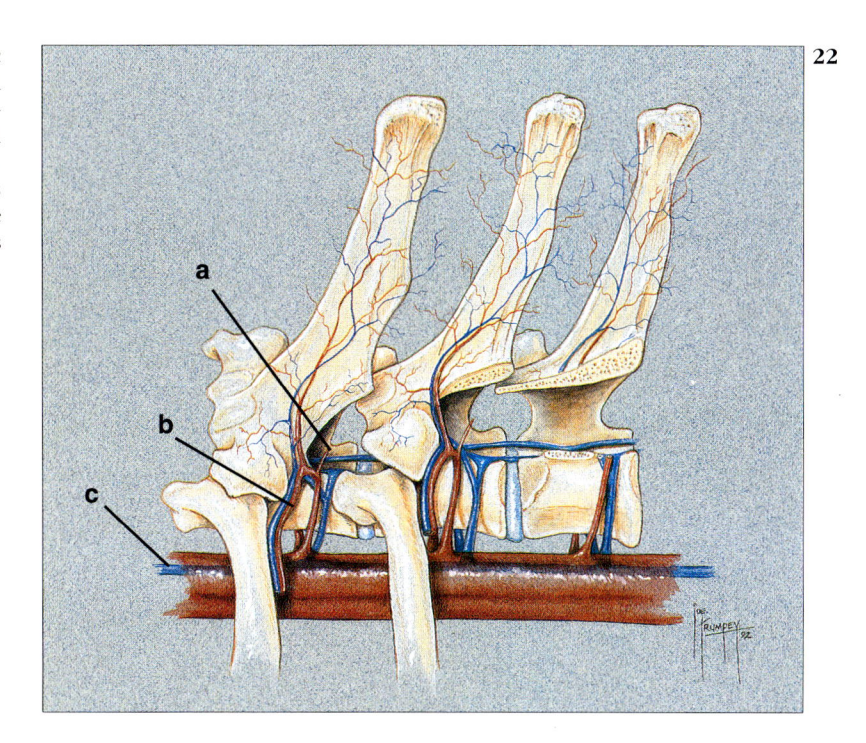

23 Blood supply to the lumbar spine. This is supplied by spinal branches (**a**) of the lumbar arteries (**b**), which arise from the aorta (**c**). A dorsal branch runs caudally behind the articular processes in the musculature (**d**). The lumbar internal vertebral venous plexus drains into major veins of the abdomen (**e**), mainly the azygous vein and the caudal vena cava.

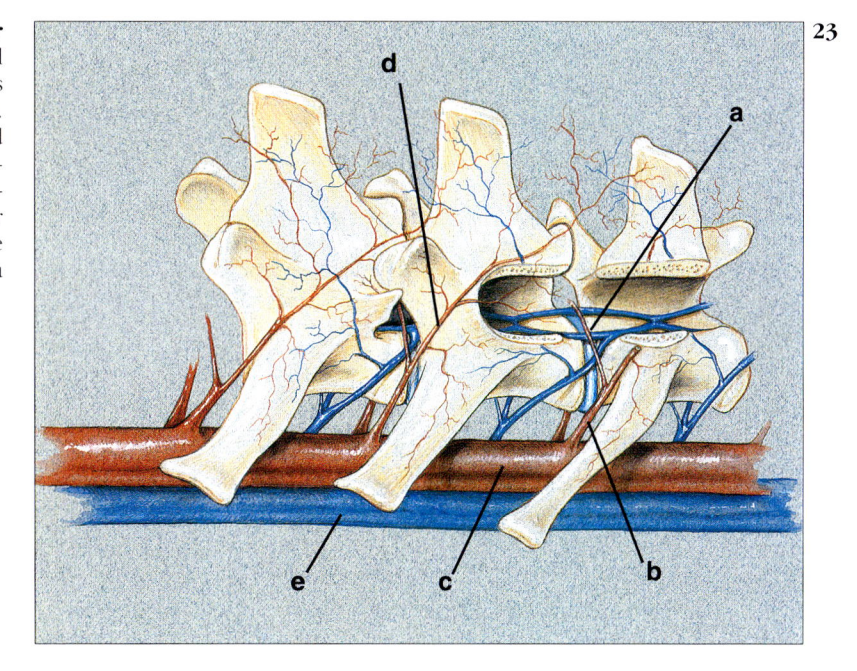

Spinal cord (24)

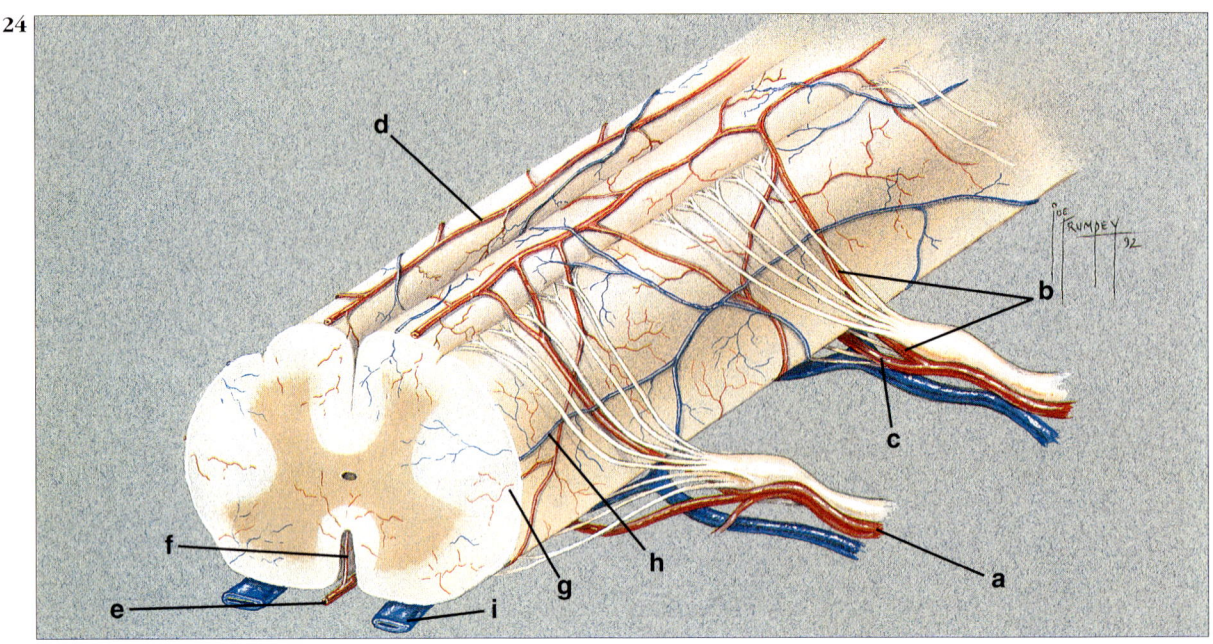

24 Blood supply to the lumbar spinal cord. This arises from the spinal arteries (**a**). These enter the vertebral canal through the intervertebral foramina and branch into dorsal (**b**) and ventral (**c**) radicular arteries, which supply an anastomotic network on the surface of the spinal cord, deep to the dura mater. Paired dorsolateral spinal arteries (**d**) run on the dorsal surface of the spinal cord and may be tortuous; they are not recognizable as a distinct entity. A ventral spinal artery (**e**) runs in the ventral fissure, and multiple anastomotic arteries connect the main vessels. Segmental arteries are inconsistently present, and several segments may be supplied by one spinal artery. The distribution is also not symmetrical. Spinal cord substance is supplied by various arteries that penetrate the surface. The vertical arteries (**f**) arise from the ventral spinal artery and pass dorsally through the ventral fissure. They supply most of the grey matter and some white matter. Radial arteries (**g**) pass centrally from the arteries on the cord surface, and enter the spinal cord substance. They supply the white matter and the peripheral grey matter. The venous drainage of the cord is also in a radial pattern, to a network of surface veins (**h**). These drain into the internal vertebral venous plexus on the floor of the vertebral canal (**i**) (these are large, valve-free vessels with occasional anastomoses in the midline). The plexus drains at the intervertebral foramina through the intervertebral veins. There are also veins draining the vertebral bodies into the plexus.

REFERENCES AND FURTHER READING

Boyd, J.S. and Paterson, C. (1991) *A Colour Atlas of Clinical Anatomy of the Dog and Cat.* Wolfe Publishing, London.

Caulkins, S.E., Purinton, P.T. and Oliver, J.E. (1989) Arterial supply to the spinal cord of dogs and cats. *American Journal of Veterinary Research* **50**, 425–430.

DeLahunta, A. (1983) *Veterinary Neuroanatomy and Clinical Neurology.* 2nd edn. W. B. Saunders Co., Philadelphia.

Evans, H.E. and Christiansen, G.C. (1979) *Miller's Anatomy of the Dog.* W. B. Saunders Co., Philadelphia.

Forsythe, W.B. and Ghoshal, N.G. (1984) Innervation of the canine thoracolumbar vertebral column. *The Anatomical Record* **208**, 57–63.

Hansen, H.J. (1952) A pathologic-anatomical study on disc degeneration in dogs. *Acta Orthopaedica Scandinavia* Suppl. **11**.

Jenkins, T. W. (1978) *Functional Mammalian Neuroanatomy.* Lea and Febiger, Philadelphia.

King, A. S. (1987) *Physiological and Clinical Anatomy of the Domestic Mammals. Vol. 1: Central Nervous System.* Oxford University Press, Oxford.

Parker, A.J. (1973) Distribution of spinal branches of the thoracolumbar segmental arteries in dogs. *American Journal of Veterinary Research* **34**, 1351–1353.

Worthman, R.P. (1956) The longitudinal vertebral venous sinuses of the dog. I. Anatomy. *American Journal of Veterinary Research* **17**, 341–348.

Worthman, R.P. (1956) The longitudinal vertebral venous sinuses of the dog. II. Functional aspects. *American Journal of Veterinary Research* **17**, 349–363.

2: PATIENT EXAMINATION

The clinical syndromes seen in animals with spinal disease are generally recognized from the history or the physical findings. However, this is not always the case. Examples when spinal disease should be suspected include nonspecific pain, and lameness not caused by orthopaedic disease. This chapter discusses the approach to a patient in which spinal disease is suspected.

APPROACH TO THE PATIENT

The aims of patient examination are as follows.
- Determine whether the problem is spinal in origin.
- Locate the site of the disorder.
- Assess the severity of the neurological deficit.
- Identify the disease process.
- Determine the most appropriate form of treatment.
- Predict the prognosis.

Knowledge of the breed incidence of spinal diseases is useful in the initial assessment, but it is a mistake to use such information as the only basis for diagnosis. Similarly, age should be considered, but again this information must be used with care.

HISTORY

Taking a history and performing a full clinical examination are prerequisites to the neurological examination. The history often leads to a provisional diagnosis. Of particular note are evidence of trauma, whether the condition is progressive, static, or episodic, previous episodes of disease, signs of pain, vaccination status, and urinary function.

PHYSICAL EXAMINATION

A general physical examination must be made in all patients. If there has been trauma or if anaesthesia is contemplated, involvement of other systems must be determined. Also, some patients in which spinal disease is suspected have disorders of other body systems. It is not at all unusual for orthopaedic disorders to mimic spinal conditions; examples are given in **Table 1**. Careful clinical examination should identify such problems, and particular note should be made of joint pain or enlargement, as these signs are present in many dogs misdiagnosed as having neurological disorders. The presence of any spinal pain or deformity should also be noted. The quality of the femoral pulse must be determined, particularly in acutely paralysed cats.

It is straightforward to perform a screening neurological examination as part of the physical examination (**Table 2**). If abnormalities are detected, carry out a complete neurological examination.

Table 1 Disorders that may mimic spinal disease

Type of disorder	Disorder
Bilateral orthopaedic disorder	Osteochondritis dissecans Cranial cruciate ligament rupture Tibial crest avulsion Fractures Coxofemoral osteoarthritis Patellar luxation
Generalized orthopaedic disorder	Hypertrophic osteodystrophy Polyarthritis Panosteitis
Muscle disorder	Infraspinatus contracture Gracilis contracture Achilles tendon rupture Myopathy

Table 2 Screening neurological examination

Observation	Mental status, posture, gait
Postural reactions	Paw position, hopping
Cranial nerves	Menace, vision, pupillary light reflex, oculovestibular response, jaw tone and temporal muscles, facial sensation, palpebral reflex, swallowing/gag
Spinal reflexes	Patellar, withdrawal, perineal
Panniculus reflex	
Spinal hyperaesthesia	
Bladder function	

HISTORY

PHYSICAL EXAMINATION

OBSERVATION

Mental status (e.g. alert, depressed, stupor, coma)

Posture (e.g. normal, paraparesis, hemiparesis, head tilt, tremor)

Gait (e.g. ataxia, circling)

POSTURAL REACTIONS

LEFT		RIGHT
	Hopping	
	Front	
	Rear	
	Paw position	
	Front	
	Rear	
	Reflex step	
	Front	
	Rear	
	Tactile placing	
	Front	
	Rear	
	Visual placing	
	Front	
	Rear	
	Hemistanding	
	Hemiwalking	
	Wheelbarrowing	
	Extensor postural thrust	

CRANIAL NERVES

LEFT	Test (Innervation)	RIGHT
	Menace response (II & VII)	
	Vision (II)	
S M L	Pupil size	S M L
	Pupillary light reflex (II & III)	
	Stimulate left eye	
	Stimulate right eye	
	Strabismus (III, IV & VI)	
	Spontaneous nystagmus (III, IV, VI & VIII)	
	Positional nystagmus (III, IV, VI & VIII)	
	Oculovestibular response (III, IV, VI & VIII)	
	Facial sensation (V)	
	Jaw tone (V)	
	Temporal muscle mass (V)	
	Corneal reflex (V, VI & VII)	
	Facial symmetry (VII)	
	Palpebral reflex (V & VII)	
	Hearing (hand clap) (VIII)	
	Swallowing or 'gag reflex' (IX & X)	
	Tongue (XII)	

EYES

Horner's Syndrome (Sympathetic)

Fundic examination

MUSCLE PALPATION

Tone

Atrophy

SPINAL REFLEXES

LEFT	Reflex (Nerve) (Spinal cord segments)	RIGHT
	Triceps (Radial) (C_7-T_1)	
	Biceps (Musculocutaneous) (C_6-C_8)	
	Extensor carpi radialis (Radial) (C_7-T_1)	
	Withdrawal (thoracic limb) (Multiple) (C_6-T_2)	
	Patellar (Femoral) (L_4-L_6)	
	Cranial tibial (Peroneal, sciatic) (L_6-L_7)	
	Gastrocnemius (Tibial, sciatic) (L_6-S_1)	
	Withdrawal (pelvic limb) (Sciatic) (L_6-S_1)	
	Perineal (S_1-S_2)	

URINARY FUNCTION

Voluntary urination?

Bladder distention?

Overflow / ease of manual expression

SPINAL HYPERAESTHESIA

PANNICULUS REFLEX

Level of cut-off (dermatome)

LEFT   RIGHT

DEEP PAIN PERCEPTION

Thoracic limb

Pelvic limb

Tail

LESION LOCALIZATION

BRAIN   Side

Forebrain

Brainstem

Cerebellum

Vestibular - peripheral

Vestibular - central

Multifocal

SPINAL CORD

C_1 - C_5

C_6 - T_2

T_3 - L_3

L_4 - S_3

MULTIFOCAL CNS

PERIPHERAL NERVE

Local

Generalised

NEUROMUSCULAR

MUSCULAR

NORMAL

KEY: ABSENT 0; REDUCED +1; NORMAL +2; INCREASED +3; CLONUS +4

25 Form for neurological examination. It is useful to follow this type of form to ensure that no aspect of the examination is missed, and it provides a permanent record.

2. PATIENT EXAMINATION

NEUROLOGICAL EXAMINATION

The neurological examination is carried out with the aims of determining the precise location of the spinal lesion and its severity. The neurological examination described here is readily performed with the animal upright in the first instance, and later placed in lateral recumbency.

It is very useful to have a form to complete with the findings of the neurological examination (**25**).

Stage 1: Patient in upright position

Assess attitude, posture, and gait
Watch the patient as it relaxes in the examination room. Let it move to the best of its ability, unless it has an acute spinal injury, when movement should be restricted. Note the degree of motor function, the gait (particularly noting any asymmetry) and the general demeanour. In cats, this part of the examination is particularly important as later parts may be difficult to perform. It is useful to listen to dogs as they walk on a hard surface; if conscious proprioceptive deficits are present, the examiner may hear the claws scuff.

Determine the locomotor status
The animal is encouraged to move, except where an acute spinal injury has occurred or if there is severe pain. Patients that appear paraplegic at rest may show some voluntary movement if supported by a sling or by the tail (see **480**). Unilateral weaknesses and sensory deficits may be revealed by hopping (**26, 27**), hemistanding, and hemiwalking tests.

Assess muscle strength, if the patient is able to stand, by pressing down on the shoulders and hips. Following these tests, the locomotor status can then be classified, for example, paraplegic, tetraparetic, hemiparetic.

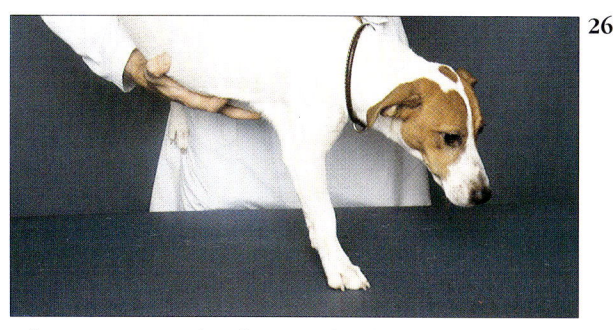

26 Hopping in the thoracic limb. The patient's body is supported with just one limb bearing weight on the ground, and it is then moved laterally. The animal will not be able to hop normally if it has a conscious proprioceptive deficit or impaired motor function.

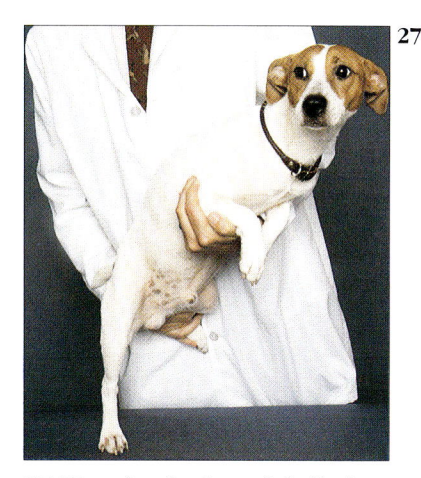

27 Hopping in the pelvic limb.

DIAGNOSIS AND SURGERY OF SMALL ANIMAL SPINAL DISORDERS

Assess conscious proprioception

This is evaluated in the standing animal by the paw position test and the reflex step (**28–34**). Animals with deficits of conscious proprioception that can walk often wear the dorsum of the claws abnormally.

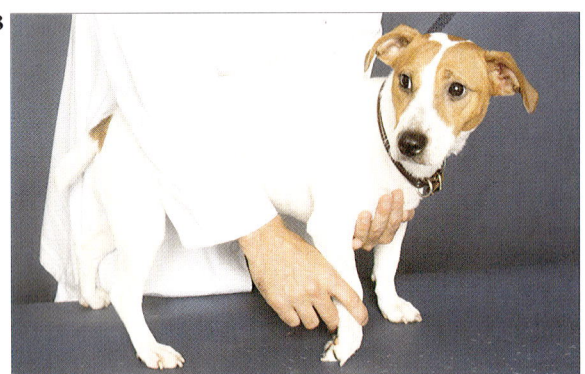

28 Conscious proprioception. The basic test is the paw position response in which the animal's body is supported and each paw individually turned over to bring the dorsal surface into contact with the ground. Normal animals return the paw to an upright position almost immediately, but those with neurological disease cranial to the limb being tested may leave the paw in the flexed position. If conscious proprioception is normal, spinal cord disease is unlikely to be present.

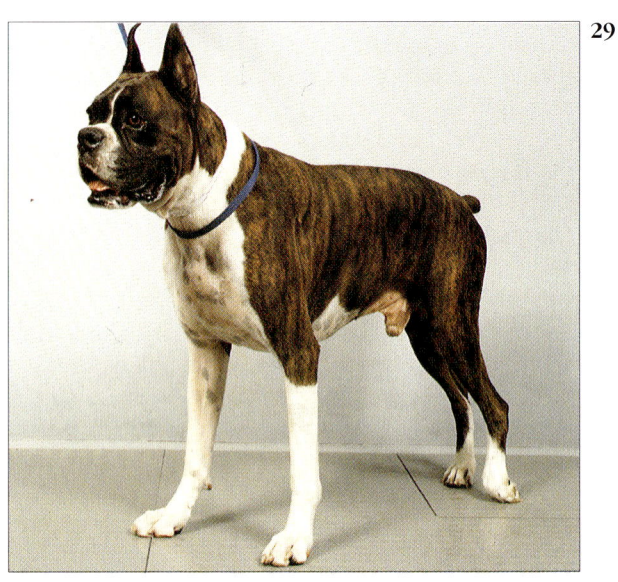

29 Conscious proprioception. Boxer dog with conscious proprioceptive deficit in the left pelvic limb.

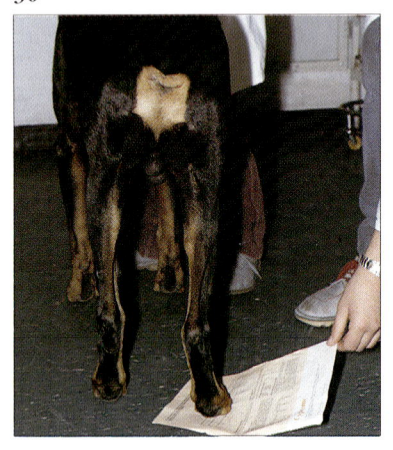

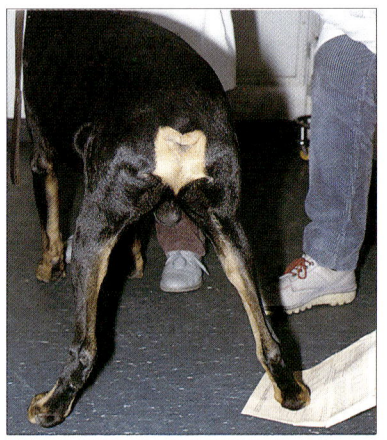

30 Conscious proprioception. This can also be tested by the 'reflex step', where a piece of paper is placed under the foot and pulled laterally. The normal animal returns the foot to the normal position.

31 An abnormal response to the test described in **30** is to let the foot be pulled away from the body.

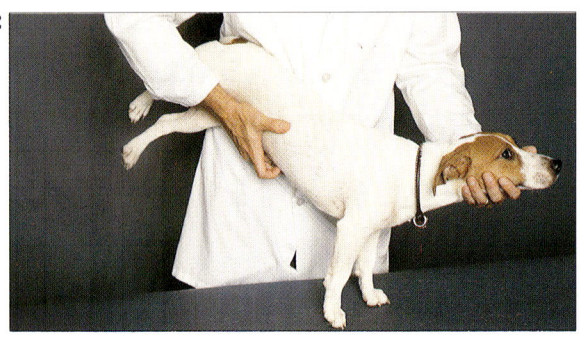

32 Wheelbarrowing test. The pelvic limbs are lifted off the ground as shown and the animal made to walk forward. This test may reveal thoracic limb paresis or asymmetrical lesions. Elevating the head on this test will sometimes reveal hypermetria.

2. PATIENT EXAMINATION

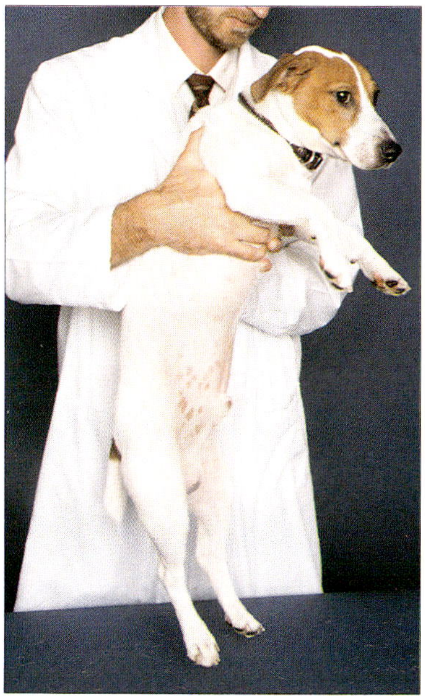

33 Extensor postural thrust. The animal is held up and lowered to the surface. Normal animals push away with their pelvic limbs and step back. This is useful for revealing pelvic limb deficits.

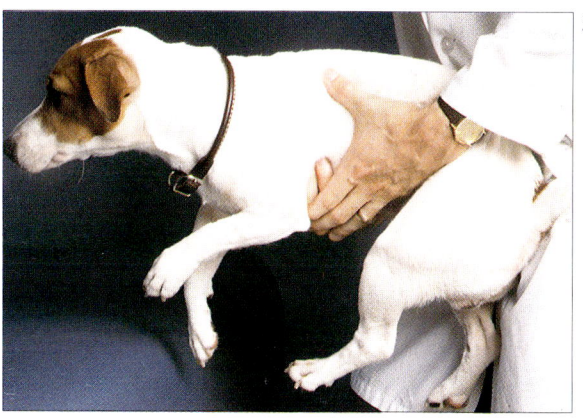

34 Placing test. Here visual placing is being evaluated as the animal can see the table edge. Before this, the test is performed with the animal's head elevated or the eyes covered, which is called tactile placing. Tactile placing evaluates sensation, proprioception, and motor function. Visual placing evaluates vision and motor function. Generally, the paw position response and hopping are more dependable.

Palpate the abdomen

Determine the degree of bladder filling, and the ease with which urine is expressed by palpating the abdomen. Urinary incontinence is often a feature of spinal disorders, and some assessment of urinary function should have been gained from the history.

If neurogenic urinary incontinence is present, it is important to determine if it is LMN or UMN in nature (see **Table 38,** page 211). The LMN bladder is typically large, flaccid, and easily expressed. This is usually associated with lesions of the sacral spinal cord segments or nerve roots. The UMN bladder is characteristically tense and difficult to express, because urethral sphincter tone is often increased. It is seen with lesions cranial to the sacral segments, usually those affecting the T_3–L_3 spinal cord region. See 'Disorders of micturition', p. 210)

The importance of determining the type of incontinence is two-fold. Appropriate drug therapy can be determined from this information (see 'Control of urinary function', page 210). Also, the prognosis for recovery of urinary function is often poor in LMN incontinence, but reasonable in most UMN lesions.

The panniculus reflex

This is tested by pinching the skin along the dorsal surface of the trunk with fine forceps and observing the twitch of the cutaneous trunci muscle on both the ipsilateral and, to a lesser extent, the contralateral side (**35, 36**).

Palpate the spine

Determine the presence of spinal hyperaesthesia by palpating the vertebral column and evaluating the patient's response (**37, 38**). This is an important step in the examination. The degree of pressure to be applied when determining the presence of pain varies between patients. In a dog with neck pain caused by a cervical disc extrusion, it is often adequate to palpate the cervical muscles gently. In some more stoical dogs, greater force either by downward pressure on the spinous processes or along the transverse processes may be required.

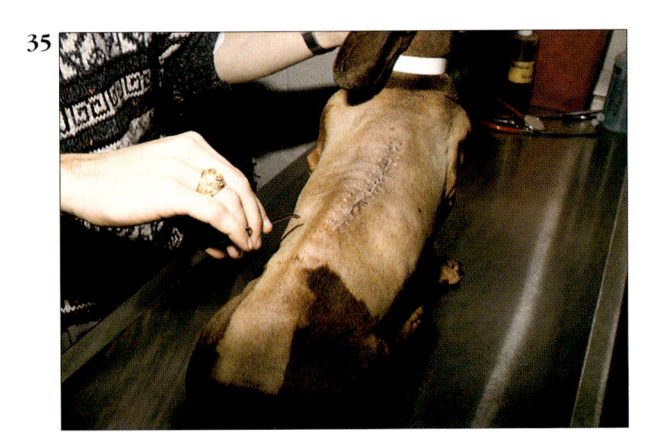

DIAGNOSIS AND SURGERY OF SMALL ANIMAL SPINAL DISORDERS

35 The panniculus reflex is activated by pinching the skin over the lumbar spine with forceps or a gentle needle prick, which leads to a twitch of the cutaneous trunci muscle. There is crossing of the pathway within the spinal cord, leading to a bilateral response after unilateral stimulation. The reflex is generally only useful in localising lesions in animals that are unable to walk on the pelvic limbs.

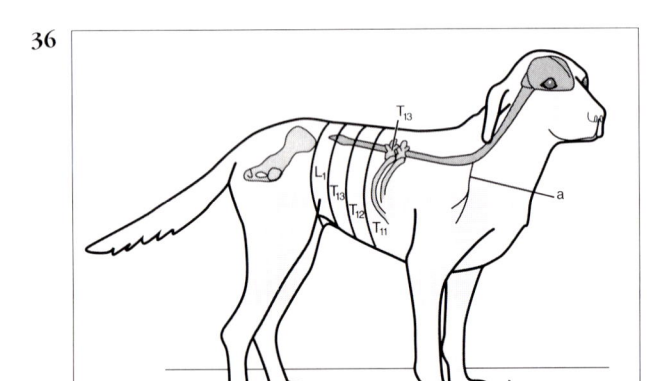

36 The panniculus reflex. Stimulation of the skin of the back activates the reflex, the efferent arm of which is the lateral thoracic nerve arising from segments C_8 and T_1 and leaving the caudal part of the brachial plexus (**a**). Thoracolumbar lesions may interfere with the afferent part of the reflex, which will be intact only in the segments cranial to a spinal cord lesion and absent in the segments caudal to it. The dermatomes are positioned caudal to their respective vertebrae as illustrated here. In cases of thoracic limb paresis, the panniculus reflex will often be absent on the affected side if the lesion involves the C_8 and T_1 spinal cord segments, roots or nerves, but will be intact on the contralateral side. This is particularly useful in differentiating radial nerve injuries (which are rare) where the panniculus reflex is intact, from brachial plexus root avulsions where it is often absent.

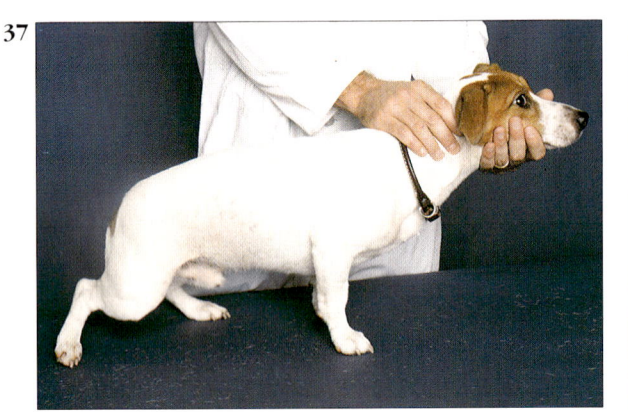

37 Examining the neck for evidence of pain. Palpating the muscles of the neck is usually adequate to reveal pain, which is apparent by tension and fasciculations in the muscles. It is not usually necessary to put the head in extreme positions to reach this conclusion.

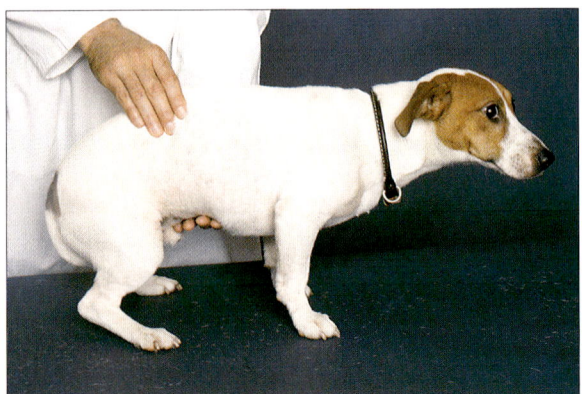

38 Palpating the thoracolumbar spine for pain.

Cranial nerve examination

Even though abnormal cranial nerve findings may not be expected in spinal disorders, it is important to include assessment of these functions in a neurological examination. Some animals with multifocal neurological disease present predominantly with signs of spinal dysfunction. Also, it adds little time to the routine clinical examination to screen cranial nerve function. The details of this examination are given elsewhere (see 'Further Reading,' page 30). Particular note should be made of the presence of Horner's syndrome (ptosis, miosis, enophthalmos, and third eyelid protrusion), which occurs with interference to the sympathetic nerve supply to the eye. This may be a feature of spinal disease if the cervical or cranial thoracic spinal cord segments or nerve roots are involved. An ophthalmoscopic examination should also be carried out.

Stage 2: Patient in lateral recumbency

The patient is then placed in lateral recumbency, and each limb evaluated with the aim of placing it into one of the following categories.
- Normal.
- LMN-type abnormality.
- UMN-type abnormality.

An understanding of the functional anatomy is required to appreciate the difference between these types of deficit (see **6**, **7**).

The effect of lesions on the LMN and UMN systems can be considered in terms of motor function, muscle atrophy, muscle tone, and local reflexes. The clinical signs that allow differentiation between UMN and LMN abnormalities are summarized in **Table 3**. LMN deficits are characterized by: paresis or paralysis; severe (neurogenic) muscle atrophy (**39**); reduced tone in the affected muscles; and depressed or absent reflexes. UMN deficits show paresis or paralysis; mild (disuse) muscle atrophy; normal or increased muscle tone; and intact, often hyperactive reflexes. There is some variation in mild cases, but from the neurological examination, it should be possible to categorize each limb as being 'normal,' 'UMN-type abnormality,' or 'LMN-type abnormality.'

Table 3 Differentiation of LMN *vs* UMN abnormalities

	LMN	UMN
Motor function	Paresis or paralysis	Paresis or paralysis
Reflexes	Absent or reduced	Intact, possibly increased
Muscle tone	Reduced	Normal or increased
Muscle atrophy	Severe, early – neurogenic	Late, mild – disuse

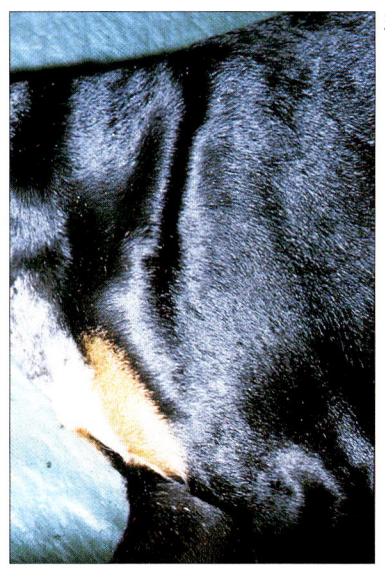

39 Neurogenic atrophy. It is useful to evaluate muscles that have a definite bony border, for example, the spinatus muscles (as shown), the cranial tibial muscle, and the muscles of the pelvis.

Motor function
This has been evaluated previously. With the animal in lateral recumbency, the examination proceeds as follows.

Muscle mass
Muscle atrophy is assessed by observing and palpating muscle masses (**39**).

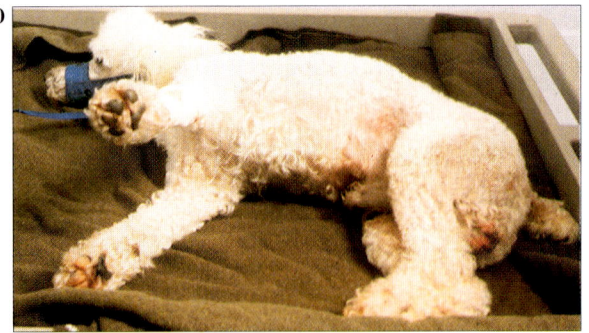

DIAGNOSIS AND SURGERY OF SMALL ANIMAL SPINAL DISORDERS

40 The Schiff–Sherrington sign. In some paraplegic dogs, increased muscle tone and hyperextension of the thoracic limbs are seen. Thoracic spinal cord lesions may interfere with inhibitory neurons that have their cell bodies in the lumbar spinal cord segments and axons that pass cranially to inhibit the thoracic limb muscles. This sign is present only in severe lesions. (See 'Ascending motor tract,' page 12).

Muscle tone

Test muscle tone by gently flexing and extending the joints. Normally there is some resistance to such manipulation. An incorrect impression of increased tone may be gained in excitable or fractious animals, or if the animal has a painful orthopaedic condition. Increased tone in the thoracic limbs is seen in the Schiff–Sherrington sign (**40**).

Reflex testing

There are a number of local reflexes available for examination, but it is usual to concentrate on the patellar and flexor (withdrawal) reflexes (**41–43**).

Other reflexes such as the triceps, biceps, cranial tibial, and extensor carpi radialis may be tested. However, they are found inconsistently in normal animals and their main significance is in finding hyperactive responses in UMN disorders. Increased

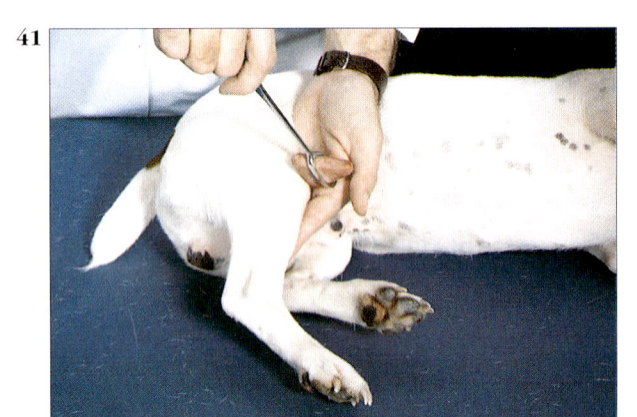

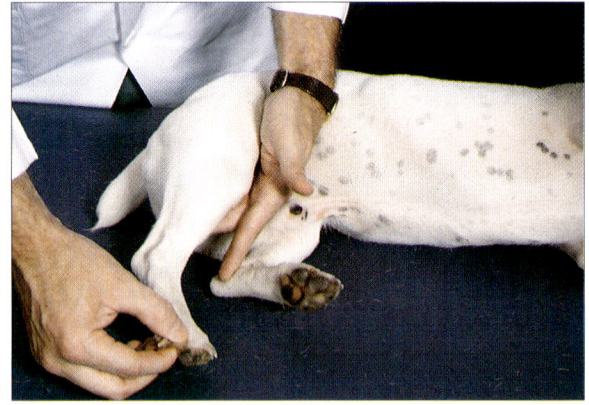

41 The patellar reflex. This is evoked by tapping the straight patellar ligament with a suitable instrument, which leads to a reflex 'kick'. Hyperactive responses seen in UMN abnormalities produce either an abnormally large kick or 'clonus', where the limb oscillates for a period after the initial reflex. In some tense patients, the patellar reflex cannot be elicited in the upper limb, but can be in the lower limb. It is still important to test both pelvic limbs by lying the dog on the opposite side and comparing the reflexes.

42 The flexor or withdrawal reflex. This is stimulated by pinching the toe, which results in flexion of the limb. It is important to persist with the stimulus until it is clear that all the limb joints are flexing. It is also important to note the animal's behavioural response to the stimulus — its deep pain perception — as this has tremendous significance in assessing the severity of lesions. While the flexor reflex is evoked, the contralateral limb should be observed for reflex extension, the crossed extensor reflex, the presence of which is of importance in assessing the severity of the lesion.

43 The flexor or withdrawal reflex. It may be necessary to stimulate the withdrawal reflex with forceps placed over the nail bed or digit in order to evoke a behavioural response.

patellar reflexes are usually seen in UMN lesions cranial to the L_4–L_6 spinal cord segments. An exception is where there is an increased patellar reflex in animals with LMN lesions involving the sciatic nerve or its origins. The muscles innervated by the sciatic nerve normally counteract the reflex kick of the patellar reflex. Interference with sciatic nerve function can reduce this effect and lead to an increased reflex. This is termed 'pseudohyperreflexia'.

Deep pain sensation

On testing the withdrawal reflex, note the patient's behavioural response to the stimulus. A turn of the head or a bark should be seen in response to the pinch, indicating that the painful stimulus has been transmitted cranially through the spinal cord to the brain. If there is no response the stimulus must be increased, usually by using large instruments (needle holders etc.) across the digit or nail bed. The reflex withdrawal of the limb must not be mistaken for a behavioural response.

Absence of deep pain sensation indicates severe spinal cord damage (see 'Assessing the severity of the lesion' (below), and 'Spinal cord nerve fibres and the effect of compression,' page 12).

LOCALIZATION OF LESIONS

On the basis of the neurological examination, it is usually possible to identify the location of the lesion in the spinal cord (**44**). Functionally, the spinal cord may be divided into four regions.

- A: C_1–C_5.
- B: C_6–T_2 (cervical intumescence).
- C: T_3–L_3.
- D: L_4–S_3 (lumbar intumescence).

Areas A and C, the cervical and thoracolumbar spinal cord, convey the UMNs. Areas B and D, the cervicothoracic and lumbosacral spinal cord, provide innervation to the thoracic and pelvic limbs respectively. Area B conveys UMNs to the pelvic limbs. It can be seen in **6** that part of the LMN lies within the spinal cord; lesions in areas B and D of the spinal cord will therefore produce LMN signs in the limbs. Variations are possible, for example, in some Dobermanns with caudal cervical spondylomyelopathy, UMN signs in the pelvic limbs predominate but the lesion is in the cervicothoracic spinal cord. The possibility of a thoracolumbar lesion in such patients should not be overlooked.

On the basis of the neurological examination, the

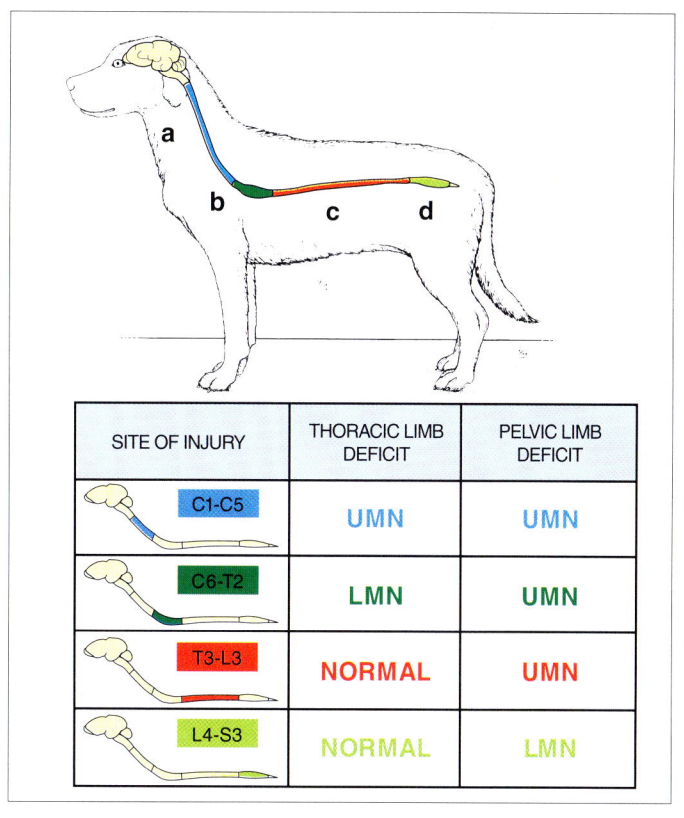

44 Lesions in specific regions will produce different combinations of neurological signs. Lesions in the cervical spinal cord (**a**) produce UMN signs in the thoracic limbs and the pelvic limbs. Lesions in the segments of the cervical intumescence (**b**) produce LMN deficits in the thoracic limbs and UMN signs in the pelvic limbs. Lesions in the thoracolumbar cord (**c**) produce UMN signs in the pelvic limbs only, with normal thoracic limbs (but the Schiff–Sherrington sign may be present in severe lesions). Lesions in the segments of the lumbar intumescence (**d**) produce LMN signs in the pelvic limbs, tail, and perineum, but the thoracic limbs are normal.

SITE OF INJURY	THORACIC LIMB DEFICIT	PELVIC LIMB DEFICIT
C1-C5	UMN	UMN
C6-T2	LMN	UMN
T3-L3	NORMAL	UMN
L4-S3	NORMAL	LMN

lesion can be localized to a particular area of spinal cord. When considering this remember that the spinal cord segments are not all contained in the vertebra of the same number, especially in the cervical and lumbar region (see **2**, **3**).

LMN deficits in all limbs generally indicate diffuse peripheral nerve or neuromuscular disease. Brain involvement is probable if there is evidence of cranial nerve dysfunction or other signs of intracranial disease.

ASSESSING THE SEVERITY OF THE LESION

Assessing the severity of the lesion plays a major part in the diagnostic procedure. In certain patients, it has as much bearing on prognosis as the aetiology; if a poor prognosis is suggested, further investigations may be deemed unnecessary. In general, patients with spinal diseases that show LMN deficits have a worse prognosis for a return to function than those showing UMN deficits.

In UMN injuries, rate of onset, duration, and degree of spinal cord damage all affect the clinical signs. For thoracolumbar lesions, the degree of dysfunction can be classified as grades 1–5.

1 Pain only.
2 Ataxia, conscious proprioceptive deficit, paraparesis.
3 Paraplegia.
4 Paraplegia with urinary retention and overflow.
5 Paraplegia, urinary retention and overflow, and loss of deep pain sensation.

(Griffiths, 1982).

The severity of the neurological deficits in UMN lesions depends on two anatomical features: the position of the tracts in the spinal cord that carry the respective function and the diameter of the fibres transmitting that function (see 'Spinal cord nerve fibres and the effect of compression,' page 12). The prognosis worsens with increasing neurological deficit, as in general this reflects an increased degree of spinal cord damage. The prognosis for patients without deep pain sensation (grade 5) is often poor, especially if it has been absent for longer than 48 hours. Animals that have lost deep pain sensation after trauma carry a poor prognosis, whatever the duration of the clinical signs. Presence of a crossed extensor reflex and the Schiff–Sherrington sign indicate severe lesions, but are not in themselves prognostic indicators.

In other grades of dysfunction, the prognosis is also somewhat dependent on the aetiology. For example, a Dachshund with grade 3 signs could possibly have a thoracolumbar disc extrusion or a spinal tumour. Clearly, the prognosis for such disorders differs.

Cervical spinal cord lesions display a similar progression of signs. However, urinary incontinence or loss of deep pain sensation are very rare. Severe cervical spinal cord lesions may result in respiratory failure caused by interference with respiratory control, although this is uncommon.

DETERMINING THE AETIOLOGY

Once the lesion has been located, a list of differential diagnoses can be made. Many components go into this, including breed and age of the patient, history, presenting signs, progression, physical and neurological findings. It is important not to depend entirely on one feature to make a firm diagnosis. It is reasonable to start from the assumption that the most common disease is the cause, but attempt to exclude less likely conditions, particularly if the patient is not progressing as expected. Differential diagnosis is discussed in Chapter 3.

FURTHER READING

DeLahunta, A. (1983) *Veterinary Neuroanatomy and Clinical Neurology*, 2nd edn. W. B. Saunders Co., Philadelphia.

Griffiths, I.R. (1982) Spinal disease in the dog. *In Practice* **4**, 44–52

Griffiths, I.R. (1989) Neurological examination of the limbs and body. In *Manual of Small Animal Neurology* (Ed. S.J. Wheeler). BSAVA Publications, Cheltenham.

McCunn, J. (1948) The clinical examination of the nervous system. *Veterinary Record* **60**, 427–433.

Oliver, J.E., Hoerlein, B.F. and Mayhew, I.G. (1987) *Veterinary Neurology*. W.B. Saunders Co., Philadelphia.

Oliver, J.E. and Lorenz, M.D. (1993) *Manual of Veterinary Neurology*, 2nd edn. W.B. Saunders Co., Philadelphia.

3. DIAGNOSIS AND DIFFERENTIAL DIAGNOSIS

On the basis of the neurological examination the lesion is localized to one of the following areas of the spinal cord (see **44**).
- A: C_1–C_5.
- B: C_6–T_2.
- C: T_3–L_3.
- D: L_4–S_3.

These areas relate to spinal cord segments. Refer to illustrations **2** and **3** to identify the location of these areas within the vertebral column.

A differential diagnosis list is then drawn up, which embraces all the disease conditions that could be present. It is usual to form this list using the DAMNIT format (**Table 4**).

Table 4 DAMNIT formula for drawing up a differential diagnosis

D	Degenerative
A	Anomalous (developmental)
M	Metabolic
N	Neoplastic Nutritional
I	Inflammatory Infectious Idiopathic Iatrogenic
T	Traumatic Toxic
(V)	(Vascular)

The list can be considerably shortened if some basic information is taken into account, such as the following.
- The age of the patient.
- Whether the condition is acute or chronic, progressive or static.
- Presence of spinal pain.
- The location of the lesion within the spinal cord can also exclude some conditions.

The breed of the patient may also indicate that certain diseases are more likely to be present, but this should not be the only information on which the diagnosis is based.

DIFFERENTIAL DIAGNOSIS

A: C_1–C_5

In adult dogs, intervertebral disc disease is the most common condition affecting this region (**Table 5**). Neck pain is prominent. In dogs less than two years of age the differential diagnosis is different. Here, atlantoaxial subluxation, inflammatory CNS disease, discospondylitis, and trauma are the most likely causes. Spinal tumours can occur in dogs of any age. The most common tumours in the cervical spine are meningiomas and nerve sheath tumours; both are more common in older dogs.

Some dogs with caudal cervical spondylomyelopathy (CCSM) have neurological signs with a C_1–C_5 pattern of dysfunction, although the lesion is more caudal in the cervical spine. Acute, non-painful, non-progressive deficits usually result from ischaemic myelopathy due to fibrocartilaginous embolism (FCE). Signs are often asymmetrical and severe.

In cats, clinical disc disease is extremely rare. The likely diagnoses are trauma, neoplasia (usually lymphoma) and inflammatory diseases, particularly feline infectious peritonitis (FIP). Atlantoaxial subluxation is rare in cats.

Table 5 Important diseases causing signs localized to C_1–C_5 (* Most likely diagnoses in immature animals)

	Acute	Chronic
Painful	Disc disease Atlantoaxial subluxation* CCSM Neoplasia Inflammatory CNS disease* Discospondylitis* Trauma*	Disc disease Atlantoaxial subluxation* CCSM Neoplasia Inflammatory CNS disease* Discospondylitis*
Non-painful	Ischaemic myelopathy	Storage diseases* Congenital vertebral malformations* Syringomyelia Neoplasia

B: C_6–T_2

Similar considerations apply in this region to those causing C_1–C_5 signs, although atlantoaxial subluxation does not occur here. Intervertebral disc disease is less frequent in the caudal cervical spine, but occasional disc extrusions are seen at this level, even at C_7/T_1 (**Table 6**).

Caudal cervical spondylomyelopathy is most prevalent in the caudal cervical spine of Dobermanns and Great Danes. Ischaemic myelopathy occurs with some frequency in this region.

C: T_3–L_3

This region of the spine accounts for most cases of spinal disease. Disc herniation is the most likely diagnosis in dogs older than one year (**Table 7**). In younger dogs, inflammatory CNS disease, discospondylitis, and trauma are common. In cats, disc disease is rare and trauma, neoplasia and inflammatory diseases are the most likely causes of thoracolumbar spinal disease.

In the large breed, older dog with chronic signs, the primary differential diagnosis is degenerative myelopathy. Chronic disc protrusion (Hansen Type II), neoplasia and discospondylitis must be eliminated before this diagnosis is reached.

Table 6 Important diseases causing signs localized to C_6–T_2 (* Most likely diagnoses in immature animals)

	Acute	Chronic
Painful	Disc disease CCSM Neoplasia Inflammatory CNS disease* Discospondylitis* Trauma*	Disc disease CCSM Neoplasia Inflammatory CNS disease* Discospondylitis*
Non-painful	Ischaemic myelopathy	Congenital vertebral malformation* Neoplasia

Table 7 Important diseases causing signs localized to T_3–L_3 (* Most likely diagnoses in immature animals)

	Acute	Chronic
Painful	Disc disease Neoplasia Inflammatory CNS disease* Discospondylitis* Trauma*	Disc disease Neoplasia Inflammatory CNS disease* Discospondylitis*
Non-painful	Ischaemic myelopathy	Degenerative myelopathy Hereditary myelopathy* Spinal dysraphism* Syringomyelia Congenital vertebral malformations* Neoplasia

D: L_4–S_3

Subacute or chronic presentations with signs localizing to this region are usually referable to the lumbosacral junction (**Table 8**). Neoplasia or discospondylitis may be present. Lumbosacral disease is common in large breeds of dog, but is rare in cats. In sacrocaudal injuries, signs referable to the bladder, perineum, and even paraparesis may be seen.

Degenerative myelopathy may appear to localize to this region if the patellar reflexes are absent. This is due to nerve root involvement; the lesion is still essentially T_3–L_3 in nature. Ischaemic myelopathy is also seen in this region. In young animals, congenital defects of the vertebrae or spinal cord are most likely. Exterior signs of spina bifida may be present, but this disease is uncommon.

The differential diagnosis list may therefore be reduced by taking the features mentioned above into account. It may be reasonable, in some circumstances, to proceed with treatment without further investigations, for example, in a middle-aged Dachshund with mild T_3–L_3 signs and where conservative treatment is planned. However, if the patient does not progress as expected, or if there is any doubt about the diagnosis, more definitive measures are required. These are covered in Chapter 4.

Table 8 Important diseases causing signs localized to L_4–S_3 (* Most likely diagnoses in immature animals)

	Acute	Chronic
Painful	Disc disease	Disc disease
		Lumbosacral disease
	Neoplasia	Neoplasia
	Inflammatory CNS disease*	Inflammatory CNS disease*
	Discospondylitis*	Discospondylitis*
	Trauma*	
	Sacrocaudal injuries	
Non-painful	Ischaemic myelopathy	Spinal dysraphism*
		Spina bifida*
		Sacrocaudal dysgenesis (Manx cats and brachycephalic dogs)*
		Syringomyelia
		Congenital vertebral malformations*
		Neoplasia

FURTHER READING

DeLahunta, A. (1983) *Veterinary Neuroanatomy and Clinical Neurology*, 2nd edn. W. B. Saunders Co., Philadelphia.

Oliver, J.E. and Lorenz, M.D. (1993) *Manual of Veterinary Neurology*, 2nd edn. W.B. Saunders Co., Philadelphia.

Oliver, J.E., Hoerlein, B.F. and Mayhew, I.G. (1987) *Veterinary Neurology*. W.B. Saunders Co., Philadelphia.

Wheeler, S.J. (Ed.) (1989) *Manual of Small Animal Neurology* BSAVA Publications, Cheltenham.

4. DIAGNOSTIC AIDS

Ancillary aids are used to reach or to confirm a diagnosis. In some circumstances one test may be all that is required; in others a combination may be necessary. The complexity of some techniques may require specialist assistance, but the majority of tests used in spinal disease investigation are readily performed in most clinics. However, some familiarity is required, particularly for the special radiological procedures, and practice is recommended.

The selection of tests varies with the circumstances. In the following chapters there are recommendations about which test is most likely to provide a diagnosis in a particular disease. Clearly, individual preference and availability of equipment will influence these decisions.

ROUTINE LABORATORY ANALYSIS

A complete blood count and chemistry profile should be checked in all patients undergoing non-emergency procedures. They rarely provide definitive diagnostic information in neurological diseases, but may be useful for detecting concurrent disorders (Evans, 1989). In emergency situations, analysis may be restricted to packed cell volume, and serum protein, glucose and urea concentrations.

Haematology

The haemogram is unremarkable in the majority of animals with spinal disease, although a stress leukogram (lymphopenia, eosinopenia, and leukocytosis) is a common finding. The haemogram is usually normal in patients with inflammatory diseases of the spinal cord and meninges, but may be inflammatory in some dogs with discospondylitis, although this is not consistent.

Biochemistry

Metabolic diseases may cause generalized weakness, which could be mistaken for spinal disease. Examples include hypoglycaemia, hypocalcaemia, hyponatraemia, and hypokalaemic polymyopathy.

Raised serum creatine kinase concentrations usually indicate muscle disease. Note that many patients will have a raised serum creatine kinase following trauma or prolonged recumbency.

Abnormal biochemical findings may occur in certain spinal diseases. Hypercalcaemia is seen in some patients with generalized bone disorders, for example primary or secondary hyperparathyroidism with skeletal involvement, and in some with lymphoma (a paraneoplastic effect). Hypergammaglobulinaemia may occur in myeloma and FIP.

Urinalysis

Urinalysis may provide specific diagnostic information or be valuable in assessing the state of the bladder where it is not functioning normally.

If bladder function is in doubt in patients with spinal disease, urinalysis should be performed on a sample collected by cystocentesis when the patient is first evaluated.

Subsequent urinalysis should be performed until normal urinary function returns (see Chapter 15). Urinary tract infection (UTI) associated with urine retention is frequently present in animals with spinal disease. Urinalysis reveals high white blood cell counts and elevated total protein, and bacteria may be present in the sediment. If so, urine culture should be performed and antibiotic sensitivity determined. For routine urinalysis, aseptic catheterization or cystocentesis is suitable. For culture, cystocentesis is preferred.

Bence–Jones proteinuria may be a feature of myeloma.

Serology

Serology is useful in many diseases, and should be considered in any spinal patient where the origin of the disorder is obscure. Specific examples include *Toxoplasma gondii* and *Neospora caninum*, and *Brucella canis* in cases of discospondylitis.

Canine distemper virus (CDV) and FIP both cause nervous system lesions, which may present with spinal involvement. The presence of serum IgG is not confirmatory of CNS involvement by these viruses. Anti-CDV IgM is indicative of recent distemper infection and thus may be useful. CSF antibody analysis may be useful in identifying CNS infections.

Microbiology

Culture and sensitivity testing of organisms has some value in neurology. Note that bacterial diseases of the CNS are very rare in dogs and cats, thus, culture of CSF is likely to be negative. Large volumes of CSF (several mls) placed in blood culture bottles are used in attempting bacterial culture.

Urine culture is indicated in patients with cystitis related to neurological disease. Sensitivity testing should also be performed to determine the most appropriate antibiotic to treat infections. However, bladder infections may only resolve when urinary function returns to normal.

In patients with discospondylitis, urine and blood culture may be attempted to isolate the causative organism.

If wound infections occur following surgery, culture from the depths of the wound should be performed (see 'Wound infection,' page 216).

Other

Other tests, for example endocrine testing, analysis of Von Willebrand's (VW) factor, and bleeding times, may be deemed necessary in the preoperative evaluation of patients (see Chapters 6 and 11).

CEREBROSPINAL FLUID

CSF analysis is an important tool in investigating neurological patients, but has many limitations. Abnormal CSF strongly indicates neurological disease, but is relatively nonspecific. Many patients with spinal disease have normal CSF (Mayhew and Beal, 1980; Evans, 1989; Chrisman, 1992a).

Collection and analysis of CSF should always be considered in patients with spinal disease, but CSF analysis alone is unlikely to provide a diagnosis. In the animal with spinal disease where radiography and myelography are normal, and in patients with multifocal signs, CSF should always be analysed.

Collection of CSF is not without hazard, and this should be made clear to owners before the procedure. It should be performed with the patient under general anaesthesia.

CSF collection

Indications
- Suspected intracranial disease (see 'Contraindications' below).
- Suspected multifocal disease.
- Spinal disease where survey radiographs are normal.
- Suspected polyneuropathy.

Contraindications
- Where general anaesthesia is contraindicated.
- If raised intracranial pressure or brain herniation could be present. This may be so in any patient with an intracranial lesion, but particularly following head trauma, space-occupying lesions, or severe inflammatory disease. Signs indicative of raised intracranial pressure include stupor or coma, respiratory depression, locomotor dysfunction, dilated pupils, and poor or absent pupillary light reflexes. Collection of CSF from either of the spinal sites in the face of increased intracranial pressure increases the likelihood of caudal brain herniation.
- Where there is a spinal injury at the proposed site of collection.
- CSF should not be collected from the cerebellomedullary cistern (CMC – 'cisterna magna') from patients who may have atlantoaxial subluxation, because of the danger associated with positioning the patient.

DIAGNOSIS AND SURGERY OF SMALL ANIMAL SPINAL DISORDERS

Collection of cerebrospinal fluid

General anaesthesia is required for CSF collection in small animals. Patients should be intubated and ventilatory support must be available. The collection site must be clipped and prepared aseptically. Sterile needles (**45**) are used for collection, and wearing of sterile surgical gloves is recommended. An assistant is required to hold the patient in the correct position.

Which collection site to use warrants some consideration. The two sites available are the CMC and the lumbar spine. Collection from the CMC is easier and is less likely to produce a sample contaminated with blood. However, as CSF flows in a cranial to caudal direction, abnormal CSF is more likely to be present caudal to a lesion. Thus, lumbar CSF is more likely to be diagnostically useful. However, lumbar collection is more difficult and blood contamination occurs more often.

If intracranial pressure is raised, lumbar collection is somewhat safer. This is not because brain herniation is any less likely, but the risk of direct damage to already-herniated tissue is not a factor with lumbar collection.

Spinal needles are preferred for CSF collection, but hypodermic needles may be used.

The CSF is collected into sterile vials; plain vials without anticoagulant are generally used.

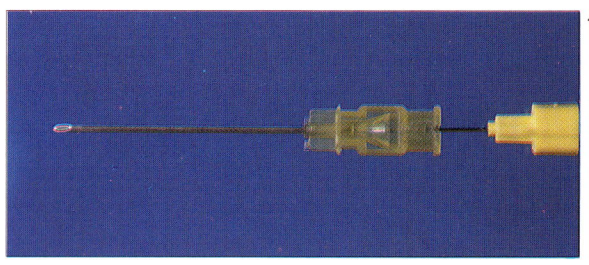

45 Spinal needles have a stilette and shallow bevel. A notch in the hub indicates the side of the bevel, which in myelography should be pointing in the direction in which contrast is intended to flow.

Collection from the cerebellomedullary cistern (**46–54**)

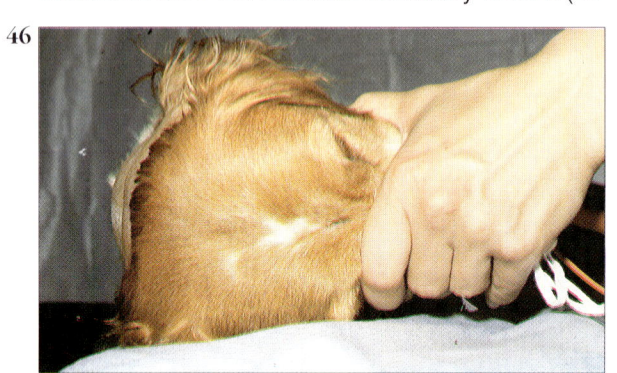

46 Patient positioned in right lateral recumbency for collection of CSF by a right-handed operator. The head is held by an assistant in 90° flexion with the nose parallel to the table top. The neck is positioned close to the edge of the table. A foam wedge may be used to support the nose.

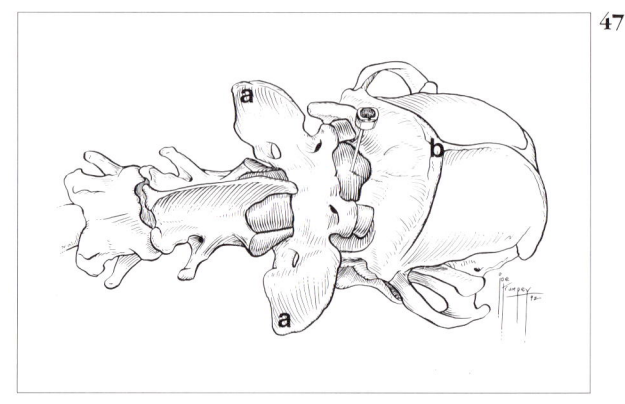

47 Diagram to show site of CMC puncture. The landmarks are the lateral margin of the wings of the atlas (**a**), the occipital protuberance (**b**), and the midline.

4. DIAGNOSTIC AIDS

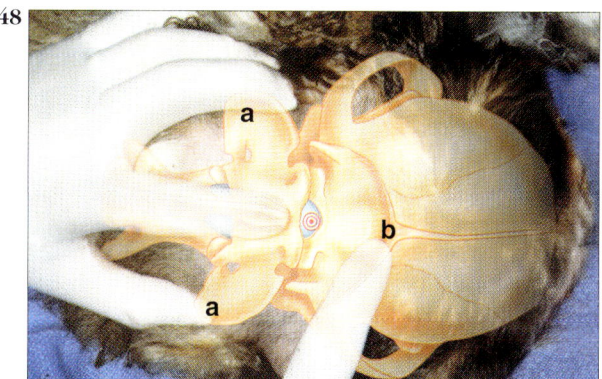

48 Landmarks for CMC puncture. These are the lateral margin of the wings of the atlas (**a**) and the occipital protuberance (**b**). An imaginary line is drawn between the wings of the atlas. The site is in the midline of the patient, half way between the occipital protuberance and the line joining the wings of the atlas. Just behind the occipital protuberance there is a slight depression in the muscles. This is not the site of needle penetration, but is cranial to it. Inserting the needle there usually leads to it striking the bone of the skull.

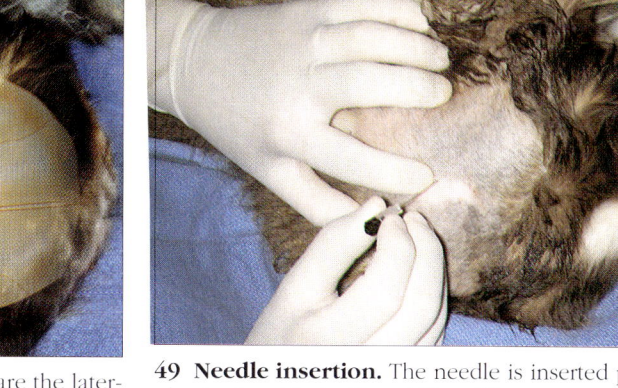

49 Needle insertion. The needle is inserted perpendicular to the skin in the midline. The operator is wearing sterile gloves, and the site has been prepared aseptically. The left hand is identifying the landmarks. The thumb and upper fingers are palpating the wings of the atlas. The index finger is on the midline, just behind the site. There are a number of methods for advancing the needle: a) Remove the stilette once the tip of the needle is in muscle. The needle is then advanced until the dura mater is penetrated and CSF appears in the hub of the needle; b) Advance the needle with the stilette still in place in small increments, removing the stilette between each movement to check whether CSF is present in the needle. A slight pop can sometimes be felt when the needle enters the subarachnoid space. We feel that method a) is the simplest and least hazardous.

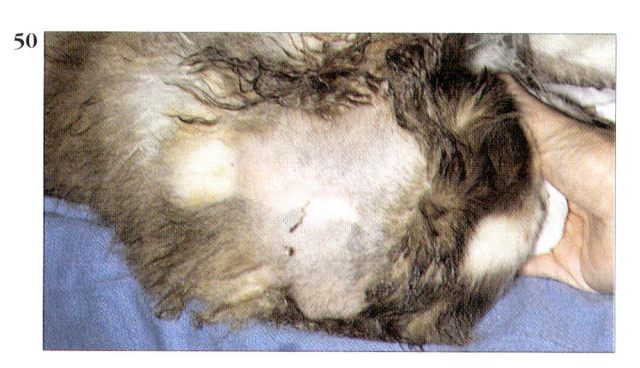

50 The needle in place with the stilette removed. A drop of CSF is seen.

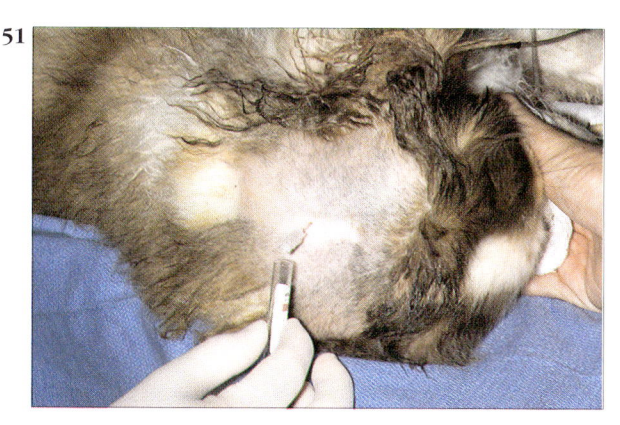

51 Fluid is collected into a sterile vial.

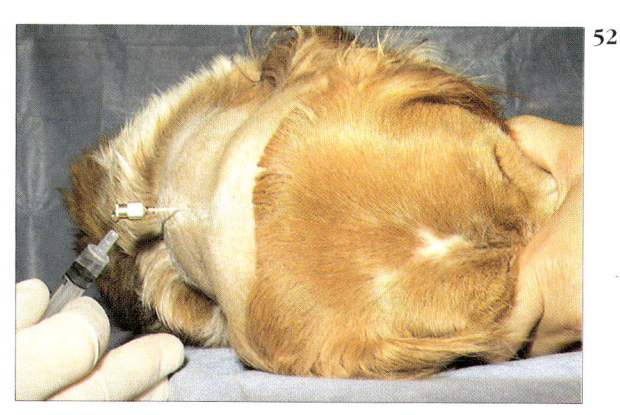

52 Alternatively fluid can be collected into a sterile syringe. The syringe is not used to aspirate CSF, just to catch it.

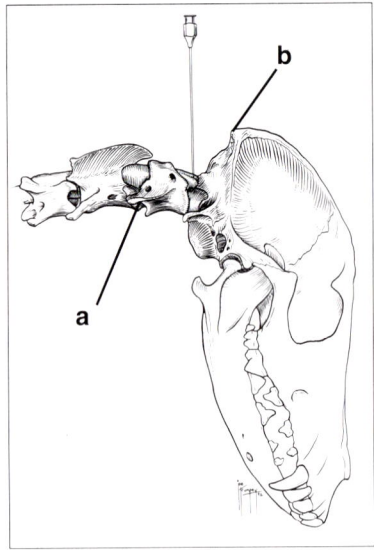

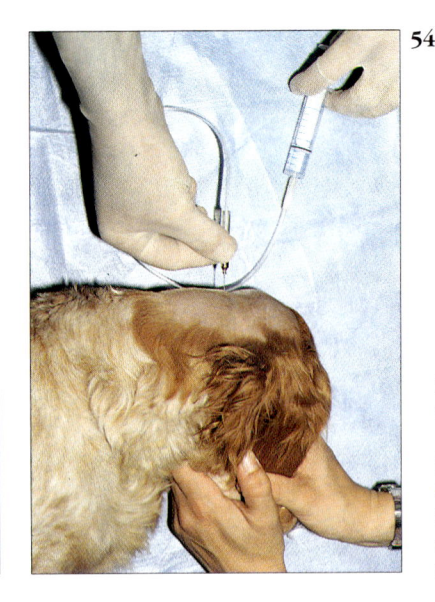

DIAGNOSIS AND SURGERY OF SMALL ANIMAL SPINAL DISORDERS

53 Diagram to show position of needle. The landmarks are as in **47**.

54 Position of patient and needle. In this patient, an extension tube has been applied to the spinal needle for the injection of contrast medium for myelography.

Because the neck is severely flexed, a kinkproof endotracheal tube should be used. Alternatively, the cuff is deflated to allow space around the tube for air flow should the tube obstruct. If CSF does not flow or is blood tinged, a number of possible complications may have arisen.

- **The tip of the needle hits bone.** The point of the needle is redirected by withdrawing it to a subcutaneous position and moving the hub.
- **If CSF flows, but is tinged with a trickle of bright red blood in the base of the hub**, a dural vessel has been penetrated. This may clear after a few seconds, then CSF may be collected. Rotating the needle may help to clear this type of haemorrhage. If a clean sample is required, it is worth removing the needle and starting again, as some red blood cells (RBC) will be present.
- **Dark venous blood flowing from the needle** indicates penetration of a venous structure, usually because the needle has strayed from the midline. It is best to start again with a fresh needle.
- **No CSF flows**, even though all the features of a successful tap appear to be present and the needle seems to have penetrated to an adequate depth may be because the needle is far off the midline, the brain has herniated, or the spinal cord has been penetrated. The latter is a significant risk if the needle is advanced with the stilette in place. The needle should be removed, the patient placed in a normal position, and the respiratory pattern observed. If respiration is normal after several minutes, the procedure may be repeated. In some patients with soft tissue lesions in the cranial cervical vertebral canal, CSF cannot be collected from the CMC.
- **If the patient moves suddenly** it is usually because the spinal cord has been damaged. The needle must be removed and the patient ventilated. This is a potentially serious situation leading to marked neurological deterioration or death. It may be useful to give the patient methylprednisolone (30 mg/kg IV) in an attempt to limit the spinal cord damage.
- **If CSF flows forcefully** from the needle it clearly indicates high CSF pressure at the CMC, but it is not always obvious why. Some dogs do not suffer any apparent deleterious effects, but others deteriorate. The needle should be removed and the precautions mentioned above taken. It may be useful to hyperventilate the patient if increased intracranial pressure is thought to be the cause. If brain herniation has occurred, mannitol and frusemide may be helpful.

4. DIAGNOSTIC AIDS

Collection from the lumbar spine (55–61)

55 Lumbar spinal puncture. The site is between L_5 and L_6. The needle is inserted alongside the spinous process of L_6 and directed cranially and ventrally through the ligamentum flavum into the vertebral canal. In the cat L_6/L_7 can be used.

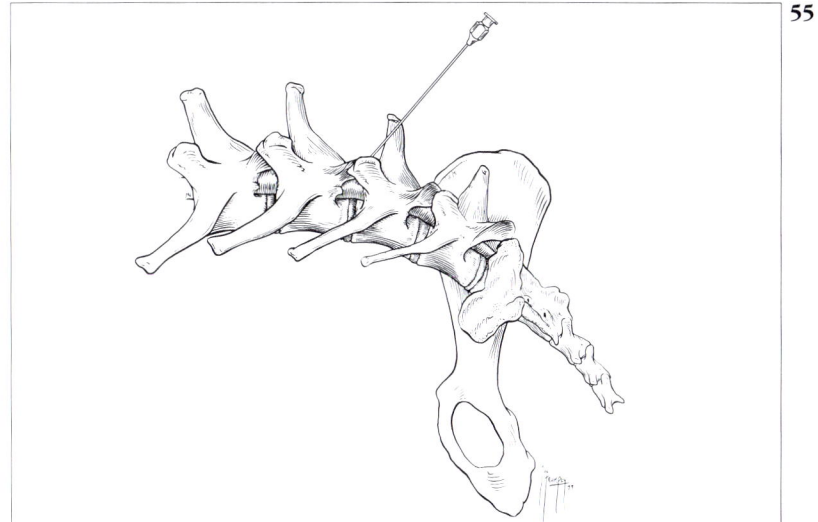

56 Here the needle is alongside the spinous process of L_6. With the patient in lateral recumbency, the pelvic limbs are pulled cranially under the abdomen. It is useful to place a foam wedge under the lower thigh.

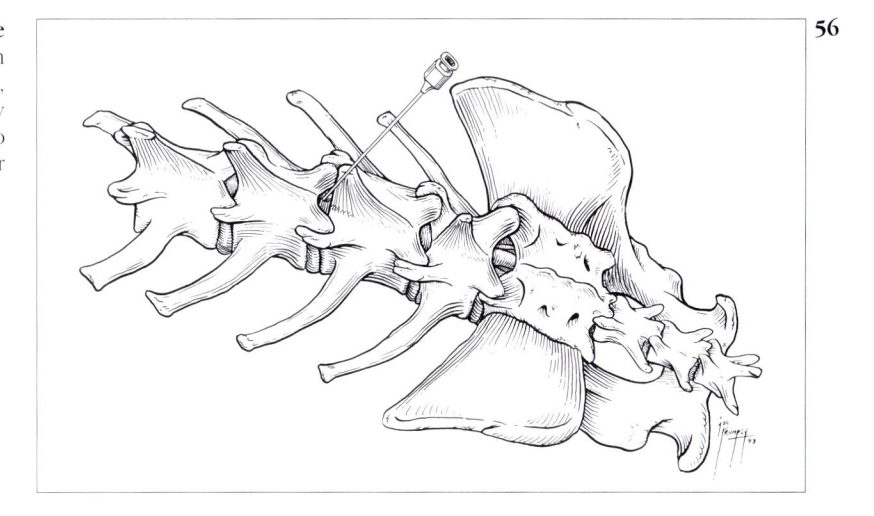

57 The tip of the L_6 spinous process is palpated. The needle is inserted alongside the caudal edge of the spinous process, slightly lateral to the midline. It is advanced in a cranioventral direction such that the point meets the midline as it reaches the vertebral lamina. It may be necessary to step the needle off the lamina into the ligamentum flavum. This ligament may be tough and require considerable force to penetrate it. The stilette is removed intermittently to check progress. On penetrating the subarachnoid space, CSF will flow. Flow of CSF is slower in the lumbar spine than at the CMC. Also, blood contamination is more likely. Sometimes, there is a perceptible twitch of the tail and pelvic limbs as the needle touches or even penetrates the neural tissues. Aspiration of CSF with a syringe is possible, but blood contamination is more likely.

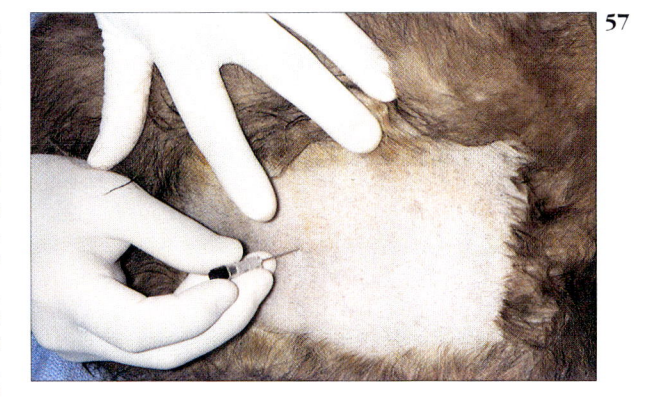

39

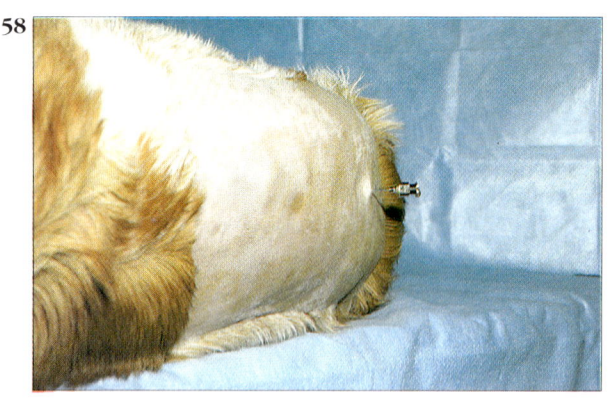

DIAGNOSIS AND SURGERY OF SMALL ANIMAL SPINAL DISORDERS

58 Needle *in situ*. Another method of lumbar puncture is to find the cranial edge of the spinous process and insert the needle vertically into the ligamentum flavum.

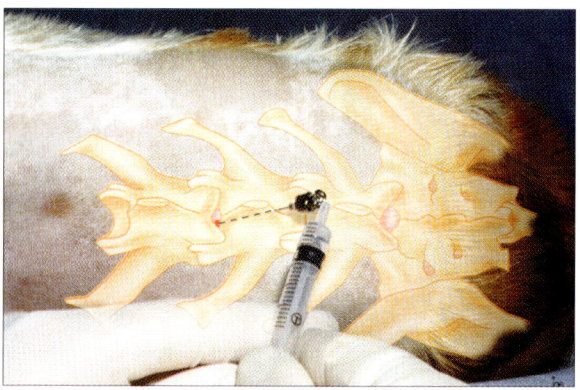

59 Collection of CSF using a syringe.

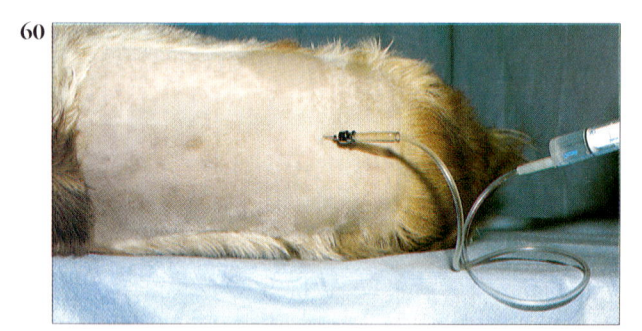

60 Contrast injection using an extension tube. Contrast injection should be slow to avoid epidural leakage.

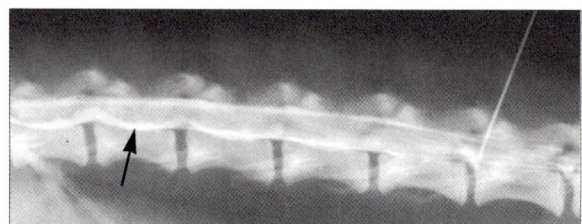

61 Radiograph to show position of needle for lumbar puncture. A myelogram has been performed here; contrast can be seen in the subarachnoid space. Note in the cranial lumbar vertebrae that there is epidural contrast (arrow). This is a common complication in lumbar myelograms and it makes interpretation difficult when present.

Collection of CSF from the lumbar site (**55–61**) is more likely to fail than from the CMC.

Contamination is also more frequent. If CSF does not flow or is blood tinged, a number of possible complications may have arisen.
- **The needle has struck bone.** The space available for penetration of the vertebral canal is relatively small, and may be particularly so in large dogs with significant vertebral new bone formation. Also, the ligamentous tissue may be mineralized and have the feel of bone. Repeated attempts may be required to position the needle and, in some patients, the technique may fail.
- **Considerations for haemorrhage** are similar to those mentioned above.

Sample handling and laboratory analysis
The routine analyses performed on CSF are gross examination, total and differential white cell (WBC) count and total protein; these are the most useful in spinal diseases. Other analyses performed include immunology and electrophoresis.

White cell analysis must be performed on fresh CSF within 30 minutes of collection as the cells deteriorate rapidly. If this is not possible, the specimen should be preserved with an equal volume of 4% formalin solution (Evans, 1989).

Gross examination

Normal CSF is clear and colourless. Colour change and turbidity may be noted in some diseases. The most frequent colour changes are due to haemorrhage or to xanthochromia (see **62**).

Cell counts

These are performed using a haemocytometer; the cell numbers are too low to be accurately counted by automatic means. Undiluted CSF is used, unless cell counts are particularly high. If this is so, the CSF will appear turbid. Normal CSF is free of red blood cells. Normal WBCs vary by laboratory, but are generally less than 5 cells per µl. An increase in WBCs is termed pleocytosis.

Cell counts and blood contamination

Small amounts of blood contamination have little effect on WBC counts in CSF. There are formulae for correcting CSF cell counts that take the peripheral blood WBC count into consideration. However, contaminating RBCs do not greatly alter markedly elevated WBC counts (Wilson and Stevens, 1977). It is probably adequate to remember that WBCs and RBCs are in a ratio of approximately 1:500 in blood, and to take this into account when viewing cell counts in blood contaminated CSF.

Differential white cell counts and cytology

This is an important part of the examination of CSF, even in the face of a normal total WBC count. The WBCs must be concentrated either by centrifugation or sedimentation, mounted on a slide and stained (Mayhew and Beal, 1980). Most WBCs in CSF are mononuclear lymphocytes, monocytes, and occasional macrophages. Occasional neutrophils are seen.

The differential WBC count is most useful in distinguishing acute and chronic inflammation, for example, between granulomatous meningoencephalitis and noninfectious suppurative meningoencephalitis.

Bacteria may occasionally be seen in CSF. These may be pathogenic, but if present in the absence of a neutrophilic pleocytosis, they are most likely the result of contamination. Bacterial meningoencephalomyelitis is very rare in the dog and cat.

Abnormal cells suggestive of neoplasia are rarely found in CSF. Lymphoma will occasionally be evident on cytology.

Protein content

Protein content of CSF is estimated by a number of methods; use of a professional laboratory is best. Normal CSF collected from the CMC has a protein concentration of less than 30 mg/dl; it may be up to 45 mg/dl at the lumbar site. Total protein may be increased in many diseases but is nonspecific. Increased protein in the absence of pleocytosis is usually indicative of non-inflammatory disorders.

Electrophoresis provides information regarding the composition of the CSF protein.

Microbiology

Examination for the presence of bacteria may be by microscopy of stained samples and by culture. Care should be exercised in interpreting positive results in the absence of pleocytosis, as bacteria may be contaminants. Intracellular bacteria should always be viewed as being significant.

Normal CSF findings

Normal CSF findings are given in **Table 9**.

Table 9 Normal values for commonly evaluated CSF parameters

Parameter	Normal
Colour	Clear, colourless
Specific gravity	1.004–1.006
White cell count	< 5/µl
Differential white cells	Mostly mononuclear
Total protein	
CMC	10–30 mg/dl (0.1–0.3 g/litre)
Lumbar	10–45 mg/dl (0.1–0.45 g/litre)

Abnormal CSF findings

Abnormal CSF is indicative of CNS or nerve root disease.

- High numbers of RBCs in the CSF generally indicates contamination at collection. Haemorrhage in the CNS may be inferred from the presence of either xanthochromia (**62**) or erythrophagocytes (macrophages containing RBCs).
- Mononuclear pleocytosis usually indicates chronic inflammation such as canine distemper infection or granulomatous meningoencephalomyelitis (**63**).
- Neutrophilic pleocytosis is seen mostly with infectious or noninfectious meningoencephalomyelitis (aseptic meningitis, **64**).
- Mixed pleocytosis is nonspecific, but can be seen in some tumours, particularly meningiomas.
- Identification of neoplastic cells in CSF is unusual. It is most likely in lymphoma and choroid plexus tumours.
- Increased protein in the absence of pleocytosis (albuminocytological dissociation) usually indicates neoplasia or extradural spinal cord compression.

Normal findings in the face of disease

Many animals with CNS disease, including spinal diseases, have normal CSF. This is particularly so if the CSF sample is collected cranial to the lesion, that is, from the CMC in thoracolumbar and lumbosacral lesions. Thus, finding normal CSF does not exclude the possibility of a lesion.

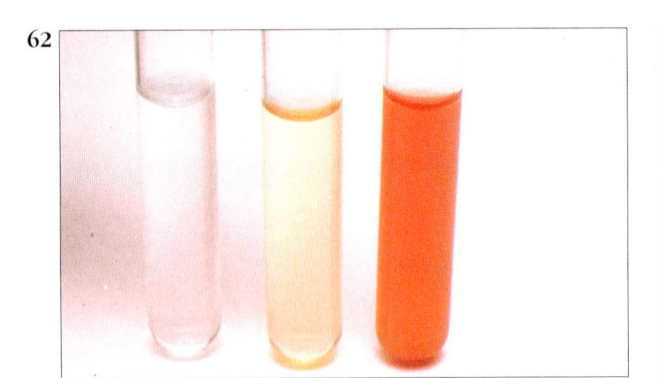

62 Specimens. Left to right: normal CSF; xanthochromia, which is caused by haemoglobin breakdown products and indicates previous intrathecal haemorrhage; haemorrhage at collection.

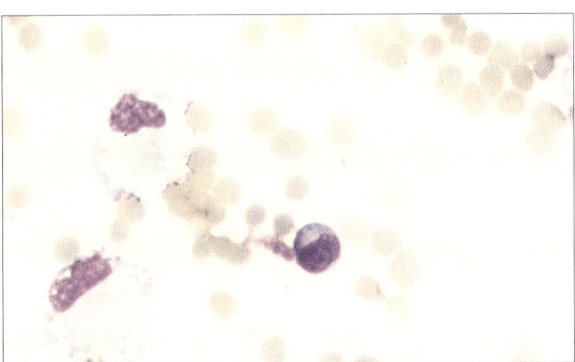

63 Slide cytospin preparation of CSF. This shows macrophages and lymphocyte from a patient with granulomatous meningoencephalomyelitis.

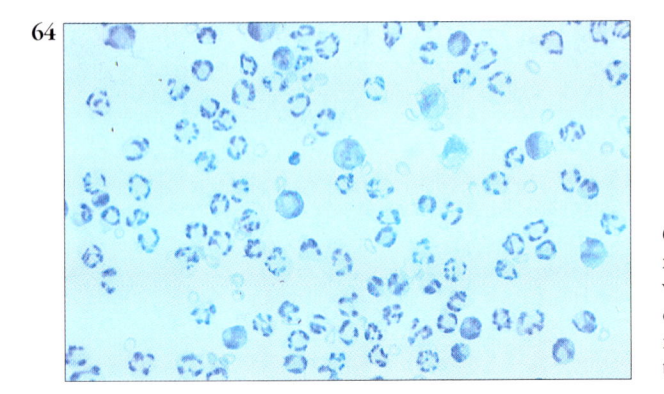

64 Slide preparation of CSF sample from a nine-month-old Bernese mountain dog with severe cervical pain. The CSF total white cell count was 179 cells/µl. The differential was 80% neutrophils, 20% mononuclear cells. The diagnosis was aseptic suppurative meningitis.

4. DIAGNOSTIC AIDS

RADIOGRAPHY

Survey radiographs

Radiography is the most valuable diagnostic aid for spinal patients. Good quality survey radiographs will provide the diagnosis in many cases. To obtain diagnostic radiographs of the spine, general anaesthesia is usually necessary to position the patient correctly and to minimize radiation exposure of personnel. In many animals with spinal disease, the radiological features are subtle, thus, accurate positioning is essential. An exception is in acute spinal injuries, where general anaesthesia or manipulation could worsen the neural damage.

The area of interest must be well centred and the beam collimated closely. Survey radiographs of large areas of the spine are rarely useful.

Radiographic positioning and normal spinal radiographs

Various positioning aids facilitate spinal radiography (**65**). Techniques for radiographing the spine are given in the following section.

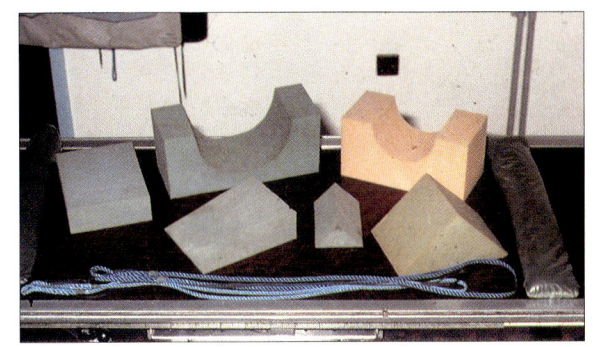

65 Radiographic positioning aids. Radiolucent foam wedges, floppy sandbags, and ties.

Cervical spine (**66–70**)

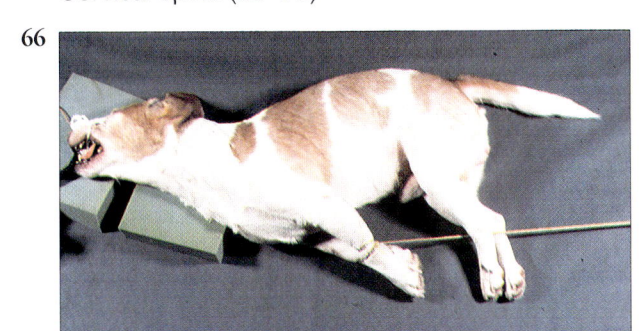

66 Lateral cervical spine. The patient is in lateral recumbency, with the head extended and the thoracic limbs pulled caudally. A wedge is placed under the sternum to prevent rotation. It is usually best to take two views, one centred at C_2 and one at C_6.

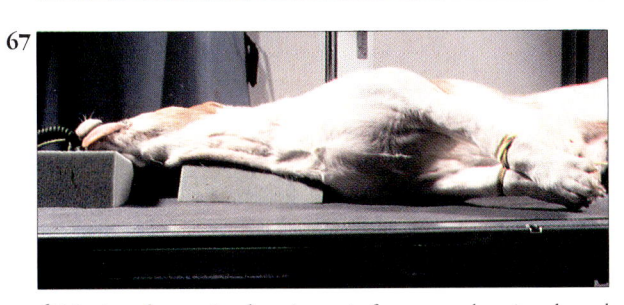

67 Lateral cervical spine. A foam wedge is placed under the middle part of the neck to avoid sagging, which could result in distortion of the intervertebral spaces.

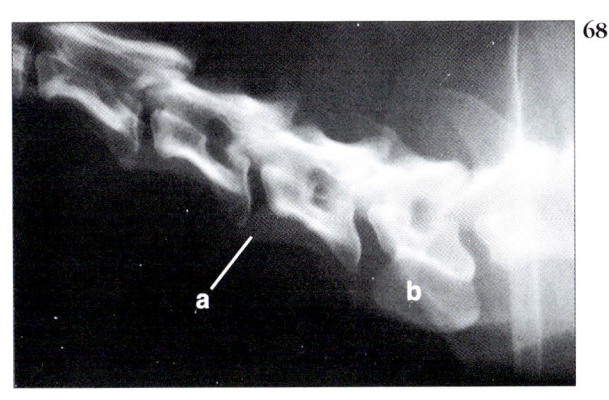

68 Lateral cervical radiograph of a normal dog. Note that the transverse processes are superimposed (**a**), and the intervertebral spaces near the middle of the film are clear and parallel. The transverse processes of C_6 are large and project ventrally (**b**). See **71** for cranial cervical radiograph.

43

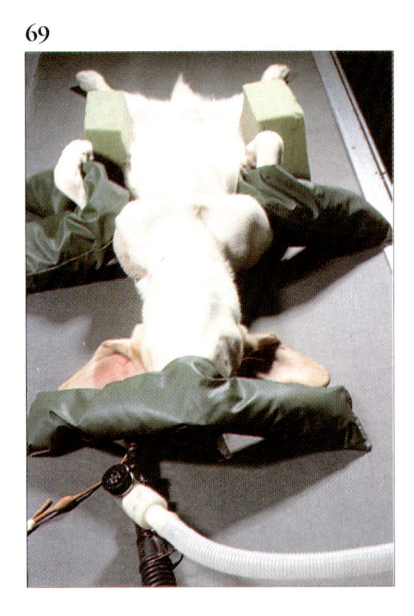

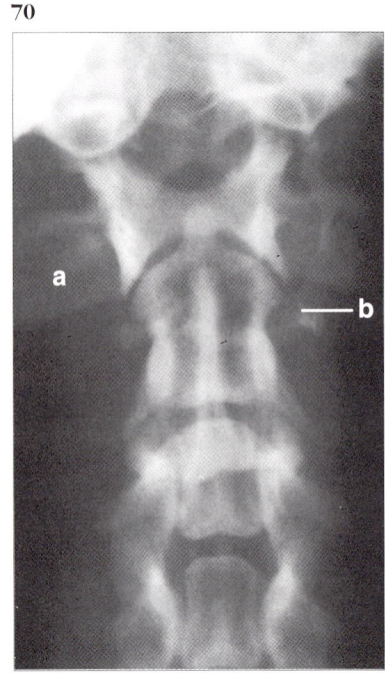

DIAGNOSIS AND SURGERY OF SMALL ANIMAL SPINAL DISORDERS

69 Ventrodorsal cervical spine. The patient is placed in dorsal recumbency, with the whole body aligned vertically. The beam is centred on the area of interest. It is useful to remove the endotracheal tube for this view, particularly in myelography.

70 Ventrodorsal cervical radiograph of a normal dog. The wing of the atlas is seen (**a**), as is the hyoid (**b**).

Stressed survey views of the cervical spine are not generally of value, but they are useful in myelography; see below.

Atlantoaxial joint (71, 72)

Projections are as for the cervical spine, with the beam centred appropriately. For the lateral projection a mild degree of flexion may be used to demonstrate subluxation, but must not be excessive. The open-mouth view to radiograph the dens is not recommended; the flexed position required can be dangerous and the ventrodorsal projection is adequate. The spinal deviation in many patients with atlantoaxial subluxation can make positioning difficult. Cervical extension alleviates the cord compression, and positioning in this way is therefore unlikely to be harmful.

A common error is to try to evaluate the atlantoaxial joint in poorly positioned films taken of a conscious patient, with the area of interest near the edge of the film. Accurate interpretation is not possible. Normal radiographs are shown in **71** and **72**.

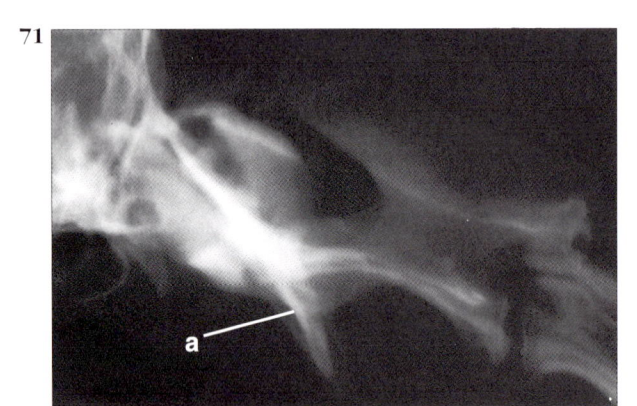

71 Lateral atlantoaxial radiograph of a normal dog. Note the normal relationship between the dorsal arch of C_1 and the spinous process of C_2. (**a**) wings of atlas.

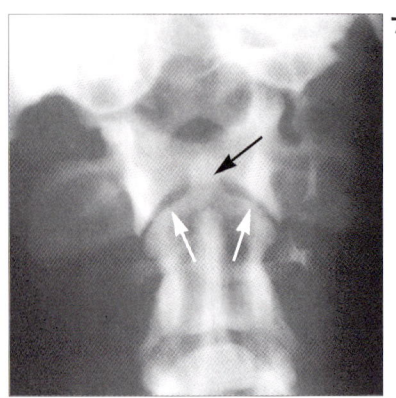

72 Ventrodorsal atlantoaxial radiograph of a normal dog. The dens is arrowed. Note the atlantoaxial articulations also (white arrows).

4. DIAGNOSTIC AIDS

Thoracolumbar spine (73–76)

73 Lateral thoracolumbar spine. The patient is in lateral recumbency with the thoracic and pelvic limbs extended cranially and caudally respectively. A foam wedge is placed under the sternum to prevent rotation; wedges placed between the limbs also help this (see **77**). A wedge is placed under the lumbar vertebrae to avoid sagging. The beam is centred on the area of interest. It is important to collimate the beam closely to the spine; this reduces scatter from the soft tissues and greatly improves radiographic quality. A common error is to centre the beam in the midlumbar region when evaluating the spine for disc disease. Most herniations occur in the T_{11}–L_1 region, and the beam should be centred accordingly.

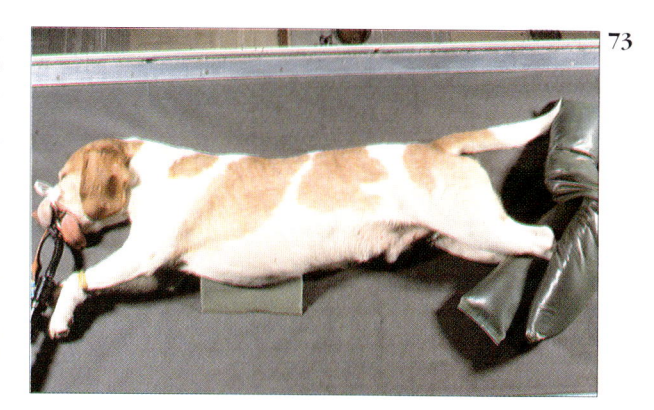

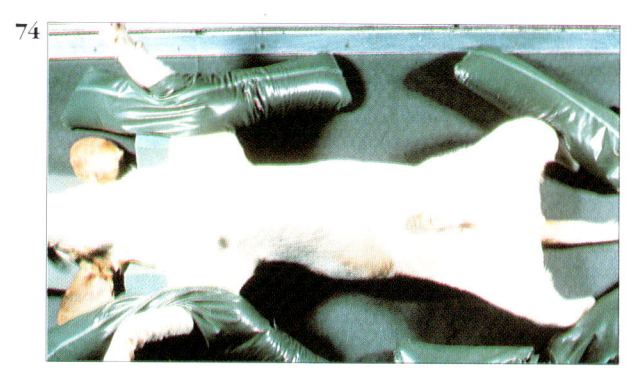

74 Ventrodorsal thoracolumbar spine. The patient is in dorsal recumbency with the limbs extended. It is important that the body is upright and that the beam is collimated.

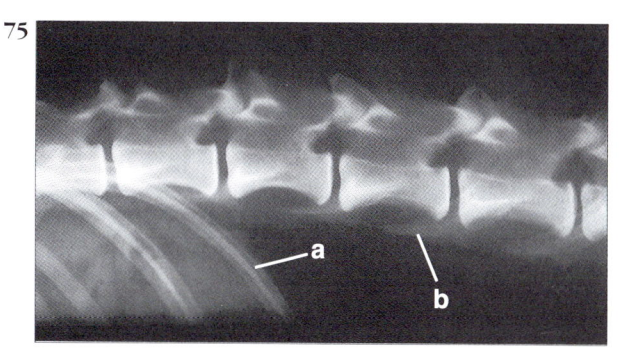

75 Lateral thoracolumbar spinal radiograph of a normal dog. The dog is well positioned, with the ribs (**a**) and transverse processes (**b**) superimposed. The intervertebral spaces in the middle of the image are parallel, but note how the space near the right edge is not clear.

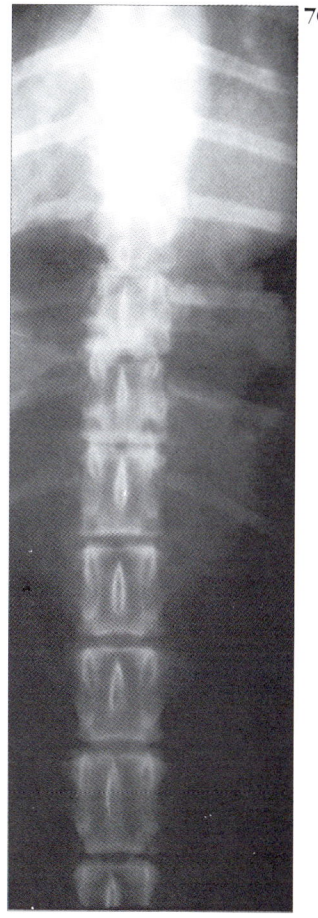

76 Ventrodorsal thoracolumbar spinal radiograph of a normal dog.

Lumbosacral spine (77–78)

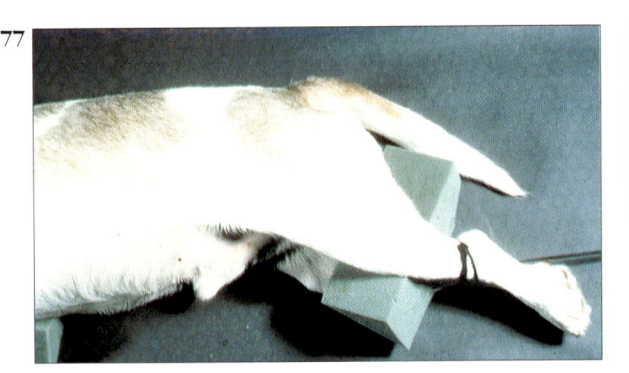

77 Lateral lumbosacral spine. Positioning is crucial as rotation may induce artefacts. The patient is positioned as for the thoracolumbar spine, taking particular care to keep both the pelvic limbs parallel to the table top.

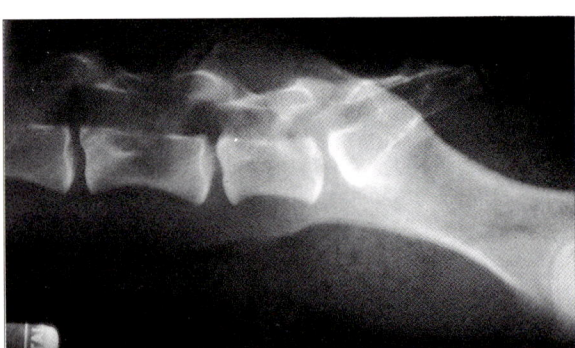

78 Lateral lumbosacral radiograph of a normal dog. In a well-positioned radiograph, the wings of the ilium will be directly superimposed.

SPECIAL RADIOGRAPHIC PROCEDURES

Myelography

In myelography the spinal cord is outlined by positive contrast medium injected into the subarachnoid space. The indications for myelography are as follows.

- Where the neurological examination indicates a spinal lesion, but none is visible on survey radiographs.
- To determine the significance of multiple lesions identified on survey radiographs.
- To determine the presence of spinal cord compression.
- To assist in deciding the indications for surgery and type of procedure to be performed.

This procedure is contraindicated if general anaesthesia or spinal puncture are unsafe (see 'Cerebrospinal fluid,' page 35), or where inflammatory disease of the CNS is present. The existence of CSF pleocytosis is not in itself a contraindication, as it is present in many compressive spinal diseases, including disc herniation (Thomson *et al.*, 1989, 1990).

The choice of contrast medium is important, as many are extremely irritant to the neural tissue. A non-ionic, water soluble contrast medium must be used; Iohexol (Omnipaque, Nycomed) is the contrast medium of choice (Wheeler and Davies, 1985; Allan and Wood, 1988).

Concentrations in the range of 180 mgI/ml–350 mgI/ml are used, most often 240 or 300 mgI/ml. The contrast medium should be warmed to body temperature before injection. Performance of a myelogram does not preclude the need to take high quality survey radiographs. The practice of using the survey films only to establish radiographic exposure factors is deplored, as significant information that would be visible on good survey films may be masked by the myelogram.

Technique

Myelography is carried out with the patient under general anaesthesia. Injection of contrast medium is either at the CMC or in the lumbar subarachnoid space. The techniques for spinal puncture are described above in CSF collection. Contrast is injected following collection of the CSF sample (see **54** and **60**). As a guide, a dose of contrast medium of 0.25–0.5 ml/kg patient body weight is used, although this can vary with the site of the injection and the expected location of the lesion.

Cervical myelography (**79, 80**)
If possible the table is tilted by 5–10° at injection. The bevel of the needle (indicated by a notch on the hub) should be directed caudally. Injection may be performed directly by applying a syringe to the spinal needle, or via a flexible tube, which is prefilled with contrast before injection. It is vital

4. DIAGNOSTIC AIDS

that the needle is not advanced into the spinal cord substance; use of the tube avoids needle movement during injection.

After injection the needle is removed and the patient's head is elevated. The legs and maxilla are tied to the table top with a noose. Initially, the patient is tilted at 15–20° with the head up and an immediate radiograph taken, further films being taken depending on the progress of the column. If the X-ray tube can be tilted parallel to the table, films may be taken in this position. The angle of tilt may be increased to 45° or more and further films taken until a lesion is demonstrated or the column ceases to flow. When the lesion is delineated, a ventrodorsal view should be taken.

If a tilting table is not available, the patient must be held up by the thoracic limbs, with the head above the body. This can be difficult in large dogs and use of a tilting table is recommended.

In normal dogs, the column will usually reach the lumbosacral joint in a maximum of 10 minutes on a suitably tilted table. Occasionally, the column stops in a totally unexpected position, often the low cervical region, and this should not be considered diagnostic until further time has elapsed and the table tilted to a steeper angle.

Lumbar myelography (81–83)

This is required in some circumstances, the most common being where an acute disc extrusion has

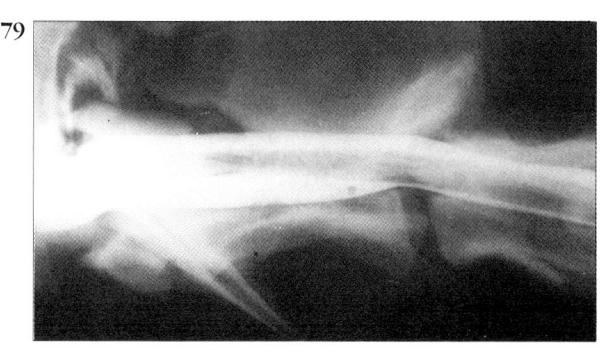

79 Normal cranial cervical lateral myelogram. Note that the columns are wide in C_1 and C_2. The ventral column thins and is elevated over the C_2/C_3 intervertebral space and to a lesser degree over the other spaces.

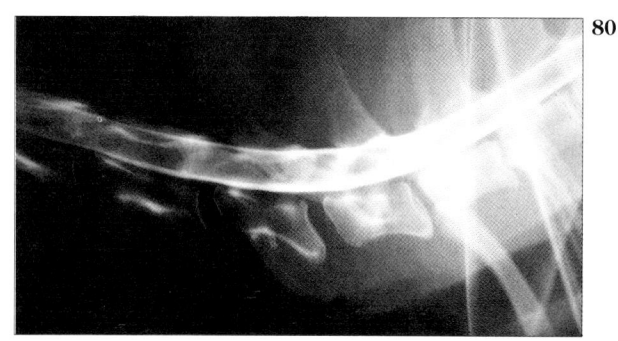

80 Normal caudal cervical lateral myelogram.

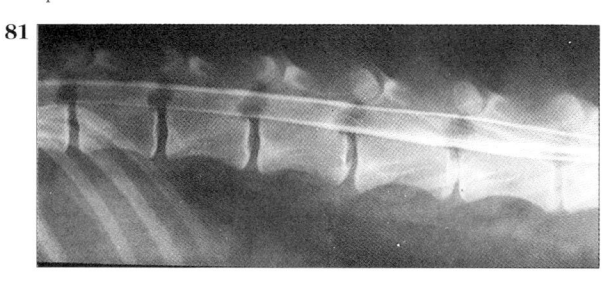

81 Normal lumbar lateral myelogram. Note the streaked appearance of the contrast medium where it outlines the nerves of the cauda equina.

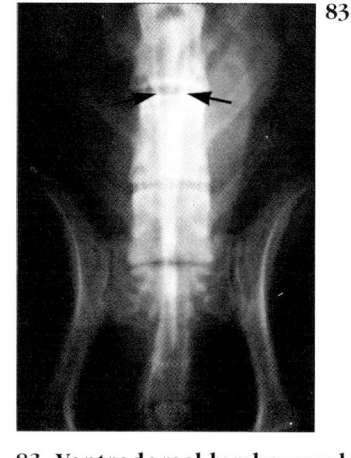

83 Ventrodorsal lumbosacral myelogram of a normal dog. The separate contrast columns can be seen in L_5 (arrows). The columns converge and cross the lumbosacral junction. Superimposition of the spinous processes and the presence of colonic contents can make interpretation difficult.

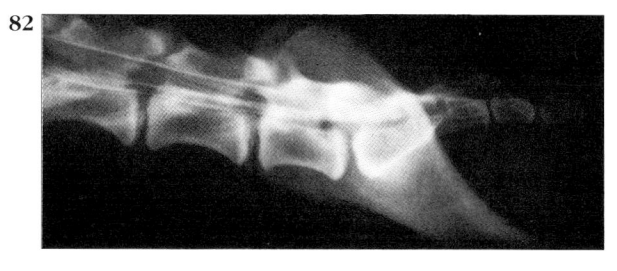

82 Lateral lumbosacral myelogram from a normal dog. Note the contrast column passes well into the sacrum.

occurred. Here, the injection of contrast medium requires relatively high pressures to delineate the lesion, as the spinal cord is often swollen. Some radiologists prefer lumbar myelography for all patients.

Epidural leakage is often a problem in lumbar myelography, which makes interpretation of the study very difficult (see **61**). Slow injection of the contrast medium reduces the chance of epidural leakage.

Special myelographic positions

Oblique projections may be useful in myelography. They help to determine which side a lesion is on, and may occasionally reveal lesions not apparent on lateral or ventrodorsal views. Obliques from the ventrodorsal position are most helpful, but interpreting these projections can be challenging.

In some circumstances, special stressed positions may give more information about a lesion seen in a neutral position, or reveal a lesion not previously apparent. These views are not often useful in survey radiographs (see **412**, **413**).

Cervical spine
In caudal cervical spondylomyelopathy special positions during myelography may be useful.
- The traction view, where tension is applied to the cervical spine. It can indicate whether the lesion is dynamic or static, which has a bearing on surgical planning (see **317**, **316**).
- The extension view, where the neck is extended dorsally, can reveal other lesions that may become significant in the future – the domino effect (see **315–318**).

Lumbosacral spine
Flexion and extension myelography may reveal lumbosacral lesions not apparent on neutrally positioned myelography (see Chapter 10), but it is possible to obtain false positive results from these positions.

Complications of myelography

Several untoward complications may occur, but the incidence is low when iohexol is used (Wheeler and Davies, 1985; Widmer *et al.*, 1992; Lewis and Hosgood, 1992).

Seizures occur infrequently on recovery from anaesthesia. The site of injection appears not to influence the frequency of seizures, but Dobermanns with CCSM may be prone to this problem. It is best managed by intravenous diazepam. Thus, it is prudent to leave an intravenous catheter in place in any patient recovering after a myelogram to facilitate medication. The patient must be observed until conscious and the head kept elevated.

Neurological deterioration is rare following myelography but can occur. Large breed dogs with significant cervical cord lesions, patients with meningitis or extradural tumours, and those with degenerative myelopathy seem to be most affected. Fortunately, this deterioration is usually transient, most patients returning to pre-myelogram status within a few days. Clearly, if the spinal puncture or injection technique is at fault, significant neurological damage may result. Injection of contrast into the central canal can occur in cisternal myelography; the effect on the patient varies but is generally serious. Cardiovascular effects are usually seen, and neurological deterioration is likely. Central canal injection in the lumbar spine is not usually associated with problems. Lumbar myelography at sites cranial to L_5/L_6 may damage the lumbar intumescence and should not be performed.

It is not clear whether the manipulations involved in obtaining flexion, extension or traction films during myelography lead to neurological deterioration, but it is wise not to position the patient in this way for excessive periods, particularly in extension of the cervical spine.

Epidurography

In epidurography, positive contrast medium is introduced into the epidural space. For some radiologists, this is the preferred method for evaluating the lumbosacral region (Feeney and Wise, 1981; Selcer *et al.*, 1988) (see **286**).

Discography

In discography, positive contrast medium is injected into the nucleus pulposus of the intervertebral disc. Normally, only a very small amount can be introduced (0.1–0.2 ml in the lumbosacral disc). If there is damage to the anulus fibrosus, more contrast can be injected and the leakage will be evident on subsequent radiographs. Indications are limited, but the technique is useful in lumbosacral lesions. (Sisson *et al.*, 1992).

4. DIAGNOSTIC AIDS

PRINCIPLES OF SPINAL RADIOLOGY

It is important to take a systematic approach to evaluating spinal radiographs. The clinician has the advantage of having similar adjacent structures with which to compare the suspected lesion. The quality of the interpretation is limited by the radiographs, and it is well worth paying attention to obtaining good films as discussed above. Also, knowledge of the normal radiographic anatomy is required, as discussed in this chapter and in Chapter 1.

One system used to evaluate lateral radiographs is to start ventrally on the spine and work from cranial to caudal, assessing each structure in turn. For ventrodorsal films, start on the left side and work cranial to caudal. This technique should be employed even if there is an obvious lesion, to avoid overlooking other important features or other lesions.

General radiological principles dictate that images are evaluated for the following features: number, position, size, shape, opacity and margination. Spinal diseases can demonstrate examples of alterations to all these features, and many are illustrated in this book (see also Davies, 1989).

Myelographic interpretation

From the myelogram, it is usually possible to gain an impression of the location of the lesion relative to the spinal cord (**84**). Note that lesions in all locations may give the appearance of an expanded or swollen cord if the film is taken face on to the lesion. For this reason, it is essential that two perpendicular projections (lateral and ventrodorsal) are made.

Interpretation is relatively straightforward if there are changes in the skeleton at the site of the myelographic abnormality, for example, in disc herniation or vertebral tumours.

Generally, it is possible to make some estimate of the location of the lesion as shown in **84**.

Causes of these compression patterns are given in **Table 10**.

Extradural lesions are shown in **85–88**, intradural extramedullary lesions in **89–91**, and intradural intramedullary lesions in **92–94**.

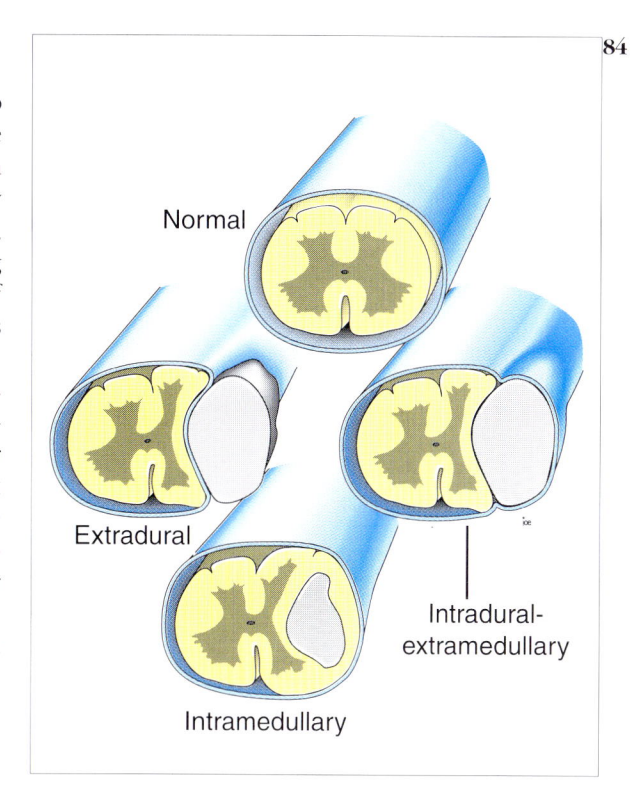

84 Spinal lesions are classified according to their location relative to the spinal cord and the dura mater. Examples of potential causes are given in **Table 10**.

Table 10 Causes of myelographic abnormalities

Location	Cause
Extradural	Disc herniation Congenital abnormality Neoplasia (vertebral, soft tissue e.g. metastatic, lymphoma) Discospondylitis Vertebral osteomyelitis Trauma (disc, bone fragments, haematoma)
Intradural-extramedullary	Neoplasia (meningioma, nerve sheath, neuroepithelioma)
Intramedullary	Ischaemic myelopathy (acute) Neoplasia (glioma, metastatic) Inflammatory CNS disease Haematoma

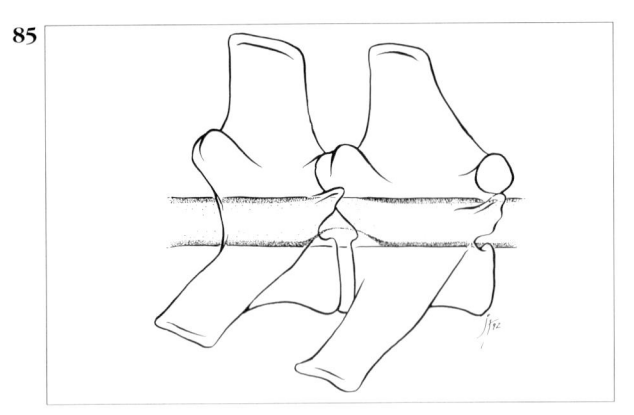

DIAGNOSIS AND SURGERY OF SMALL ANIMAL SPINAL DISORDERS

85 Extradural lesion. Diagram of the myelographic pattern of an extradural lesion.

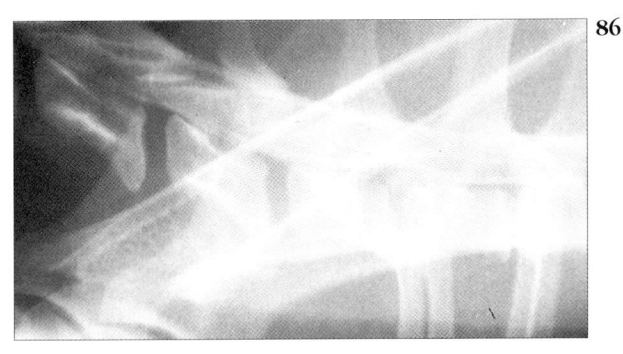

86 Extradural lesion. Myelogram of Beagle with neck pain, showing extradural compression of the myelogram at C_7/T_1. This was caused by a disc extrusion, an unusual site for this problem.

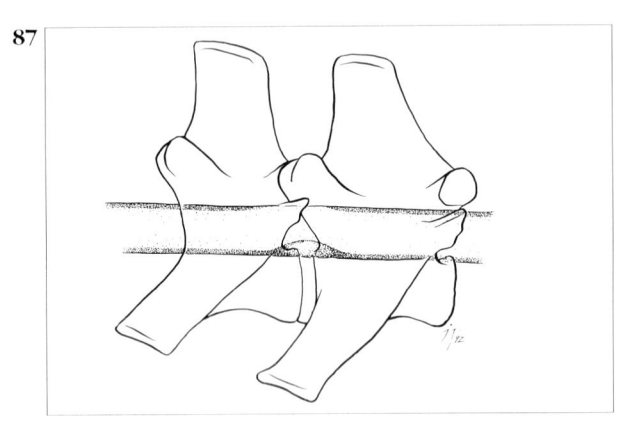

87 Extradural lesion causing column splitting. Diagram of column splitting, which generally indicates an asymmetrical extradural lesion.

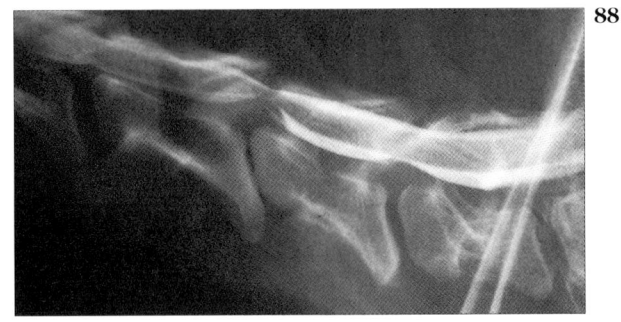

88 Extradural lesion causing column splitting. Myelogram of a Dobermann with neck pain and tetraparesis. The intervertebral spaces at C_5/C_6 and C_6/C_7 were narrow on the survey radiographs. The myelogram shows extradural compression at both sites with column splitting at C_5/C_6. A large disc extrusion was removed via a ventral approach at this site. The other lesion was not operated on, and the dog made a full recovery.

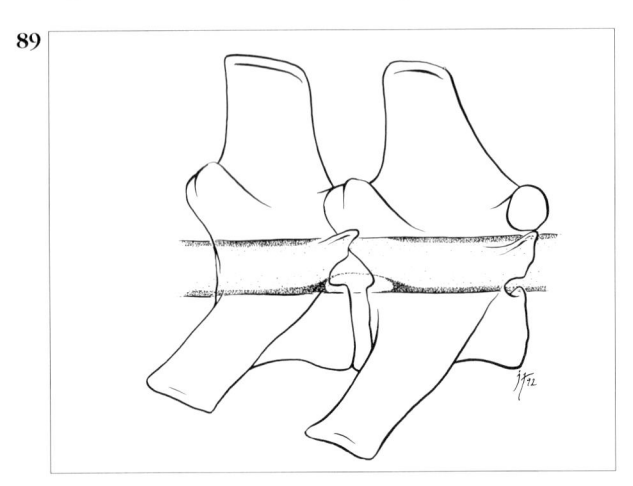

89 Intradural-extramedullary lesion. Diagram of the typical 'golf tee' pattern.

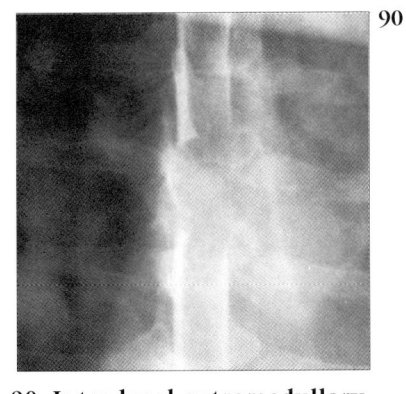

90 Intradural-extramedullary lesion. Myelogram of mixed breed dog with signs of thoracic spinal cord compression. A dorsal laminectomy was performed and a nerve sheath tumour resected.

4. DIAGNOSTIC AIDS

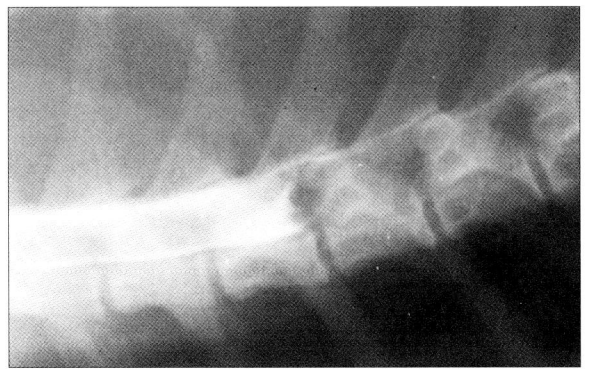

91 Intradural-extramedullary lesion. Myelogram of a cat with thoracic spinal pain and paraparesis. Diagnosis following surgical resection was meningioma.

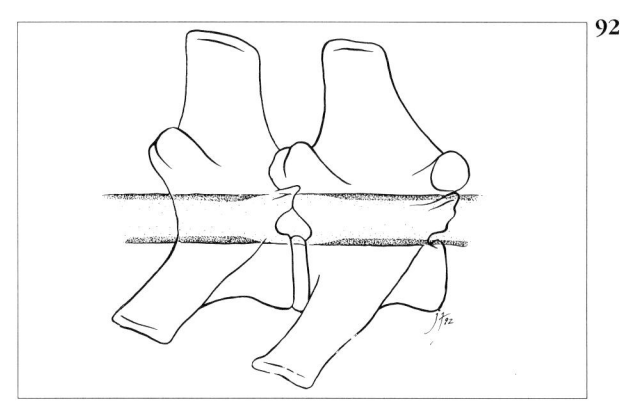

92 Intramedullary lesion. Diagram showing spinal cord swelling.

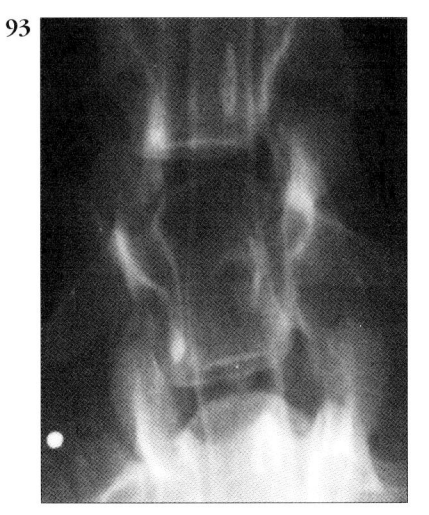

93 Intramedullary lesion. Myelogram of a Golden retriever with chronic progressive tetraparesis, but no spinal pain. The myelogram columns diverge in this ventrodorsal view, as they did in the lateral view. Diagnosis was a glioma.

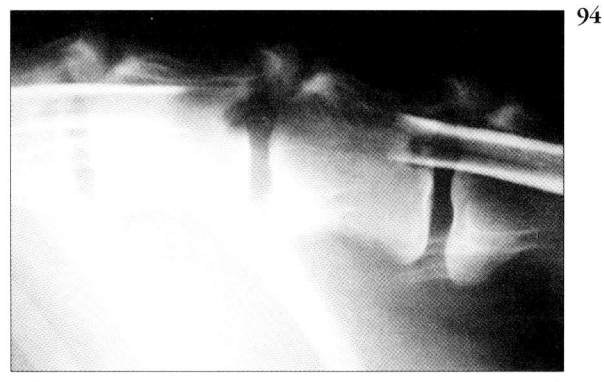

94 Intramedullary lesion. Lateral myelogram of five-year-old mixed breed dog with paraparesis without spinal pain. A similar divergent pattern was seen on the ventrodorsal myelogram. Diagnosis was astrocytoma.

OTHER IMAGING TECHNIQUES

Computed tomography

Computed tomography (CT) of the vertebral column is useful in the investigation of spinal diseases in certain circumstances, particularly vertebral tumours and caudal cervical spondylomyelopathy. Contrast enhancement by myelography (rather than intravenous contrast administration as performed in intracranial imaging) is most useful. A much lower dose of contrast medium is required for CT myelography than for conventional myelograms. If only a CT study is planned, the dose of iohexol is reduced to about one quarter of the dose for conventional myelography. If the CT study is performed directly after a conventional myelogram, the natural dilution and absorption of the contrast medium is adequate to reduce the contrast concentration usually after 1 or 2 hours. Alternatively, the patient can be positioned to allow the contrast to run away from the site of the lesion (but not into the head).

Vertebral tumours (see Chapter 12)

CT can provide greater information than survey radiography or myelography in some patients with spinal tumours. The lesion is first located by survey radiography or myelography. The CT images are then made in the appropriate region (**95–99**).

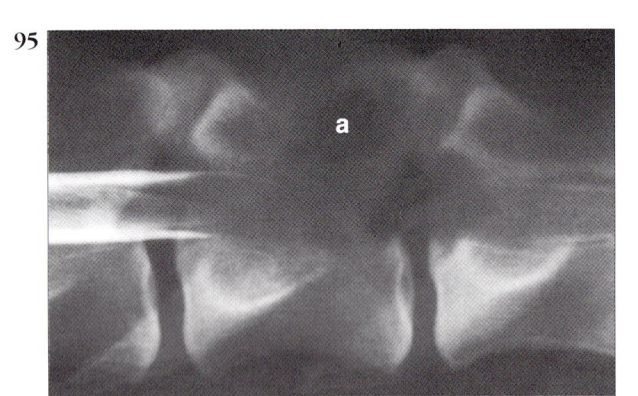

95 Myelogram of nine-year-old Rottweiler with lumbar pain and severe paraparesis (Grade 2 deficit). There is loss of bony detail in the vertebral arch (**a**) and dorsal extradural compression of the myelogram in the mid lumbar region.

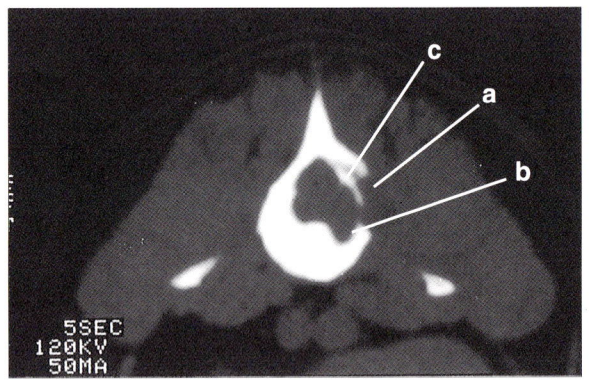

96 CT performed immediately after the myelogram. Loss of the pedicle (**a**) and part of the vertebral body (**b**) on the right side is seen. The extent of bony involvement was clearer on this and adjacent scans than on the myelogram. The subarachnoid contrast is almost obliterated on this slice, but part can be seen (**c**).

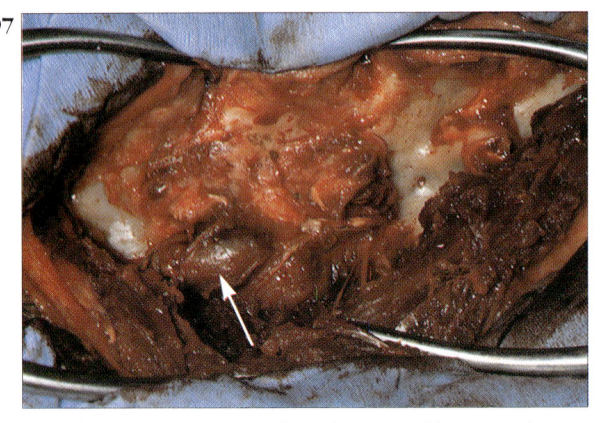

97 The region was explored surgically via a dorsolateral approach (see Chapter 8). Exposure of the vertebral column revealed a mass of abnormal tissue on the surface of one vertebra (arrows). The patients head is to the right in these illustrations.

4. DIAGNOSTIC AIDS

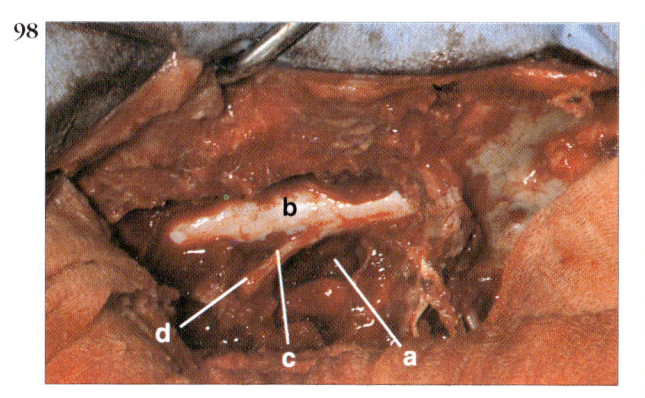

98 A hemilaminectomy was performed. Much of the vertebral arch was absent. Debulking of the soft tissues revealed a large defect in the vertebral body (**a**). The spinal cord (**b**), spinal nerve (**c**), and spinal ganglion (**d**) are seen. The dog recovered well from surgery, being able to walk within two days. In the interim the pathology report indicated a diagnosis of a highly malignant carcinoma. Attempts to find the primary tumour failed, and the dog was again paraparetic in four weeks, when it was euthanatized.

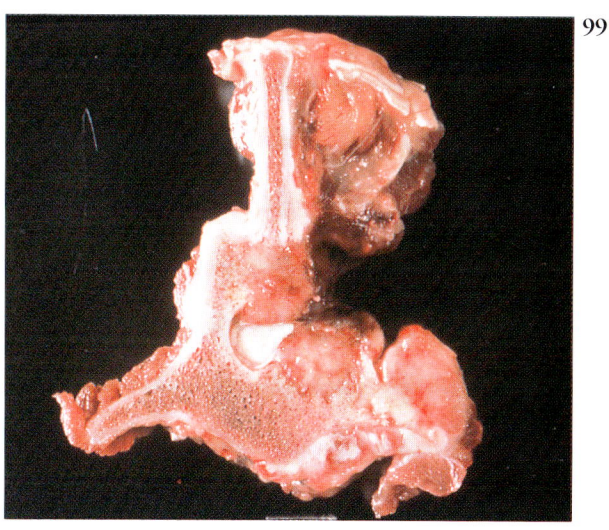

99 Section through the lumbar vertebra revealed the extent of the tumour regrowth, particularly involving the vertebral body and the lamina. The CT image in **96** is very similar to this picture.

Caudal cervical spondylomyelopathy (see Chapter 11)

CT is particularly useful in surgical planning as it provides information about the site of compression in the vertebral canal (that is, dorsal, ventral, lateral). Also, the size of the spinal cord can be seen; cord atrophy, if present, may be a poor prognostic sign (see **319–321**).

Magnetic resonance imaging

Magnetic resonance imaging (MRI) has an important role in intracranial imaging and has value in spinal diseases, particularly in lumbosacral disease (**100**) and in parenchymal cord lesions (DeHaan *et al.*, 1993).

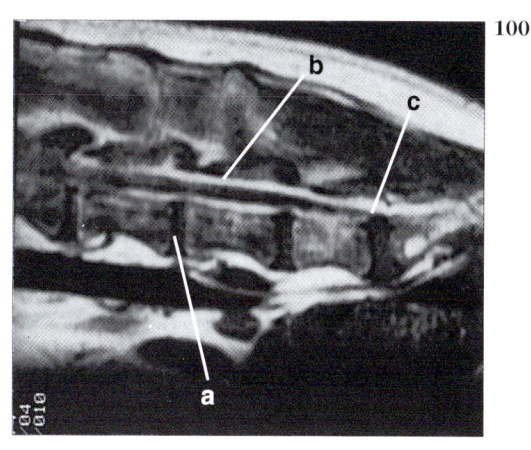

100 MRI image of dog with lumbosacral disease (T1-weighted scan). (**a**) intervertebral disc; (**b**) epidural fat in vertebral canal appears white; (**c**) protruded lumbosacral disc.

DIAGNOSIS AND SURGERY OF SMALL ANIMAL SPINAL DISORDERS

Scintigraphy

Bone scintigraphy evaluates some functional aspects of bone (**101**). Certain types of lesions will produce a hot spot on a bone scan; this may be evident before radiographic changes are visible. Particular uses of bone scintigraphy include discospondylitis and vertebral tumours (Lamb, 1987; Stefanacci and Wheeler, 1991).

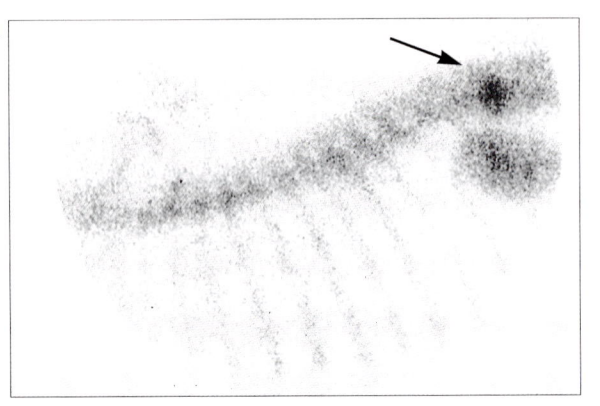

101 Bone scan. This is the scan of a seven-year-old Golden retriever, which had undergone limb-sparing surgery for an appendicular osteosarcoma three months earlier. No sign of spinal disease was present when this bone scan was performed, which revealed a lesion in the cranial lumbar region (arrow). Within several weeks, the dog was showing pain and paraparesis, and was euthanatized. Post-mortem examination confirmed the presence of metastatic osteosarcoma in the lumbar spine.

CLINICAL ELECTROPHYSIOLOGY

Electromyography

Electromyography is the method by which the electrical activity of muscle is studied and analysed. It can assist the neurosurgeon by helping to localize some of the more subtle lesions as either UMN or LMN. If LMN deficits are present, they will generally be associated with spontaneous electrical activity in the muscles supplied by the injured spinal cord segment or nerve root (**102**). This spontaneous activity takes about 5–7 days to appear, which is the time taken for the axons to degenerate from the site of injury to the neuromuscular junctions (Duncan, 1989). Two broad categories of LMN lesions can be seen.

- The first relates to lesions that are restricted to either the brachial or lumbosacral regions in isolation, such as brachial plexus avulsion injury or damage to the cauda equina. In this case, the spontaneous activity will be restricted to a discrete muscle group or groups.
- The second category is when the animal has a generalized peripheral neuropathy or myopathy, in which case spontaneous activity will be widespread and not restricted to any particular muscle group.

If an UMN lesion is present, electromyography of the paraspinal muscles can sometimes be very useful to help localize the lesion. Although UMN deficits are evident mainly through their effects on white matter tracts, they also impair neurons in the local grey matter at the same level. Damage to these neurons usually results in spontaneous activity in epaxial and hypaxial spinal muscles adjacent to the injured spinal cord segment. This activity seems to occur as a result of both degenerative and irritative effects, and so the latter may be evident on an acute basis (Chrisman, 1992b).

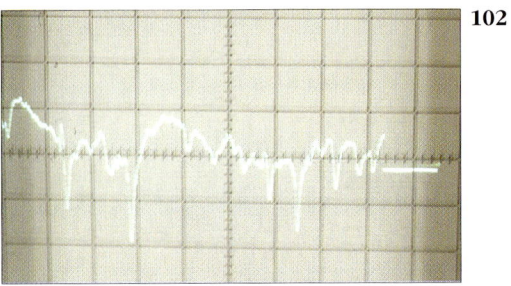

102 Spontaneous electrical activity. This was recorded from the gastrocnemius muscle of a dog that had a severe sciatic neuropathy secondary to a pelvic fracture.

4. DIAGNOSTIC AIDS

Spinal cord evoked response

A recording electrode is placed on the dorsal lamina of a cervical, thoracic, or lumbar vertebra in order to detect an electrical response travelling in the spinal cord. The impulse is created by stimulating a peripheral sensory nerve caudal to the recording electrode. The impulse or evoked response needs to undergo signal averaging to remove background information, much like a brain stem auditory-evoked response. The spinal cord-evoked response has the potential to give information about the functional state of the spinal cord after trauma.

Various parameters can be recorded from the evoked waveforms travelling in the spinal cord, but no single one has proved predictive of the eventual outcome in dogs with acute spinal cord injuries. Mathematical manipulations of the data may provide useful information but it can be difficult to identify and interpret the waveforms accurately in dogs with severe spinal cord injuries, as the waveforms are often small and dispersed. It would be a tremendous advantage for the neurosurgeon to have a more objective criterion than deep pain sensation to predict the eventual outcome in an animal with severe spinal cord injury. Further study is required before the spinal cord evoked response can make a significant contribution to the management of clinical cases (Shores *et al.*, 1987; Holiday, 1992).

BIOPSY

Most biopsies of spinal tissue will be performed following surgical exposure of the lesion. Neoplasms are most likely to be biopsied and are discussed in Chapter 12. Surgical exposure can sometimes be avoided. Fine needle aspiration of tissue from within the vertebral canal or vertebral body can be attempted, preferably under fluoroscopic control (Irving and McMillan, 1990) (**103–105**).

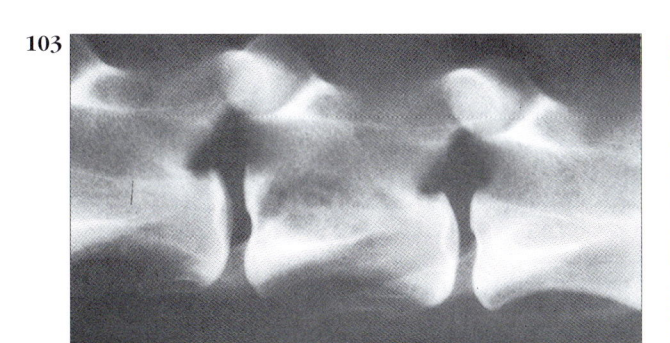

103 Radiograph of the lumbar spine. This radiograph of the lumbar spine of a six-year-old Golden retriever with lumbar pain and asymmetrical paraparesis shows loss of bone within the vertebral body.

104 Myelogram of the dog in **103** showing ventral extradural compression. A spinal radiographic survey, bone scan and thoracic radiographs revealed no other lesions.

105 Fine needle aspiration. A fine needle aspiration was performed under fluoroscopy. The material collected indicated a diagnosis of myeloma. The dog was treated on the basis of this diagnosis by radiation and chemotherapy and was still in remission two years later.

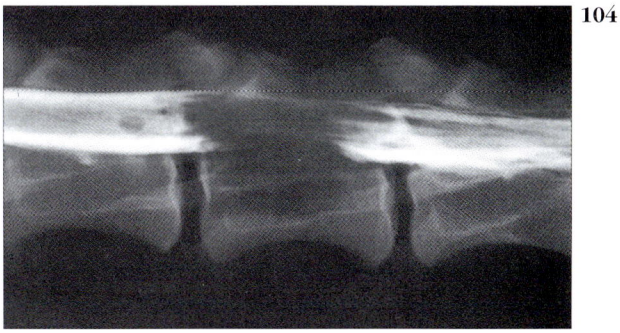

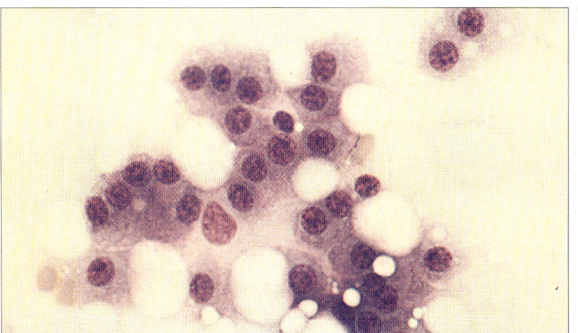

REFERENCES

Allen G.S. and Wood, A.K.W. (1988) Iohexol myelography in the dog. *Veterinary Radiology* **29**, 78–82.

Chrisman, C.L. (1992a) Cerebrospinal fluid analysis. *Veterinary Clinics of North America, Small Animal Practice* **22**(4), 781–810.

Chrisman, C.L. (1992b) *Problems in Small Animal Neurology*, 2nd edn, pp 89–100. Lea and Febiger, Philadelphia.

Davies, J.V. (1989) Radiology. In *Manual of Small Animal Neurology* (Ed. S.J. Wheeler), pp 85–106. BSAVA Publications, Cheltenham.

DeHaan, J.J., Shelton, S.B. and Ackerman, N. (1993) Magnetic resonance imaging in the diagnosis of degenerative lumbosacral stenosis in four dogs. *Veterinary Surgery* **22**, 14.

Duncan, I.D. (1989) Electrophysiology. In *Manual of Small Animal Neurology* (Ed. S.J. Wheeler), pp 63–65. BSAVA Publications, Cheltenham.

Evans, R.E. (1989) Haematology, biochemistry, cerebrospinal fluid analysis and other clinicopathological investigations. In *Manual of Small Animal Neurology* (Ed. S.J. Wheeler), pp 49–62. BSAVA Publications, Cheltenham.

Feeney, D.A. and Wise, M. (1981) Epidurography in the normal dog: technic and radiographic findings. *Veterinary Radiology* **22**, 35–39.

Holiday, T.E. (1992) Electrodiagnostic examination: somatosensory evoked potentials and electromyography. *Veterinary Clinics of North America, Small Animal Practice* **22**(4), 833–857.

Irving, G. and McMillan, M.C. (1990) Fluoroscopically guided percutaneous fine needle aspiration biopsy of thoracolumbar spinal lesions in cats. *Progress in Veterinary Neurology* **1**, 473–475.

Kornegay, J.N. (1981) Cerebrospinal fluid collection, examination and interpretation in dogs and cats. *Compendium on Continuing Education for the Practicing Veterinarian* **3**, 85–90.

Lamb, C.R. (1987) Bone scintigraphy in small animals. *Journal of the American Veterinary Medical Association* **191**, 1616–1621.

Lewis, D.D. and Hosgood, G. (1992) Complications associated with the use of iohexol for myelography of the cervical vertebral column in dogs: 66 cases (1988–1990). *Journal of the American Veterinary Medical Association* **200**, 1381–1384.

Mayhew, I.G. and Beal, C.R. (1980) Techniques of analysis of cerebrospinal fluid. *Veterinary Clinics of North America, Small Animal Practice.* **10**, 155–176.

Selcer, B.A., Chambers, J.N., Schwensen, K. and Mahaffey, M.B. (1988) Epidurography as a diagnostic aid in canine lumbosacral compressive disease: 47 cases (1981–1986). *Veterinary and Comparative Orthopaedics and Traumatology* **2**, 97–103.

Shores A., Redding R.W. and Knecht C.D. (1987). Spinal-evoked potentials in dogs with acute compressive thoracolumbar spinal cord lesions. *American Journal of Veterinary Research* **48**, 1524–1530.

Sisson, A.F., LeCouteur, R.A., Ingram, J.T., Park, R.D. and Child, G. (1992) Diagnosis of cauda equina abnormalities by using electromyography, discography, and epidurography in dogs. *Journal of Veterinary Internal Medicine* **6**, 253–263.

Stefanacci, J.D. and Wheeler, S.J. (1991) Skeletal scintigraphy in canine discospondylitis. *Proceedings, American College of Veterinary Radiology Annual Scientific Meeting*, p. 66

Thomson, C.E., Kornegay, J.N. and Stevens, J.B. (1989) Canine intervertebral disc disease: Changes in the cerebrospinal fluid. *Journal of Small Animal Practice* **30**, 685–688.

Thomson, C.E., Kornegay, J.N. and Stevens, J.B. (1990) Analysis of cerebrospinal fluid from the cerebellomedullary and lumbar cisterns of dogs with focal neurologic disease: 145 cases (1985–1987). *Journal of the American Veterinary Medical Association* **196**, 1841–1844.

Wheeler, S.J. and Davies, J.V. (1985) Iohexol myelography in the dog and cat: a series of one hundred cases, and a comparison with metrizamide and iopamidol. *Journal of Small Animal Practice* **26**, 247–256.

Widmer, W.R., Blevins, W.E., Jakovljevic, S., Teclaw, R.F., Han, C.M. and Hurd, C.D. (1992) Iohexol and iopamidol myelography in the dog: a clinical trial comparing adverse effects and myelographic quality. *Veterinary Radiology and Ultrasound* **33**, 327–333.

Wilson, J.B. and Stevens, J.B. (1977) Effects of blood contamination on cerebrospinal fluid analysis. *Journal of the American Veterinary Medical Association* **171**, 256–258.

5. INSTRUMENTATION

Spinal surgery requires some special instruments and many of the items are illustrated in this chapter (**106–127**)*. However, the starting point is a well-equipped general surgical pack, as would be used for most soft tissue and orthopaedic procedures (Nieves *et al.*, 1993). With experience, surgeons find which instruments they prefer for spinal surgery, but there is no doubt that certain instruments make the tasks easier and, thus, more efficient.

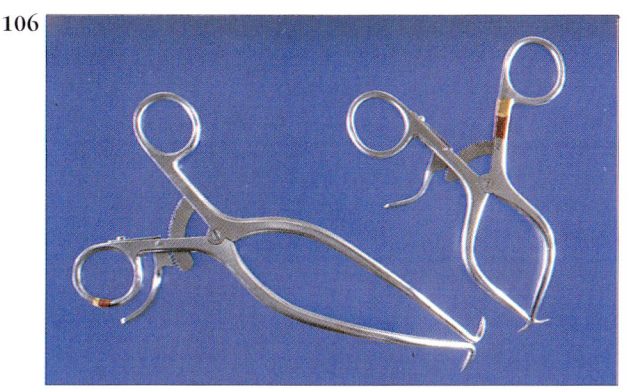

106 Gelpi self-retaining retractors. These are particularly useful in all dorsal and dorsolateral approaches to the spine.

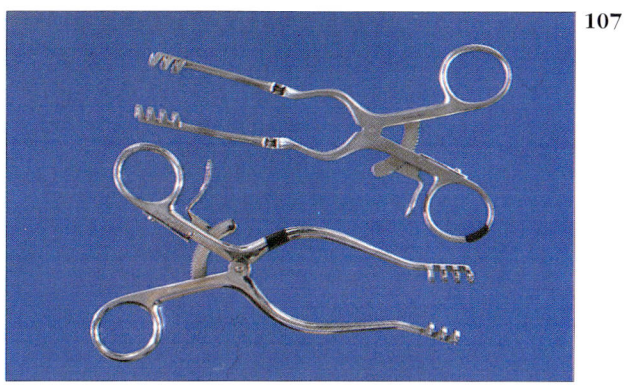

107 Multi-toothed self-retaining retractors. Here illustrated are Weitlander and Adson–Baby (top) retractors. West retractors are similar.

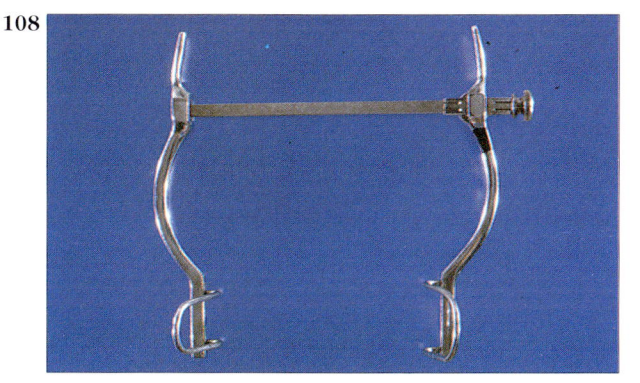

108 Blunt self-retaining retractors. These are invaluable in the ventral approach to the cervical spine, either Gosset (illustrated) or paediatric Balfour.

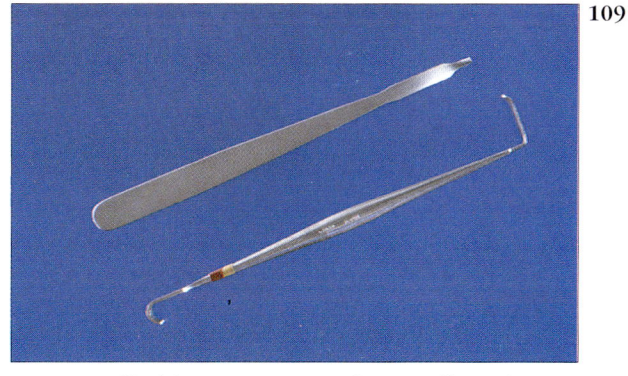

109 Handheld retractors. The small Hohmann retractor (above) is useful in ventral repair of atlantoaxial subluxation. The Senn (below) or Langenbeck retractor is useful in dorsal, dorsolateral and lateral approaches to the spine.

* The instruments described here are available from Veterinary Instrumentation, 62 Cemetery Road, Sheffield, S11 8FP, United Kingdom; tel: 0742 700078; fax: 0742 759471.

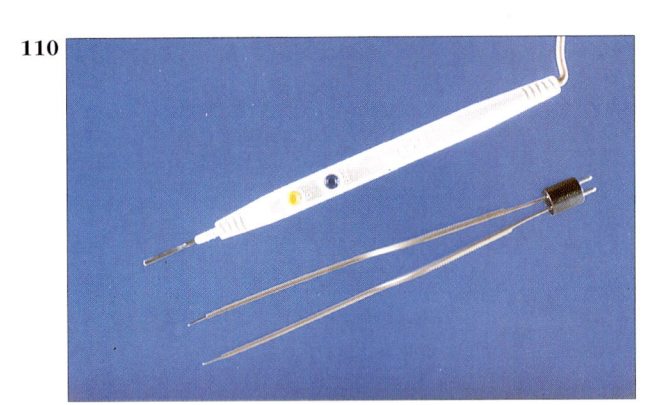

DIAGNOSIS AND SURGERY OF SMALL ANIMAL SPINAL DISORDERS

110 Electrosurgical instruments. The monopolar system (top) is used for coagulation and for incising tissues (see **188**). Monopolar cautery should not be used in close proximity to the spine, as the current travels through the patient, and this can lead to spinal cord damage. Close to the spinal cord, bipolar cautery (lower) must be used for coagulation (see **196**).

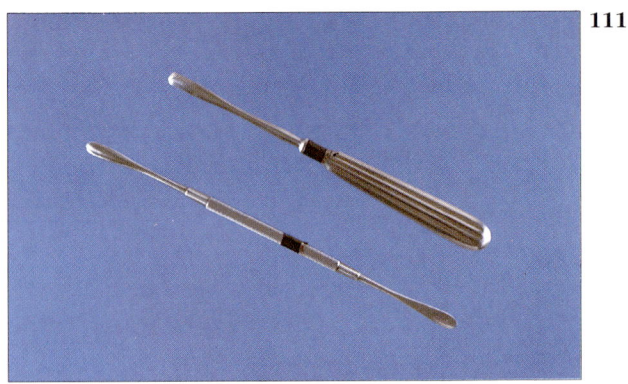

111 Periosteal elevator (top) and freer. For removal of muscle from the vertebrae.

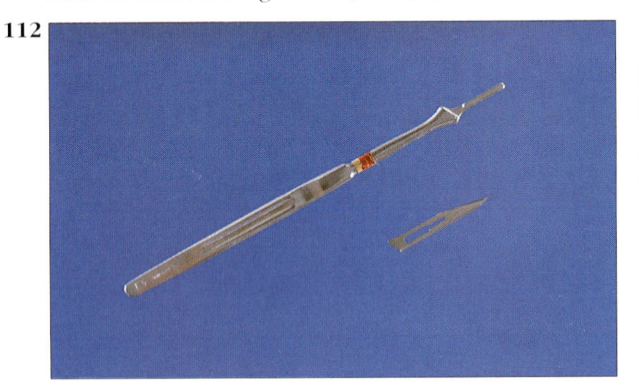

112 #7 scalpel handle with #11 blade. This is particularly useful for procedures such as disc fenestration and ligament removal.

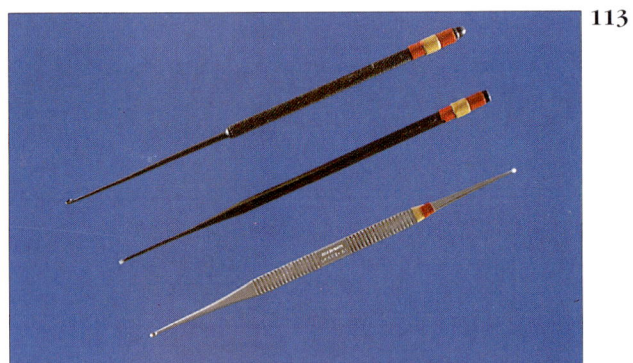

113 Instruments for fenestration and disc removal from the vertebral canal. From top: Shea curette; Rosen mobilizer; House curette. The latter is also very useful for removal of bone during the final stages of laminectomy and ventral spinal decompression.

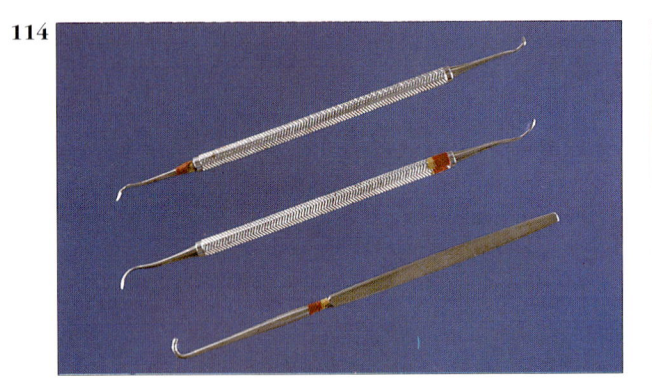

114 Nerve hook (below) for retraction of spinal nerves. Dental tartar scrapers (blunt and pointed) for fenestration and removal of disc material from the vertebral canal.

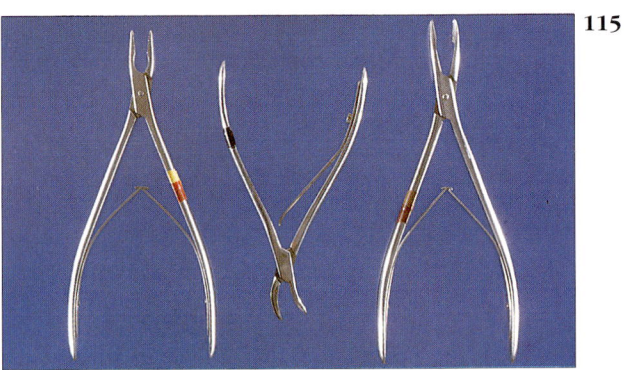

115 Rongeurs. These delicate rongeurs are used for fine bone removal. Larger, double action rongeurs are available for heavier bone removal.

5. INSTRUMENTATION

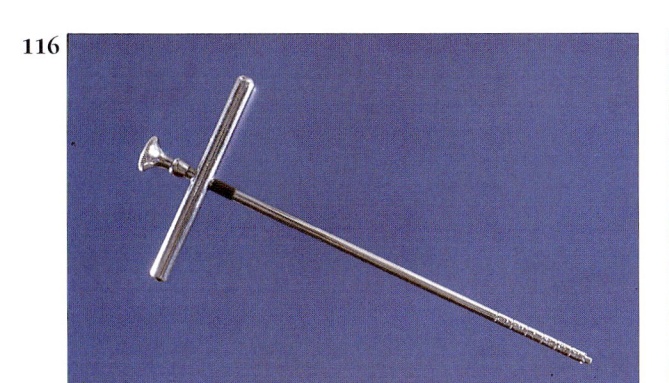

116 Mitchel trephine. This may be used for removal of bone in approaches to the spinal cord, but is less satisfactory than powered instruments.

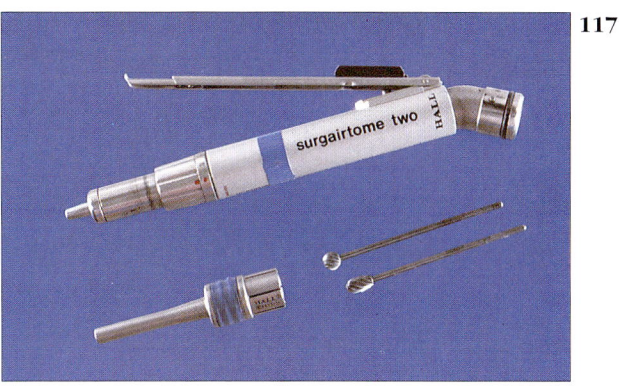

117 Pneumatic systems. These are preferable for bone removal in neurosurgical procedures. Illustrated here is the Hall Surgairtome 2 with long bur guard, and round and oval burs.

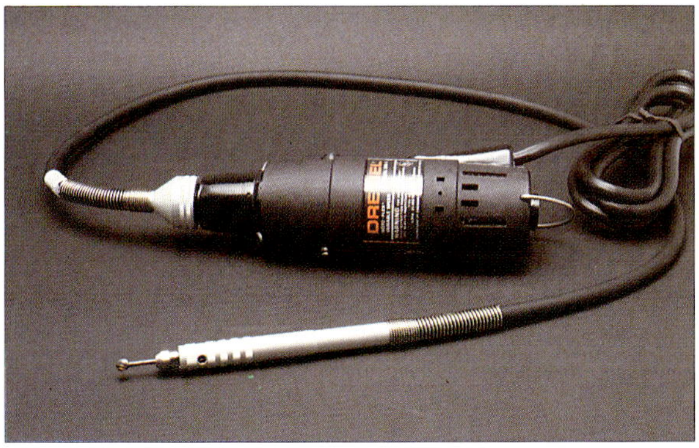

118 Electric drill. Alternatively, an electrical drill may be used, for example, the Dremel model drill. It is considerably less expensive than the pneumatic system and does have acceptable performance (Walker *et al.*, 1981). Sterilization is a problem; ethylene oxide systems can be used but their availability is restricted. Methods of wrapping the instrument in sterile drapes are available, but are less satisfactory, and we do not recommend them in view of the requirement for asepsis in spinal surgery.

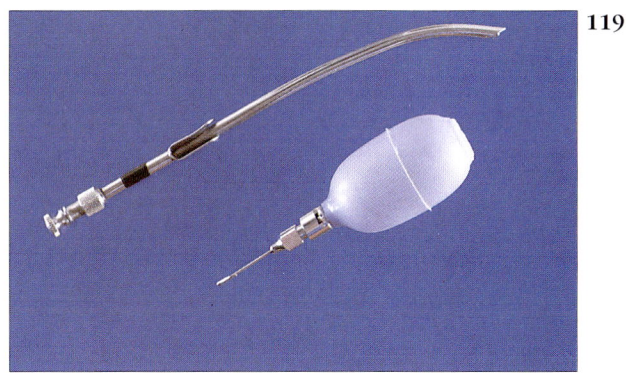

119 Adson suction tip and bulb syringe for bur irrigation.

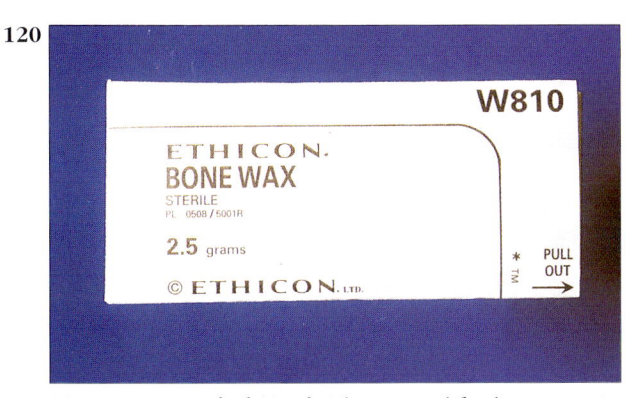

120 Bone wax (Ethicon). This is used for haemostasis; it is used to plug small vessels in bone by pressing over the bleeding site.

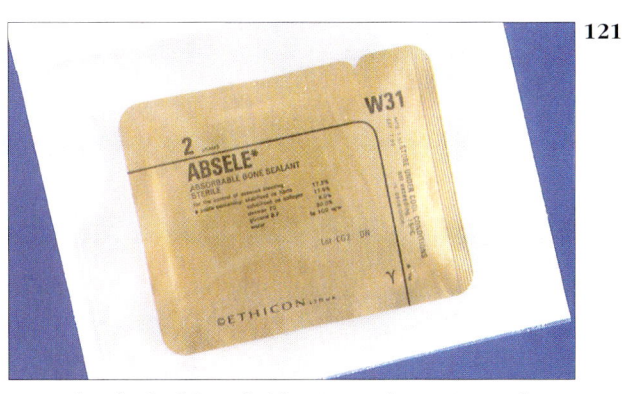

121 Absele (Ethicon). This is an alternative to bone wax, with the advantage that it is absorbable.

59

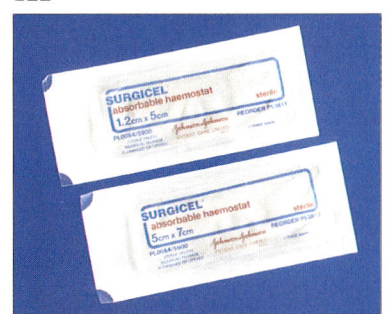

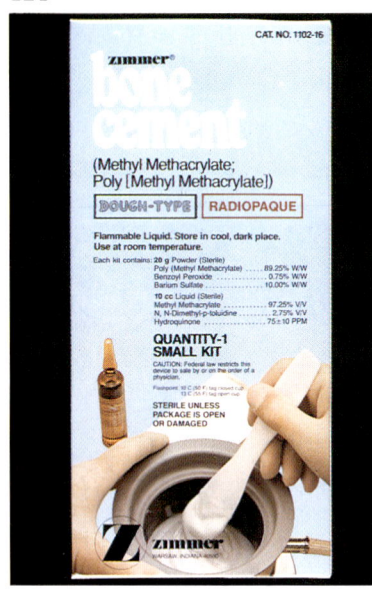

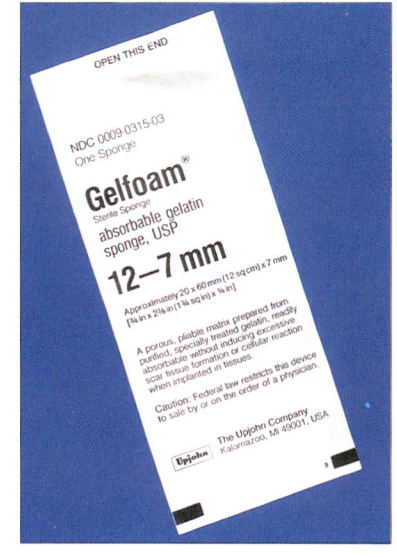

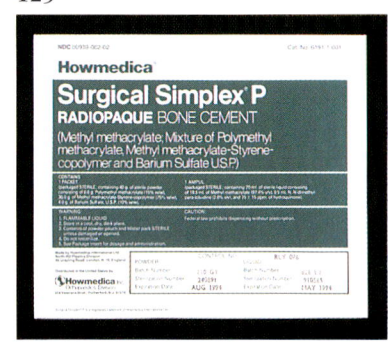

DIAGNOSIS AND SURGERY OF SMALL ANIMAL SPINAL DISORDERS

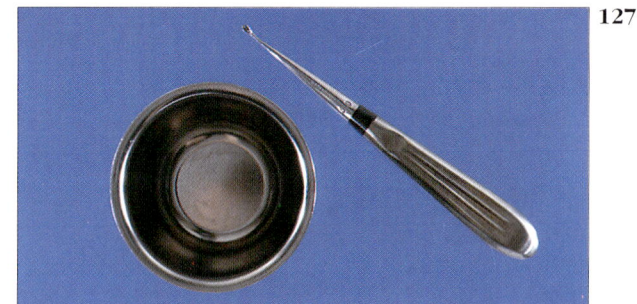

122 Surgicell (Ethicon) surgical cellulose. This is useful for haemostasis and covering defects in the vertebral canal.

123 Gelfoam (Upjohn). This is an alternative product.

124, 125 Methylmethacrylate bone cement. This is used in several of the procedures described in this book. It is worth emphasising the requirement for sterility when using these products.

126 The distractor and washers used for vertebral distraction and fusion in caudal cervical spondylomyelopathy (see Chapter 11).

127 Bone graft is used in several situations to promote vertebral fusion. Illustrated is a curette and bowl for graft collection.

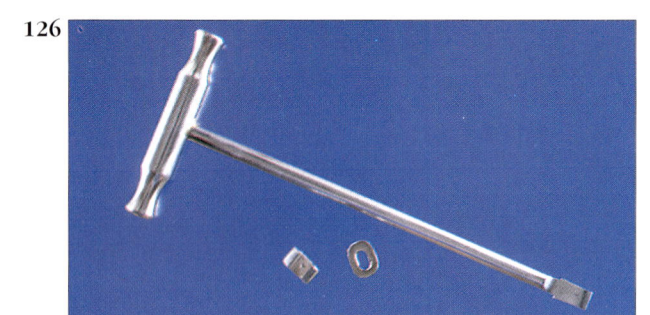

REFERENCES AND FURTHER READING

Knecht, C.D. (1987) Instruments and equipment. In *Veterinary Neurology* (Eds. J.E. Oliver, B.F. Hoerlein and I.G. Mayhew), pp 411–412. W.B. Saunders Co., Philadelphia.

Nieves, M.A., Merkley, D.F. and Wagner, S.D. (1993) Surgical Instruments. In *Textbook of Small Animal Surgery*, 2nd edn, pp 154–168, (Ed. D. Slatter). W.B. Saunders Co., Philadelphia.

Walker, T.L., Roberts, R.E., Kinkaid, S.A. and Bratton, G.R. (1981) The use of electric drills as an alternative to pneumatic equipment in spinal surgery. *Journal of the American Animal Hospital Association* **17**, 605–612.

6. PREOPERATIVE ASSESSMENT

The preoperative assessment of the neurosurgical patient is extremely important in view of the time, expense, and complexity of the procedures performed. Important aspects are considered in this chapter.

CLINICAL ASSESSMENT

It can be all too easy to overlook concurrent subclinical or clinical disorders that may have an important bearing on the case (**Table 11**). This is particularly true for older patients, those that have suffered trauma (see **Table 29**, page 171), and dogs with caudal cervical spondylomyelopathy (see **Table 23**, page 139).

Table 11 Conditions that may complicate management of a neurological patient

Skin or periodontal disease
Cushing's disease
Orthopaedic disease
Hypothyroidism
Cardiac disease
Diabetes mellitus
Hepatic disease
Disorders of haemostasis
Renal disease
Urinary tract infection
Neoplasia (undetected primary or metastatic disease)
Prostatic disease
Pyometra

Concurrent disease

The physical examination must be thorough. Skin disorders may necessitate delaying elective surgery, because pyoderma, clipper rash, or povidone-iodine reactions may predispose to wound infection. Fleas should be eliminated to prevent them entering the surgical field.

Osteoarthritic joints may significantly interfere with rehabilitation after neurological deficits, especially in large or obese dogs.

Laboratory evaluation should include a haematological and biochemical profile and a urinalysis. In cats, the feline leukaemia virus (FeLV) and feline immunodeficiency virus (FIV) status should be determined. If there is suspicion of cardiac dysfunction in large or giant breed dogs, suitable investigations should be performed, such as an electrocardiogram (ECG) or ultrasound. Chest radiographs are essential following trauma or in suspected neoplasia, and are recommended for recumbent, tetraparetic patients where pneumonia is possible. Endocrine disorders may also predispose the patient to many complications, for example, UTI and poor wound healing in Cushing's disease and diabetes mellitus (Muller *at al.*, 1989).

Neuropathies or myopathies associated with hypothyroidism may complicate the patient's neurological status. The assessment and, if possible, stabilization of endocrine disorders is always recommended before any neurosurgical procedure.

Haemostasis

Haemostasis is divided into primary and secondary events. Primary haemostasis depends on platelet aggregation and adhesion, and usually causes most concern to the neurosurgeon. It may be disturbed in the following conditions.
- Von Willebrand's disease.
- Severe thrombocytopenia (platelet count < 20,000/ml).
- Azotaemia (serum creatinine > 5.6 mg/dl).
- Non-steroidal anti-inflammatory drug (NSAID) induced platelet dysfunction, especially aspirin at doses above 25 mg/kg.

Disorders of primary haemostasis should be identified by a platelet count and bleeding time evaluation (see **324**, **325**). Problems include nuisance bleeding for the surgeon, postoperative bruising (see **472**), haematoma formation, or other more serious complications (see **322**). Haematoma formation with its risk of wound infection warrants appropriate surgical drainage (see 'Surgical drains page 65).

PHARMACOLOGICAL CONSIDERATIONS

Antibiotics

Most neurosurgical procedures can be classified as clean and uncontaminated, and will not require prophylactic antibiotics unless sterility is broken, or one or more of the factors in **Table 12** apply (Daly, 1985). Cephazolin (20 mg/kg IV) is recommended for its good tissue penetration and broad-spectrum of activity against staphylococci and other Gram-positive organisms (Richardson *et al.*, 1992).

Amoxycillin or trimethoprim-sulpha are preferable for many urinary tract infections, but antibiotic selection is best based on urine culture and sensitivity (Aronson and Aucoin, 1989).

Table 12 Some factors that can predispose to wound infections

Skin infection or severe inflammation
Periodontal disease
Urinary tract infection
Obesity
Shock or sepsis
Use of a surgical implant
Cushing's disease
Surgical time over 90 minutes
Excessive use of electrocautery

A short, decisive window for prophylactic antibiotic use extends from the start of surgery to a maximum of three hours afterwards. It is at this time that bacterial contamination of tissue can be suppressed by antimicrobial therapy. There is no advantage to using IV antibiotics before the start of surgery, or for continuing them beyond its completion, except in concomitant diseases such as pyoderma or UTI (Rosin, 1988).

Corticosteroids

Corticosteroids can cause gastrointestinal bleeding in as many as 15% of neurosurgical patients, with mortality rates of up to 2% (Moore and Withrow, 1982; Toombs *et al.*, 1986). Dexamethasone is most likely to cause these problems, yet there is little evidence that this drug has benefit in CNS injury and it is of doubtful value in experimental acute spinal cord trauma (Rucker *et al.*, 1981; Hoerlein *et al.*, 1983, 1985; Brown and Hall, 1992). Thus, routine dexamethasone therapy in spinal patients is strongly discouraged.

Methylprednisolone sodium succinate

After acute injury, the blood supply to the spinal cord is progressively reduced. When the injured tissue is reperfused, massive amounts of highly reactive chemicals called free radicals are liberated. These are especially damaging to the cell membrane by the process of lipid peroxidation. Free radical-induced lipid peroxidation is now recognized as a key pathophysiological mechanism for irreversible tissue loss following spinal cord trauma and ischaemia (Brown and Hall, 1992).

Some corticosteroids can exert a powerful protective effect against reperfusion injury by acting as free radical scavengers. These benefits are not, however, due to glucocorticoid activity and only occur in doses far higher than those normally used. The optimal neuroprotective dose of methylprednisolone sodium succinate has been determined to be 30 mg/kg, whereas doses of 60 mg/kg were detrimental and doses of 15 mg/kg had no effect.

Benefit has only been observed in humans with spinal cord injury who received treatment within eight hours of injury (Bracken *et al.*, 1990). Further follow-up has confirmed that the gains are limited (Bracken *et al.*, 1992).

In animals, the suggested dosage regimen is an initial IV bolus of 30 mg/kg methylprednisolone sodium succinate, followed by 15 mg/kg IV two and six hours later, then 2.5 mg/kg IV per hour for a further 24–48 hours (Brown and Hall, 1992). The bolus doses should be given slowly to avoid vomiting and hypotension. This regimen may also have some beneficial effects when spinal cord decompression is performed on lesions that have been present for longer than eight hours (**128**).

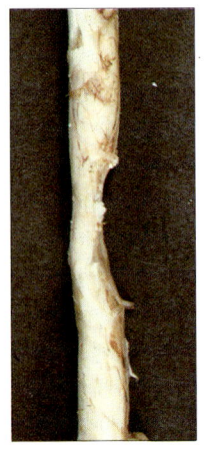

128 Post-mortem appearance of the spinal cord from a dog with a large intervertebral disc extrusion. Regardless of how many hours previously such a lesion occurred, reperfusion injury may occur when the spinal cord is decompressed. For this reason, some surgeons advocate high-dose methylprednisolone sodium succinate therapy at the time of decompressive surgery.

However, this hypothesis has not yet been adequately tested.

No serious side-effects were reported using high-dose methylprednisolone sodium succinate therapy in dogs with thoracolumbar disc disease (Seimering and Vroman, 1992). Caution is advised, however, because the effect of previous treatment with other corticosteroids prior to methylprednisolone sodium succinate is not known. A further note of caution is also necessary. Although high dose methylprednisolone therapy may be an advance in the management of acute spinal cord injury, it is not a panacea. Despite clinical improvement, all human spinal injury patients remained in their original category of either tetraplegic, tetraparetic, paraplegic or paraparetic (Bracken *et al.*, 1990, 1992). The subtle improvement seen in humans may not translate into useful benefits in animals. Methylprednisolone sodium succinate therapy must be looked upon as a way to compliment, but not replace, current veterinary neurosurgical techniques.

ANAESTHETIC CONSIDERATIONS

Many neurological patients will be dehydrated at presentation. They must be adequately rehydrated before anaesthetic induction, because of the detrimental effect of hypotension on spinal cord perfusion.

Premedication
Pethidine (meperidine) (3–5 mg/kg IM) or butorphanol (0.1–0.2 mg/kg IM) are recommended premedicants to relieve pain and anxiety (Court *et al.*, 1990). Glycopyrrolate (0.01 mg/kg) is the preferred anticholinergic as it does not induce tachycardia, although atropine (0.005–0.01 mg/kg) may still be required to treat severe bradyarrhythmias (Stauffer *et al.*, 1988). Diazepam (0.1–0.4 mg/kg IM) or acepromazine (0.025–0.05 mg/kg IM) can be added to provide sedation, if loss of protective muscle tone and hypotension are acceptable side-effects.

Anaesthesia
Induction should be rapid; thiopentone sodium is the usual agent of choice. Intubation should employ a laryngoscope and be performed with as little movement of the spine as possible, especially for dogs with cervical lesions. An armoured endotracheal tube is recommended if CSF is to be taken from the cerebellomedullary cistern, if stress radiographs are to be taken, or if a ventral approach to the neck is to be used.

Isofluorane is the inhalation agent of choice, because it is both less depressant to the cardiovascular system and less arrhythmogenic than halothane (Dodman, 1992).

Methoxyfluorane provides good muscle relaxation and better postoperative analgesia than isofluorane, but is contraindicated in animals receiving opioids or NSAIDs, or in those with renal disease (Cribb, 1992). Maintenance of anaesthesia should be at a depth sufficient to prevent movement of the patient, which could be very dangerous during surgery. Isofluorane at 1.5 minimum alveolar concentration has been recommended, combined with mild hyperventilation to keep the $PaCO_2$ between 25–35 mm Hg (Gilroy, 1985). Muscle relaxation can help in laminectomies or fracture repairs, and will tend to lower the requirement for inhalation agents. Atracurium is probably the safest agent for neurological patients (Jones, 1992). Nitrous oxide should not be used if the patient will be temporarily disconnected from the gas supply during CSF collection or radiography, as this may rapidly result in hypoxia.

Potential complications
Myelography may cause cardiac arrhythmias, and hypothermia is a potential problem, particularly in small patients or if the anaesthetic period is prolonged. In one study, six out of 66 dogs developed bradycardia, one died, and two also developed bradycardia during recovery following iohexol injection (Lewis and Hosgood, 1992). However, other studies have shown it to be a very safe contrast agent for myelography (Wheeler and Davies, 1985; Allan and Wood, 1988). The risks may be higher for other contrast agents. It is recommended that the patient be at an adequate depth of anaesthesia

before the injection is made, and that the contrast be used at body temperature, and injected at a steady rate. The ECG must be monitored closely during this period and any problems treated promptly. Similar precautions should be taken during CSF collection at the CMC (Court *et al.*, 1990).

The type of surgery may also produce cardiac abnormalities. Cervical spinal surgery is associated with a much higher risk of arrhythmias and ventricular premature contractions than thoracolumbar surgery (Stauffer *et al.*, 1988). This may result from manipulation of either the spinal cord itself, or of nerves in the ventral neck. Surgery in the rostral and midthoracic spine can also impair autonomic control of cardiovascular function and should likewise be monitored very closely.

Anaesthesia must optimize both cardiovascular and respiratory function to minimize ischaemia of the spinal cord. Spinal cord blood flow is normally autoregulated in a manner analogous to cerebral blood flow; volatile anaesthetic agents depress this and trauma to the spinal cord can abolish it (Gilroy, 1985; Kobrine, 1975; Kornegay, 1985). It is important to monitor the patient for cardiac arrhythmias or hypotension and to treat these promptly.

Recovery

Recovery from anaesthesia should be smooth, and this may be helped by the use of narcotics, diazepam, or both. If the animal has undergone myelography, its head must be kept elevated during the recovery period until it regains consciousness. Seizures should be treated with diazepam (0.4 mg/kg IV), repeated as necessary. The use of iohexol for myelography means that the risk of seizures is low, although Dobermanns with caudal cervical spondylomyelopathy may be at increased risk and warrant careful monitoring (Lewis and Hosgood, 1992). It is prudent to leave an IV catheter in place until the patient is fully recovered.

SURGICAL CONSIDERATIONS

Basic surgical techniques for neurosurgery share most of the principles of soft tissue and orthopaedic surgery (Powers, 1985; McCurnin and Jones, 1993).

Draping

The patient should be completely covered by sterile, waterproof surgical drapes. Their additional expense must be weighed against the morbidity and the cost of a surgical wound infection caused by organisms penetrating a porous drape. Sew-in or clip-in drapes may be used to isolate the wound further (see **194**).

Dampened towel drapes placed on top of the waterproof drapes are very useful to prevent tissues from drying out under surgical lights. They also help self-retaining retractors to expose the surgical field (see **296**). Tissues should be regularly irrigated with sterile saline to prevent desiccation and to reduce airborne contamination.

After completion of surgery, the site must be inspected to ensure that no swabs (sponges) have been left in the field.

Vision

Good lighting is essential for neurosurgery, and the availability of some form of magnification can also be very useful.

Electrosurgery

A bipolar cautery unit (see **110**) is essential if thermocautery is to be used near the spinal cord.

Laminectomy healing

A laminectomy heals as the haematoma forms a fibrous callus, which then undergoes metaplasia to cartilage and bone. To minimize development of spinal cord compression at the laminectomy site related to wound healing, it is advisable to keep the exposed dura mater separate from the dam-

6. PRE-OPERATIVE ASSESSMENT

aged epaxial muscles. Several implants have been used for this, the best results being obtained with autogenous fat rather than a non-biological implant (Trotter *et al.*, 1988). Fat conforms well to the surface of the dura mater and lies in a position that would otherwise be occupied by haematoma. The graft should be just large enough to cover the bony defect (see **212**), and should make a good seal around the edges of the laminectomy to prevent scar tissue from entering. As a free fat graft must revascularize, it should ideally be only 3–5 mm thick. An initial inflammatory phase resolves over 8–16 weeks, when the graft has shrunk to roughly half its original size. Free-fat grafts appear to perform as well as pedicle grafts (Trevor *et al.*, 1991). However, we have seen aseptic necrosis of free fat grafts used in laminectomies (see **395**).

Durotomy

Durotomy, or incision of the dura mater, is sometimes performed after laminectomy (see **210**). It is useful for evaluating intradural lesions, and it has been suggested that it may help decompress spinal cord swelling. Although it may provide additional decompression, the relative risks and benefits of the technique are not clear. In experimental situations, it was of value when performed immediately following trauma, but was of no benefit two hours after the injury (Parker and Smith, 1972, 1974). After incision, the dural edges subsequently rejoin, but they often adhere to the spinal cord as well (Trevor *et al.*, 1991). Mild temporary deterioration has been noted after durotomy (Parker and Smith, 1972).

Pharmacological treatment of spinal cord swelling is preferable to durotomy, which should not be performed routinely. Durotomy is of value in determining the prognosis where myelomalacia is suspected (see Chapter 8).

Myelotomy

Myelotomy involves incising the spinal cord on the dorsal midline to the level of the central canal. No value has been demonstrated for this technique, and it proved difficult to perform in cats in one experimental study without causing additional injury (Hoerlein *et al.*, 1985).

Surgical drains

If the surgeon thinks a subcutaneous haematoma will form after surgery, and certainly in animals with abnormal clotting, some form of drainage should be provided.

After a ventral approach to the cervical spine, it is not possible to close dead space around the trachea. When necessary, a Penrose drain is most appropriate for this location. It must exit through a separate stab incision near the caudal end of the wound. The drain is anchored at its proximal end within the wound and attached to the skin where it emerges distally, using a tacking suture (Lee *et al.*, 1986). The lumbosacral region is also prone to haematoma formation if the surgeon does not carefully close all dead space. Should a drain prove necessary, the closed suction type is preferred in this location. This can be either a butterfly scalp needle and vacutainer, or a syringe with the plunger held at a certain level within the barrel by a needle (**129, 130**). A closed suction drain keeps wounds and dressings dry and retards ascent of bacteria along the drain. It is important that high negative pressure is not applied near the spinal cord or nerve roots.

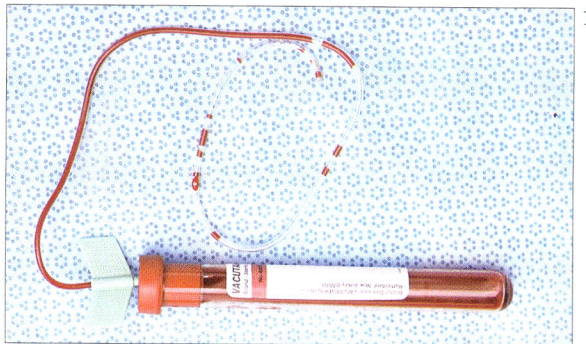

129 Continuous suction drain. Continuous suction drain made from a 19-gauge butterfly needle, from which the connector portion has been cut off and discarded. The polyethylene tubing, which can be fenestrated, is placed through a separate stab incision in the skin, and the vacutainer is then connected to the butterfly needle to provide negative pressure (Lee *et al.*, 1986). The apparatus must be covered to prevent patient interference and held in place by tapes, sutures, or both.

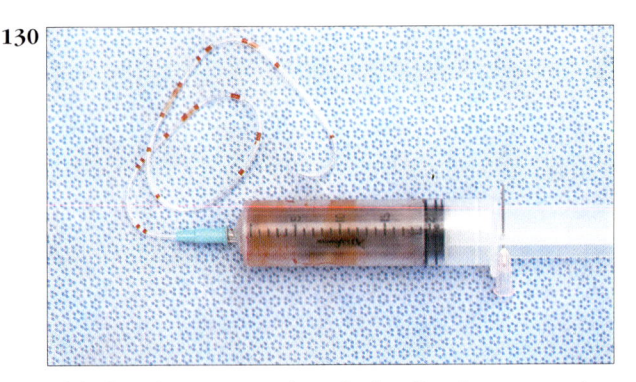

130 Continuous suction drain. Continuous suction drain made from a standard 20 ml syringe, in which the plunger has been pulled into the barrel to produce negative pressure. The plunger is kept in position by a suitably sized hypodermic needle, inserted into the plunger as shown. The size of the syringe can be varied, depending on the degree of drainage expected. This device also needs adequate protection and anchorage.

Drains must be covered by a sterile dressing to prevent external contamination, and bandages should be changed frequently to remove fluid from the wound area. A drain should be removed as soon as it is no longer beneficial. A 24-hour period of drainage is usually sufficient, although oozing associated with VW disease may last for several days. It should be remembered that the drain itself will induce some fluid production. The routine use of drains is not recommended, as no matter how well managed, they are still a potential route for bacteria to enter the wound. Penrose drains can actually increase the infection rate, especially if undrained pockets of fluid are colonized by ascending bacteria (Probst, 1993).

CLIENT COMMUNICATION

We feel that the client should always be offered the 'textbook' approach for managing a patient, in terms of the diagnostic evaluation and treatment. This should be offered regardless of the clinician's perception of whether the client will pursue treatment, even when it involves referral. In this way, the client is made aware that the very best is available for their animal, and any compromises arrived at will be seen in the proper perspective. Whenever possible, the clinical problems and the diagnostic and therapeutic options should be explained to the client in non-scientific terms. Anatomical specimens, drawings and the animal's own laboratory data and radiographs should be used to illustrate the situation.

On the other hand, care must be taken not to overload the client with excessive information, and they should be given time and the opportunity to think privately about their decision. It is also very important that the client be given as accurate a prognosis as possible, both for the degree of recovery and the time required. Giving the client prior knowledge of the probable prognosis and of the most likely complications is invaluable, should the patient suffer a protracted recovery or setbacks in its postoperative course. The client should never be pressured into consenting to a course with which they are not comfortable, even if the clinician feels that it is in the animal's best interests. If complications do arise the client may then hold the clinician responsible, not only for the decision but also for the complications.

Finally, the client should be given, and asked to sign, a consent form and a written estimate of the likely cost for the entire procedure. This estimate should include a price range to take into account any foreseeable variations in the postoperative course. If the bill begins to approach the upper end of the estimate, or if unforeseen complications develop, the client must be notified immediately.

REFERENCES

Allan G.S. and Wood, A.K.W. (1988) Iohexol myelography in the dog. *Veterinary Radiology* **29**, 78–82.

Aronson, A.L. and Aucoin D.P. (1989) Antimicrobial drugs. In *Textbook of Veterinary Internal Medicine*, 3rd edn, pp 383–412, (Ed. S. J. Ettinger). W. B. Saunders Co., Philadelphia.

Bracken, M.B., Shepherd, M.J., Collins W.F., *et al.* (1990). A randomized controlled trial of methylprednisolone or naloxone in the treatment of acute spinal cord injury. *New England Journal of Medicine* **322**, 1405–1411.

Bracken, M.B., Shepherd, M.J., Collins W.F., *et al.* (1992). Methylprednisolone or naloxone treatment after acute spinal cord injury: 1 year follow-up data. *Journal of Neurosurgery* **76**, 23–31.

Brown, S.A., and Hall, E.D. (1992) Role for oxygen-derived free radicals in the pathogenesis of shock and trauma, with focus on central nervous system injuries. *Journal of the American Veterinary Medical Association* **200**, 1849–1859.

Court, M.H., Dodman, N.H., Norman, N.M. and Seeler, D.C. (1990) Anaesthesia and central nervous system disease in small animals part II. Anaesthetic management for specific diseases and procedures. *British Veterinary Journal* **146**, 296–308.

Cribb, P.H. (1992) Advantages and guidelines for using methoxyfluorane. *Veterinary Clinics of North America, Small Animal Practice* **22**, 316–318.

Daly W.R. (1985) Wound infections. In *Textbook of Small Animal Surgery*, pp 37–51, (Ed. D.H. Slatter). W.B. Saunders Co., Philadelphia.

Dodman, N.H. (1992) Precautions when using isofluorane. *Veterinary Clinics of North America, Small Animal Practice* **22**(**2**), 332–334.

Gilroy B.A. (1985) Neuroanesthesia. In *Textbook of Small Animal Surgery*, pp 2643–2649, (Ed. D.H.Slatter). W.B. Saunders Co., Philadelphia.

Hoerlein, B.F., Redding, R.W., Hoff, E.J. and McGuire, J.A. (1983) Evaluation of dexamethasone, DMSO, mannitol, and solcoseryl in acute spinal cord trauma. *Journal of the American Animal Hospital Association* **19**, 216–226.

Hoerlein, B.F., Redding, R.W., Hoff, E.J. and McGuire, J.A. (1985) Evaluation of naloxone, crocetin, thyrotropin releasing hormone, methylprednisolone, partial myelotomy, and hemilaminectomy in the treatment of acute spinal cord trauma. *Journal of the American Animal Hospital Association* **21**, 67–77.

Jones, R.S. (1992). Muscle relaxants in canine anaesthesia 2: Clinical applications. *Journal of Small Animal Practice* **33**, 423–429.

Kobrine, A. (1975) Local spinal cord blood flow in experimental traumatic myelopathy. *Journal of Neurosurgery* **42**, 144–149.

Kornegay, J.N. (1985) Pathogenesis of diseases of the central nervous system. In *Textbook of Small Animal Surgery*, 2nd edn, pp 1022–1037, (Ed. D.Slatter). W.B. Saunders Co., Philadelphia.

Lee, A.H., Swaim, S.F. and Henderson R.F. (1986) Surgical drainage. *Compendium on Continuing Education for the Practicing Veterinarian* **8**, 94–103.

Lewis, D.D. and Hosgood, G. (1992) Complications associated with the use of iohexol for myelography of the cervical vertebral column in dogs: 66 cases (1988–1990). *Journal of the American Veterinary Medical Association* **200**, 1381–1384.

McCurnin, D.M. and Jones, R.L. (1993) Principles of surgical asepsis. In *Textbook of Small Animal Surgery* 2nd edn, pp 250–261, (Ed. D.Slatter). W.B. Saunders Co., Philadelphia.

Moore, R.W. and Withrow, S.J. (1982) Gastrointestinal hemorrhage and pancreatitis associated with intervertebral disc disease in the dog. *Journal of the American Veterinary Medical Association* **180**, 1443–1447.

Muller, G.H., Kirk, R.W. and Scott, D.W. (1989) *Small Animal Dermatology IV*, p. 646. W.B. Saunders Co., Philadelphia.

Parker, A.J. and Smith, C.W. (1972) Functional recovery following incision of the spinal meninges in dogs. *Research in Veterinary Science* **16**, 418–421.

Parker, A.J. and Smith, C.W. (1974) Functional recovery from spinal cord trauma following delayed incision of spinal meninges in dogs. *Research in Veterinary Science* **18**, 110–112.

Powers, D.L. (1985) Preparation of the surgical patient. In *Textbook of Small Animal Surgery*, pp 279–285, (Ed. D.H. Slatter). W.B. Saunders Co., Philadelphia.

Probst, C.W. (1993) Wound healing and specific tissue regeneration. In *Textbook of Small Animal Surgery*, 2nd edn, pp 53–63. (Ed. D.H. Slatter). W.B. Saunders Co., Philadelphia.

Richardson, D.C., Aucoin, D. P., DeYoung, D.J., Tyczkowska, K.L. and DeYoung, B.A. (1992) Pharmacokinetic disposition of cephazolin in serum and tissue during canine total hip replacement. *Veterinary Surgery* **21**, 1–4.

Rosin, E. (1988) The timing of antibiotic administration for antimicrobial prophylaxis in surgery. *Veterinary Surgery* **17**, 181.

Rucker, N.C., Lumb, W.V. and Scott, R.J. (1981). Combined pharmacologic and surgical treatments for acute spinal cord trauma. *American Journal of Veterinary Research* **42**, 1138–1142.

Siemering, G.B. and Vroman, M.L. (1992) High dose methylprednisolone sodium succinate: An adjunct to surgery for canine intervertebral disc herniation. *Veterinary Surgery* **21**, 406.

Stauffer, J.L., Gleed, R.D., Short, C.E., Erb, H.N. and Schlukken, Y.H. (1988) Cardiac dysrrythmias during anaesthesia for cervical decompression in the dog. *American Journal of Veterinary Research* **49**, 1143–1146.

Toombs, J.P., Collins, L.G., Graves, G.M., Crowe, D.T. and Caywood, D.D. (1986) Colonic perforation in corticosteroid treated dogs. *Journal of the American Veterinary Medical Association* **188**, 145–150.

Trevor, P.B., Martin, R.A., Saunders, G.K. and Trotter, E.J. (1991) Healing characteristics of free and pedicle fat grafts after dorsal laminectomy and durotomy in dogs. *Veterinary Surgery* **20**, 282–290.

Trotter, E.J., Crissman, J., Robson, D. and Babish, J. (1988) Influence of non-biologic implants on laminectomy membrane formation in dogs. *American Journal of Veterinary Research* **49**, 634–643.

Wheeler, S.J. and Davies, J.V. (1985) Iohexol myelography in the dog and cat: a series of one hundred cases, and a comparison with metrizamide and iopamidol. *Journal of Small Animal Practice* **26**, 247–256.

7. CERVICAL DISC DISEASE

Cervical disc disease is a frequent disorder of dogs. Small breeds, particularly those with chondrodystrophoid characteristics, are commonly affected, but it can occur in any dog. Dachshunds, Beagles, Poodles, Spaniels, Shih Tzus, Pekingese, and Chihuahuas are most often affected. Dobermanns suffer from cervical disc disease as part of the syndrome of caudal cervical spondylomyelopathy (CCSM) (see Chapter 11). Most patients are two years old or more, with a mean of six years. Disc disease is so rare in dogs less than one year old that other conditions must be considered first, for example, inflammatory CNS disease, atlantoaxial subluxation, or discospondylitis. There is no sex predilection (Denny, 1978; Dallman *et al.*, 1992).

CLINICAL SIGNS

The predominant clinical sign is severe neck pain, which may be acute or chronic (**131**, **Table 13**).

Table 13 Clinical signs of cervical disc disease

Neck pain
Low head carriage
Thoracic limb lameness or paresis
Thoracic limb nerve root signature
Hemiparesis
Tetraparesis

131

131 Dachshund with neck pain caused by cervical disc extrusion. Note low head position and thoracic limb held up. The hunched posture can be mistaken for thoracolumbar pain; physical examination differentiates the two.

Often the pain is unremitting and unresponsive to medication. This is one of very few conditions that causes dogs to scream spontaneously. Affected dogs may be reluctant to eat unless the food is raised off the floor. When examining the patient, it is usually not necessary to flex and extend the neck to demonstrate pain. Generally, it is adequate to palpate the spine and muscles of the neck, where the tension and pain are evident (see **37**).

Neurological deficits related to cervical spinal cord compression may be seen; paresis or lameness in a thoracic limb are most frequent. However, any signs related to cervical spinal cord compression can occur, including hemiparesis and tetraparesis. Nerve root signature (pain apparent on palpation or traction of the limb) is another frequent finding. An uncommon syndrome of severe, asymmetrical neurological deficits associated with large disc explosions following trauma has been described (Griffiths, 1970). Signs include hemiplegia, decreased pain sensation, and sympathetic dysfunction. Surgical treatment was not attempted in that series. In another series of asymmetrical disc extrusions, neck pain and thoracic limb lameness were seen. These dogs were treated by dorsolateral hemilaminectomy (Felts and Prata, 1983).

Disc herniation follows degeneration of the disc. Most occurrences are Hansen Type I extrusions. Hansen Type II protrusions do occur, generally in larger breed dogs (see **15**, **16**). The C_2/C_3 disc is the most frequently involved, with the incidence decreasing caudally. The C_6/C_7 disc is rarely affected, with the exception of Dobermanns and other large breeds as part of CCSM. The C_7/T_1 disc occasionally herniates.

It may be possible to determine the approximate location of the lesion in the cervical spine by identifying the site of most pain on palpation. Nerve root signature is more often a feature of caudal disc involvement.

7 CERVICAL DISC DISEASE

DIAGNOSIS

Radiography
The diagnosis is based on the clinical signs described above. Confirmation is by radiographic demonstration of narrowing of the intervertebral space and dorsal displacement of mineralized disc material (**132**).

Myelography
Myelography is required if the diagnosis is not apparent on survey films or if there are multiple discs potentially involved (**133–135**). In some lateral or intraforaminal extrusions, lateral and ventrodorsal projections of the myelogram may be normal; oblique views may reveal the offending disc. They are also useful in locating which side an asymmetrical extrusion lies.

CSF analysis
Analysis of CSF is useful to eliminate inflammatory CNS disease. Results of CSF analysis may be abnormal in disc disease, but elevations of protein and cells are usually mild (Thomson *et al.*, 1989).

The differential diagnosis to be considered is given in **Table 14**. Be particularly cautious in diagnosing cervical disc disease in dogs less than two years old or in aged animals.

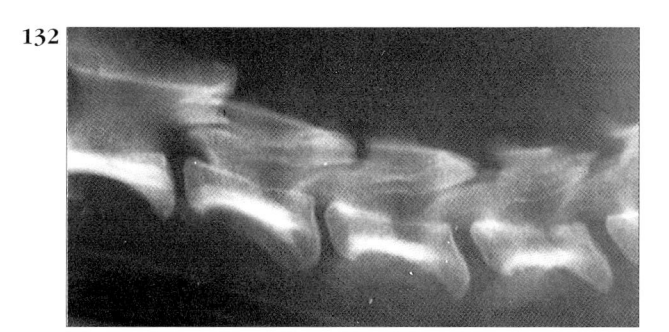

132 Lateral radiograph. Note the narrow intervertebral space at C_3/C_4.

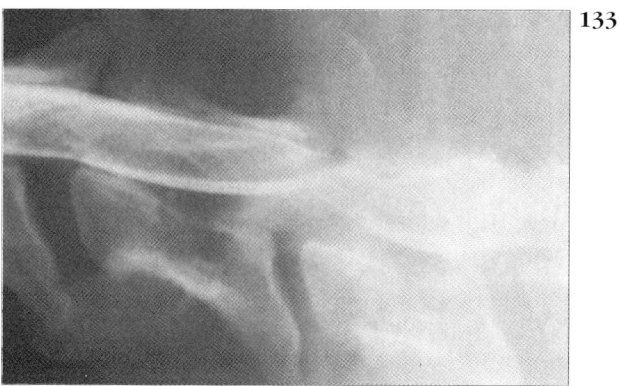

133 Myelogram demonstrating extradural compression at C_5/C_6. The intervertebral space is narrow and there is radiopaque material in the intervertebral canal above it.

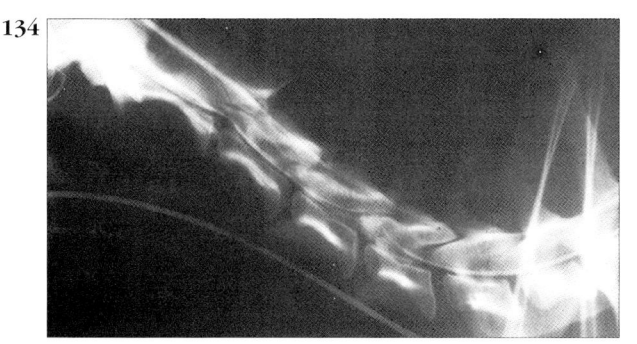

134 Lateral myelogram. Note the large extruded disc at C_4/C_5.

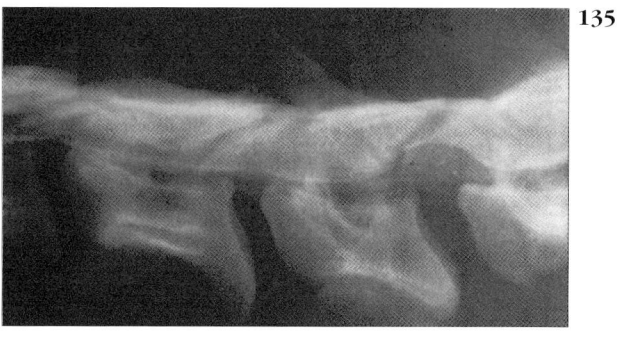

135 Lateral myelogram. Ventral spinal cord compression with split column delineating an asymmetrical lesion. Note also that the intervertebral space is not narrow. It is possible to have an extruded disc in the vertebral canal over what appears to be a normal disc space. In this patient the diagnosis was in doubt and the possibility of a nerve root tumour was considered. A dorsolateral hemilaminectomy was therefore performed. A large piece of anulus fibrosus was compressing the nerve root.

Table 14 Differential diagnosis of cervical disc disease

Clinical picture	Differential Diagnoses
Young dog with neck pain	Atlantoaxial subluxation Inflammatory CNS disease Discospondylitis Congenital disorders Trauma Neoplasia
Adult dog with neck pain	Discospondylitis Neoplasia Trauma Inflammatory CNS disease
Dog without neck pain	Ischaemic myelopathy Neoplasia

TREATMENT OPTIONS

Treatment may be nonsurgical or surgical.

Nonsurgical treatment

This entails cage rest and use of anti-inflammatory medications. It is appropriate to try this course with any patient, unless marked neurological deficits are present. Generally, NSAIDs are used (see **Table 35**, page 205). Diazepam or methocarbamol may also be of benefit (see page 205). Catastrophic worsening of the neurological status with medical treatment, which is often seen in thoracolumbar disc disease, is rare in cervical discs. Neck pain in cervical disc disease seems to be less responsive to nonsurgical treatment than does pain from thoracolumbar disc disease. Progression of signs or lack of response in one or two weeks indicate treatment failure. A dog that is responding well to nonsurgical treatment should be kept rested for at least two weeks after clinical signs have resolved. Recurrence of clinical signs after nonsurgical treatment occurs in 36% of patients (Russell and Griffiths, 1968).

Surgical treatment

Indications
- Failure of nonsurgical treatment.
- Marked neurological deficits.
- Progressive neurological deficits.
- Unremitting pain.

Ventral fenestration or ventral decompression (ventral slot) are the most frequently performed procedures. Rare cases may require dorsal laminectomy or hemilaminectomy (see Chapters 11 and 12). The choice between ventral fenestration and decompression must be made on an individual patient basis. There are advantages and disadvantages to both procedures (**Table 15**). General indications for ventral decompression are as follows.
- Presence of neurological deficits.
- Myelographic evidence of spinal cord compression.
- Failure of fenestration.

Clinicians who routinely perform myelography find that most cervical disc patients come into one of the first two categories. Current opinion is that ventral decompression is the optimal treatment (see 'Prognosis,' page 83). Dorsal or dorsolateral decompressive surgery is only required in lateral disc extrusions that cannot be reached via a ventral slot, or where there is doubt about the diagnosis on myelography (see **135**).

Table 15 Comparison of ventral fenestration and slot

	Fenestration	Decompression
Technically	Easy	Difficult
Accurate identification of disc involved	Not required	Required
Special equipment	Little	More
Potential iatrogenic change	Unlikely	Possible
Removal of disc material from vertebral canal	No	Yes
Resolution of neck pain	Slow in some dogs	Usually within a few days

7 CERVICAL DISC DISEASE

SURGERY

Ventral procedures are covered in this chapter. Dorsal techniques are covered in Chapters 11 and 12.

Ventral approach to the neck (136–153)

The ventral approach to the neck is required for both procedures described here.

136 Positioning of dog for ventral approach to neck. The cervical spine is extended over a sandbag. The thoracic limbs are positioned caudally, and tape is used to fix the head and thorax. It is important to have the dog straight to ensure that the neck is correctly aligned.

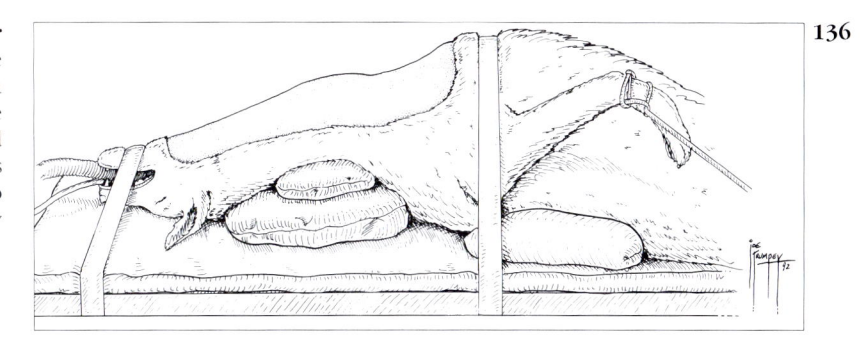

137 Positioning of dog. An oesophageal stethoscope is in position; this aids the anaesthetist and is useful in identifying the oesophagus. Landmarks are (**a**) larynx, (**b**) wing of atlas, (**c**) manubrium of sternum. Incision site is depicted on midline.

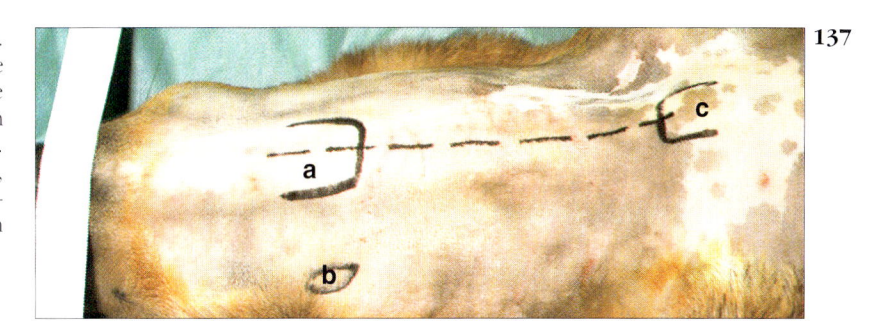

138 Landmarks can be palpated. In this illustration the surgeon is palpating the wings of the atlas (left hand) and the prominent transverse process of C_6 (see **152**).

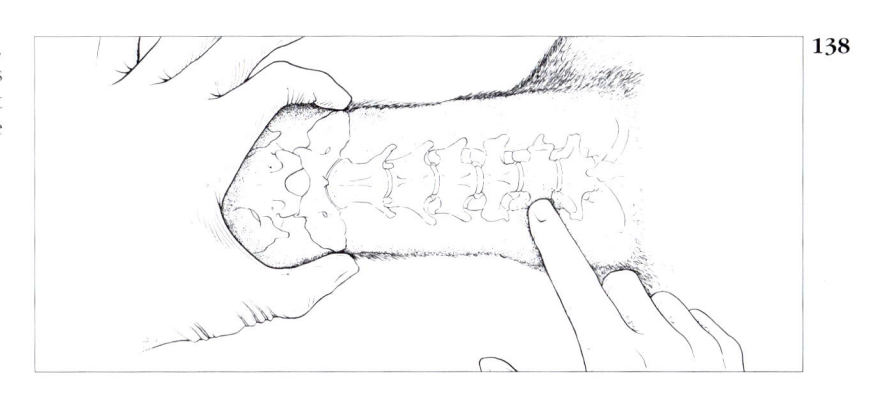

139 Incision site. The dog's head is to the left in all illustrations. Relate landmarks to **137**.

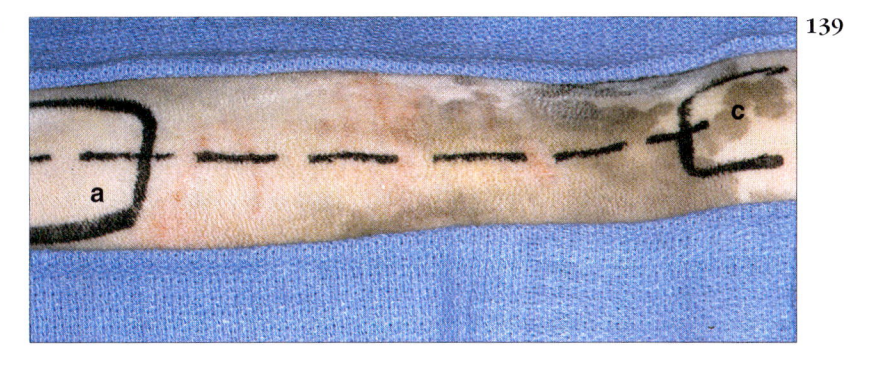

71

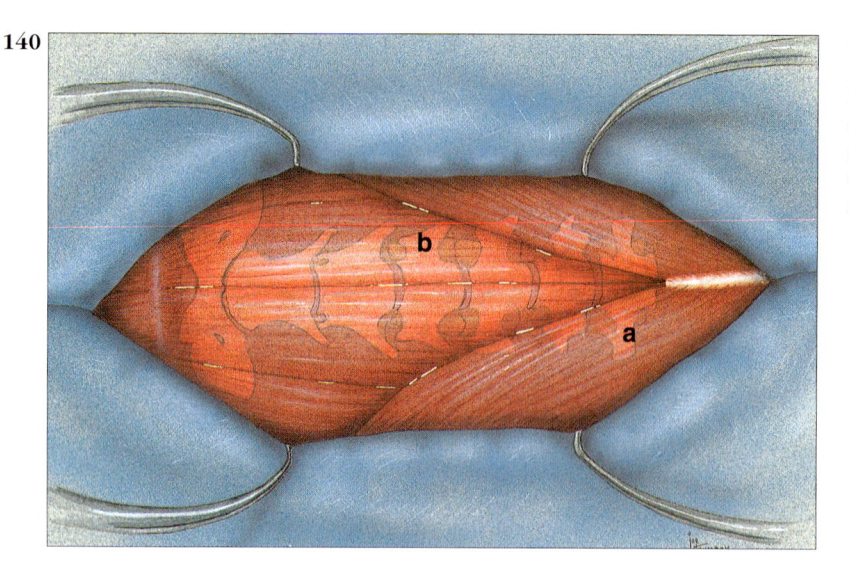

DIAGNOSIS AND SURGERY OF SMALL ANIMAL SPINAL DISORDERS

140 Superficial anatomy. See also **141**. The skin and superficial fascia have been divided. This reveals the sternocephalicus muscles (**a**) and the sternohyoid muscles (**b**). The cervical vertebrae C_1 through C_7 are seen in the background.

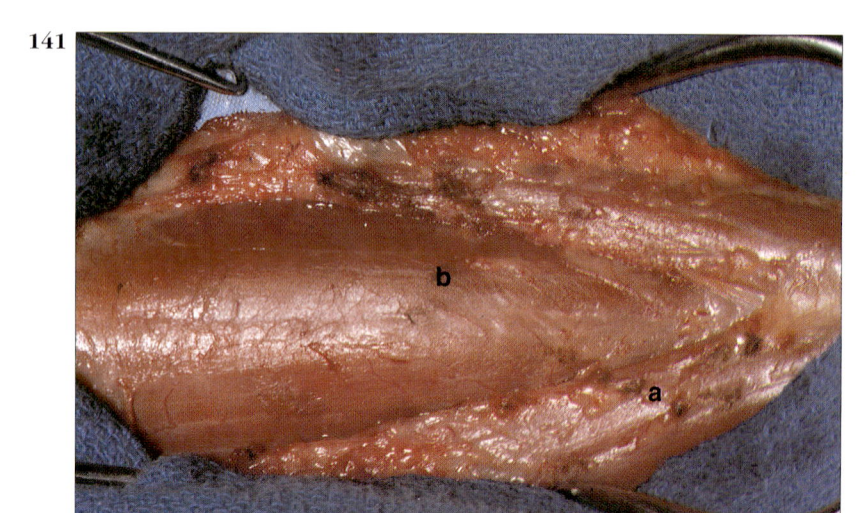

141 The skin and superficial fascia have been incised. This reveals paired sternocephalicus muscles (**a**) and sternohyoid muscles (**b**). The sternocephalicus muscles should be divided to the manubrium, particularly if access to the caudal cervical discs is required.

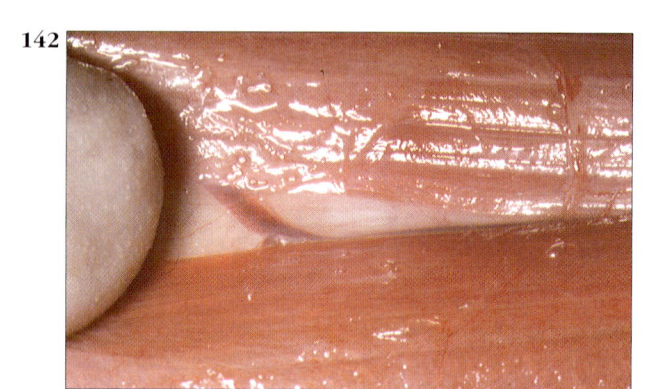

142 The sternohyoid muscles are divided in the midline. The median raphe is easiest to see in the caudal part of the incision. If not apparent, apply finger pressure to the muscles over the trachea; the raphe will become visible.

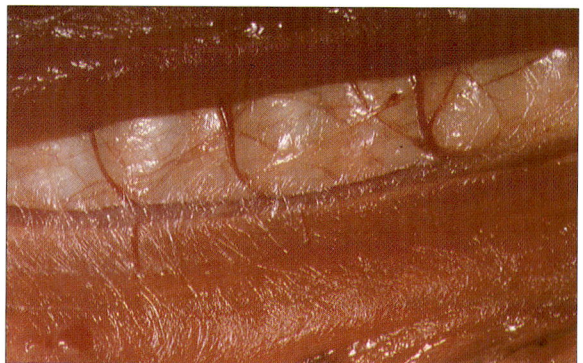

143 The caudal thyroid vein. This lies in the connective tissue with small branches on each side. It should be preserved if possible. The trachea is seen under the fascia.

7 CERVICAL DISC DISEASE

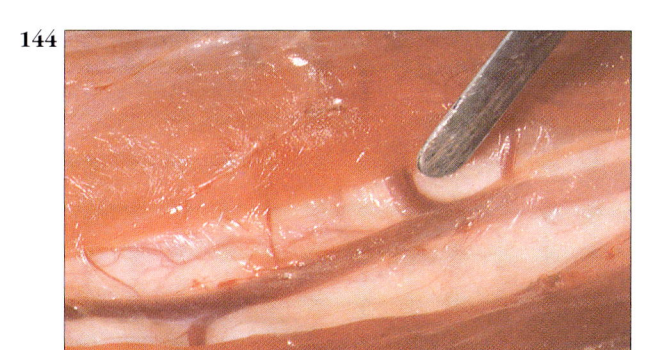

144 The branches of the vein may be cauterized.

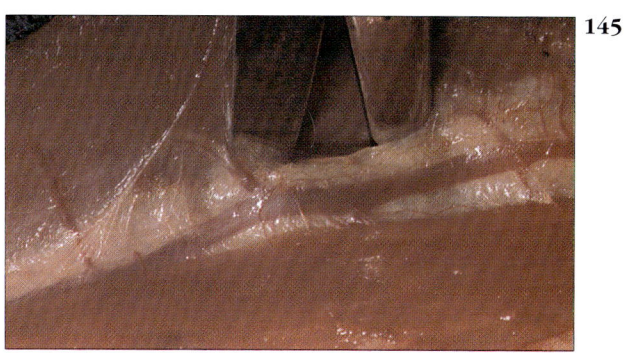

145 Making a small incision and then bluntly dissecting the fascia usually avoids bleeding.

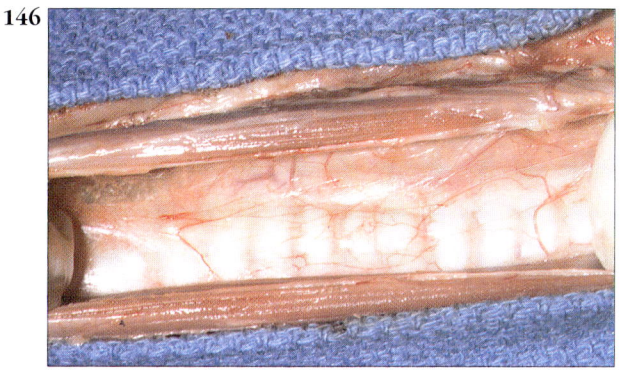

146 Once the sternohyoid muscles have been divided the trachea is visible. Here the separation has been made with fingers.

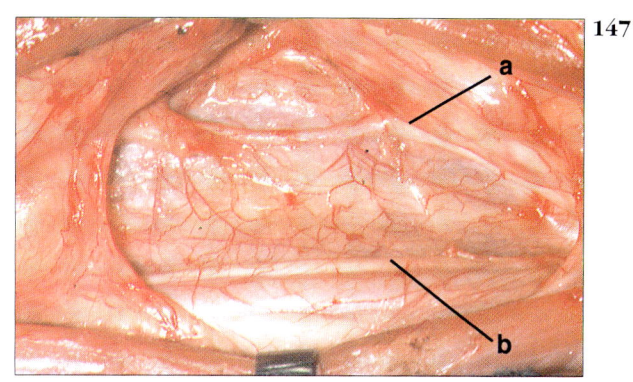

147 There are various layers of fascia deep to the sternohyoid muscles. The structures are shown in a similar position as in **148**. See **148** for labels.

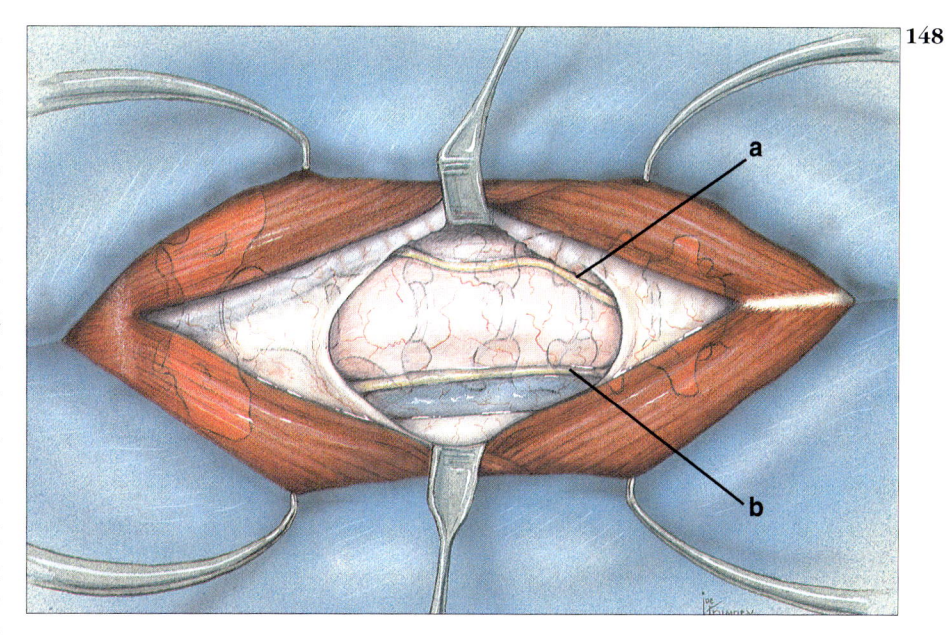

148 Deep anatomy including vital structures: carotid sheath, recurrent laryngeal nerve, oesophagus. The oesophagus is identified by its pinker appearance compared to the darker red of the longus colli muscles; identification is aided by having an oesophageal stethoscope in place. Careful dissection of these fascial layers in a longitudinal direction will expose these structures. Again, blunt finger dissection is safe and effective. Note recurrent laryngeal nerve (**a**) and carotid sheath containing carotid artery and vagosympathetic trunk (**b**). The trachea and oesophagus have been retracted away from the surgeon, upward in the photograph; they are kept together on the same side of the incision. (The recurrent laryngeal nerve has been separated from the trachea. This is for illustration only and is not normally done). Further dissection of the deep fascia reveals the longus colli muscles, which lie ventral to the cervical vertebrae (see **149**, **150**).

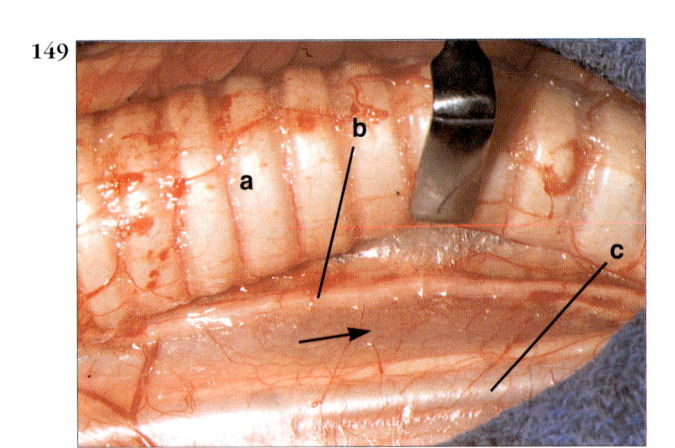

DIAGNOSIS AND SURGERY OF SMALL ANIMAL SPINAL DISORDERS

149 Close-up view of the trachea (a), recurrent laryngeal nerve (b), and carotid sheath (c). The approach is between the recurrent laryngeal nerve (which stays with the trachea) and the carotid sheath. Arrow shows site of approach.

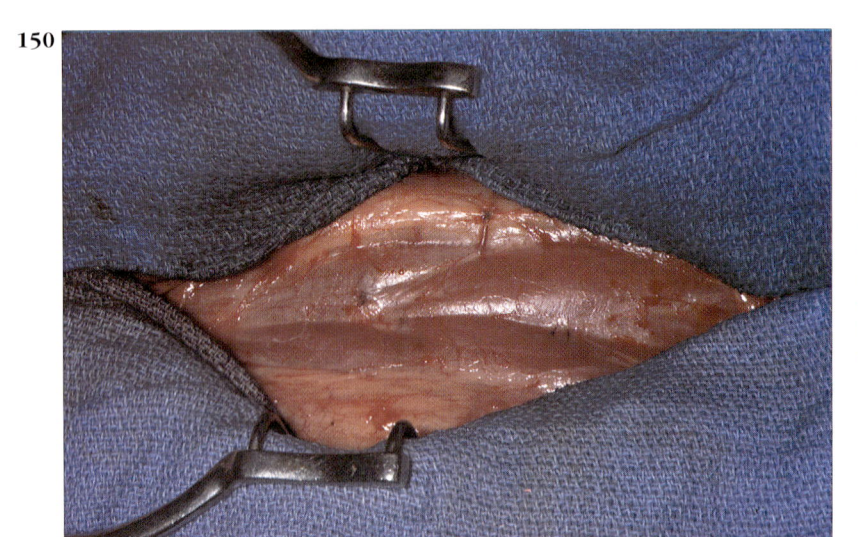

150 Retraction of the vital structures exposes the longus colli muscles. Blunt-jawed self-retaining retractors (Gossett or Balfour) are used to maintain exposure. The retractors must not interfere with gas flow in the airway. Palpate the end of the endotracheal tube and ensure that it is distal to the retractors. Moist towels or sponges are used to protect the tissues. These towels must be kept moist with saline. The pattern of the longus colli muscles is visible. They join in the midline and insert on the ventral process of the vertebrae, thus overlying the intervertebral discs (see **153**).

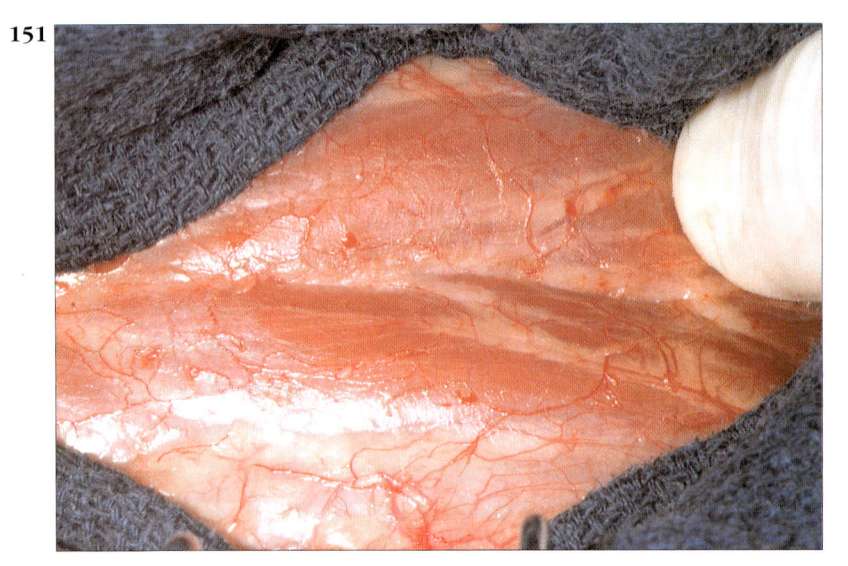

151 Accurate identification of the intervertebral discs is important. The transverse processes of C_6 are large and are directed ventrally; they are readily palpated as shown here. The ventral process of C_5 lies in the midline between the cranial border of the transverse processes of C_6; the C_5/C_6 intervertebral disc lies immediately behind this ventral process. The ventral process of C_1 is particularly prominent and sharp. This also should be palpated. There is no intervertebral disc at C_1/C_2.

7 CERVICAL DISC DISEASE

152 Lateral radiograph illustrating ventrally directed transverse processes of C$_6$ (arrow).

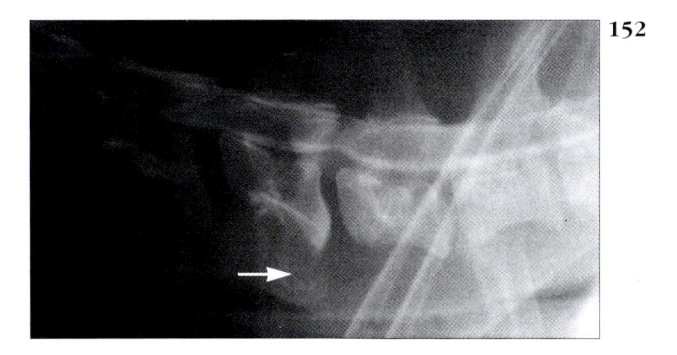

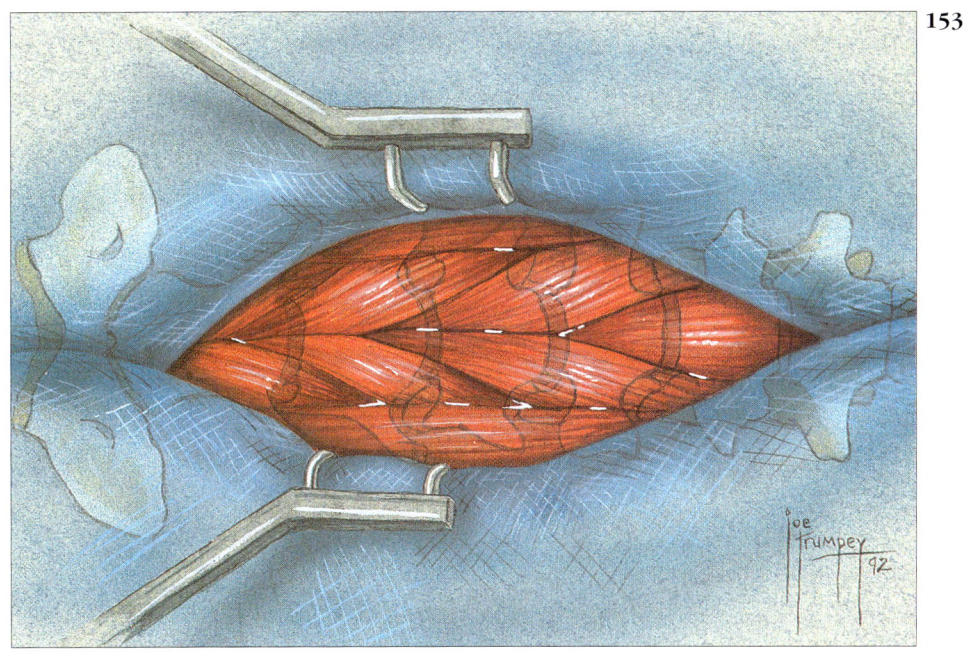

153 Deep anatomy. Note the pattern of longus colli muscle bellies running cranially. Relate to **150** and **151**.

Fenestration (154–161)

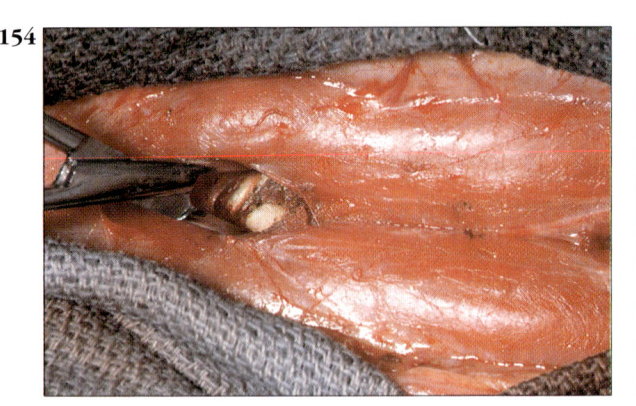

154 To gain access to the disc, the longus colli muscles are divided in the midline immediately caudal to the ventral process. This may be achieved with a small curved haemostat. It is important not to confuse the ventral process with the transverse processes of the C_2–C_5 vertebrae. The longus colli muscles run cranially to insert on the ventral process in the midline. The transverse processes can be palpated lateral to the ventral process. The three rows of structures (ventral processes in the midline, transverse processes laterally on each side) should be identified.

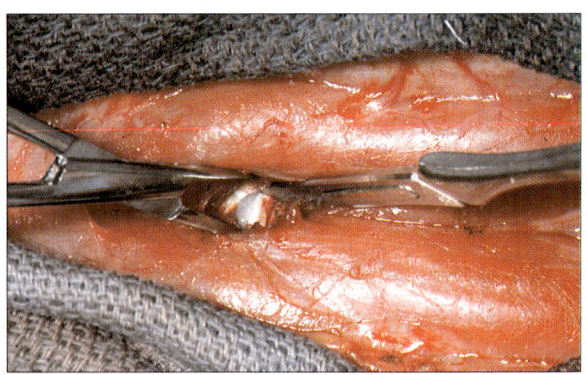

155 Fenestration is achieved by cutting a hole in the ventral anulus fibrosus with a #11 blade. Nucleus pulposus can be seen oozing from the intervertebral space.

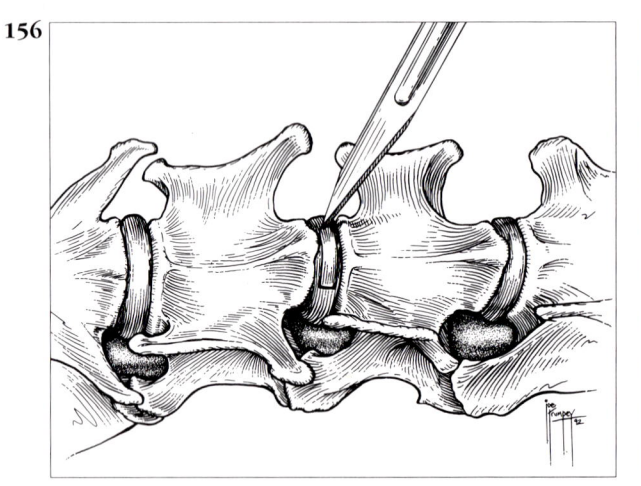

156 Method of fenestration. The anulus fibrosus is cut in the form of a window to allow access to the nucleus pulposus.

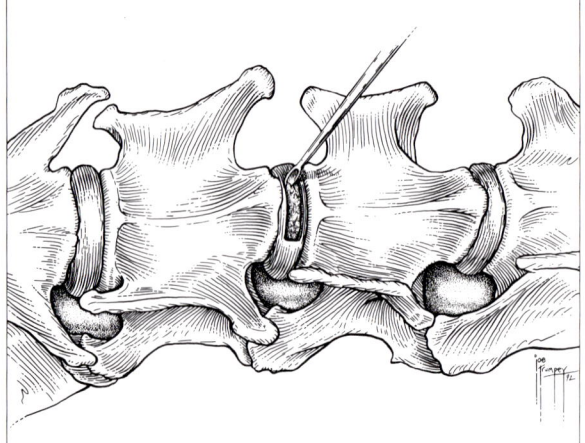

157 The nuclear material is removed with a small curette, tartar scraper or Rosen mobilizer. It is important to evacuate the nucleus pulposus thoroughly, by using a sweeping motion with the instrument. Also, it is important not to push the instrument deeply into the vertebral canal. Some guide as to the depth of the intervertebral space should be judged from the radiographs. The window in the anulus fibrosus must be significantly larger than the instrument to avoid creating a piston effect, which could force disc material dorsally into the vertebral canal.

7 CERVICAL DISC DISEASE

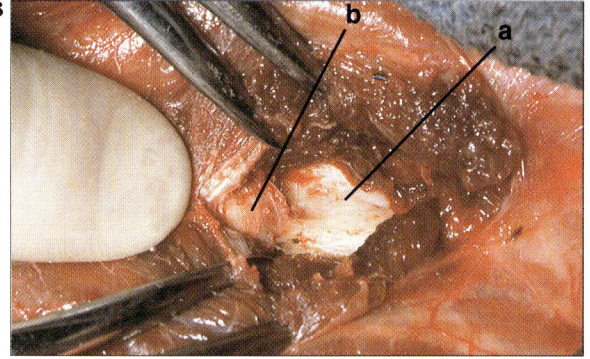

158 If greater exposure of the disc is required, the muscle separation is maintained by self-retaining retractors (Gelpi or Weitlander). The longus colli muscles can be seen separated. The ventral surface of the vertebra (**a**) and the ventral anulus fibrosus (**b**) can be seen. The surgeon's finger is on the ventral process of the vertebra cranial to the disc.

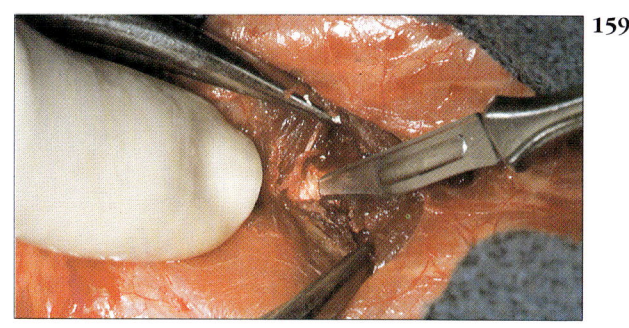

159 Access for the fenestration is gained by cutting a hole in anulus fibrosus. The hole should be as large as possible, to allow complete evacuation of the nucleus pulposus. A sharp #11 scalpel blade is used to make the opening, either by making four cuts in a rectangular pattern in the anulus fibrosus, or by continuously cutting in an oval pattern until the piece of anulus is free. The surgeon's finger is on the ventral process.

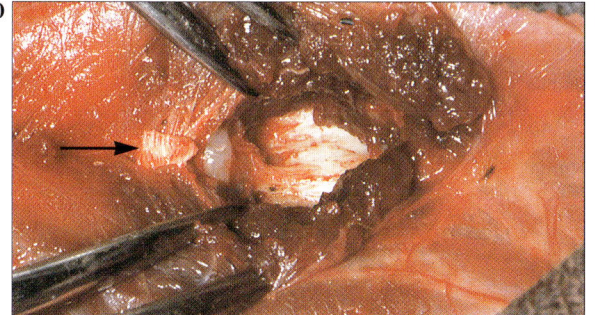

160 Disc fenestrated. Nucleus pulposus is oozing from the intervertebral space. The removed piece of anulus fibrosus lies cranial to the disc space (arrow). A small curette (Shea) or blunt instrument (tartar scraper or Rosen mobilizer) is used to remove the nucleus pulposus by penetrating the space, dragging towards or away from the surgeon and then lifting the material out. This manoeuvre should be repeated until there is a reasonable certainty that all the nuclear material has been removed, as healing processes will not remove this. Clearly, care must be taken to avoid penetrating the vertebral canal dorsally.

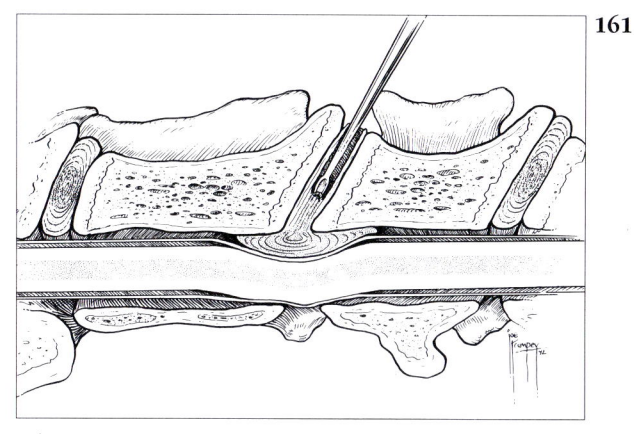

161 Sagittal diagram shows that fenestration only allows access to disc material in the intervertebral space. Extruded disc in the vertebral canal cannot be removed by fenestration.

It is usual to fenestrate the discs from C_2/C_3 to C_5/C_6. The disc at C_6/C_7 is fenestrated if there is evidence of disease. Some surgeons question the value and desirability of such widespread fenestration (Fingeroth, 1989), but others believe it is useful in treatment and prophylaxis. Some dogs will experience very rapid improvement following fenestration, and some dogs with profound neurological disabilities recover after this procedure (see 'Prognosis,' page 83). A well-executed fenestration should prevent further herniation of disc material into the vertebral canal.

DIAGNOSIS AND SURGERY OF SMALL ANIMAL SPINAL DISORDERS

Ventral decompression (162–178)

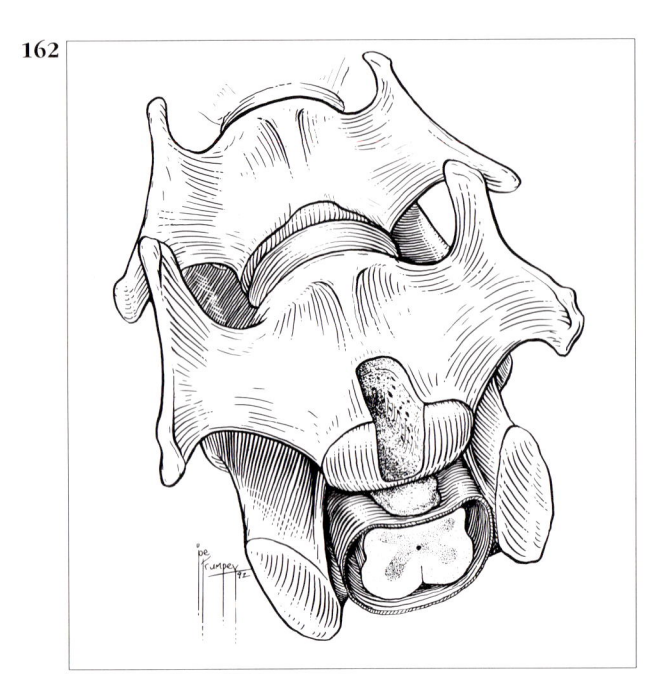

162 Ventral aspect of cervical vertebrae showing ventral decompression by slot. The procedure allows access to the vertebral canal through the vertebral body.

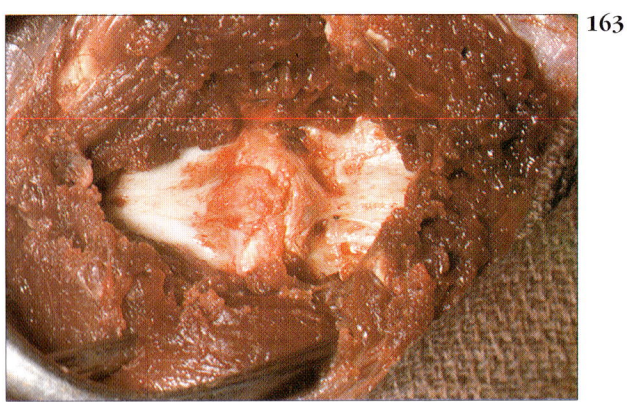

163 The site for the ventral slot is prepared by removing the musculature from the vertebrae in the midline on both sides of the disc. This is a cranial extension of the exposure in **158**. The longus colli muscles are separated from their attachment on the ventral process. This can lead to bleeding; it is useful to remove the muscles with bipolar cautery (which should be used in preference to diathermy in close proximity to the spine). Hemostasis at this stage is important, as excessive bleeding will obscure the site of the slot. Muscle separation is maintained with self-retaining retractors.

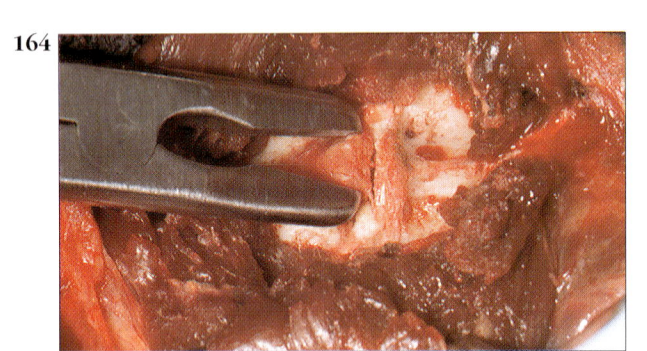

164 The ventral process is removed with rongeurs. The muscles are protected with moist swabs or sponges.

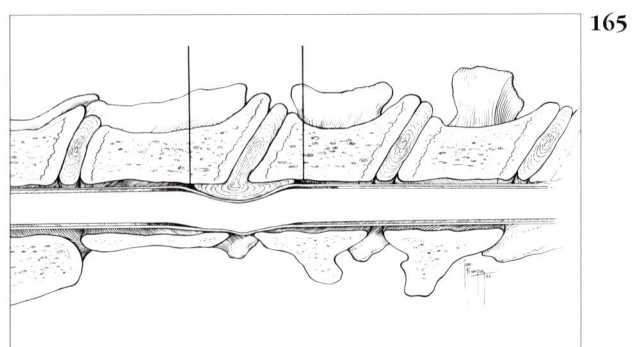

165 Sagittal section. This shows that the slot must be started more in the vertebra cranial to the disc than the one caudal, because of the orientation of the discs relative to the vertebral canal. As in all this series of surgical illustrations, the left side of the picture is cranial.

7 CERVICAL DISC DISEASE

166 The slot is commenced in the position described in 165. The cortical bone has been penetrated to reveal purple cancellous bone. The intervertebral disc is seen caudal to this. Haemorrhage from the bone is controlled with bone wax. It is important to keep the bur irrigated and the site free of debris. It is useful to stop drilling periodically to clean the site and to assess progress. The aim is to create a slot approximately one third of the width of the vertebra and one third of its length, each side of the disc space (see **162**, **167**). This size of slot will avoid the internal vertebral venous plexus and not create instability. It is important that the slot stay in the midline, to avoid the venous plexus (see **169**).

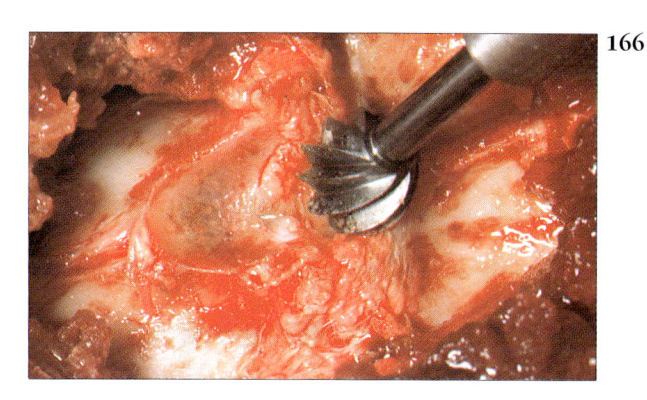

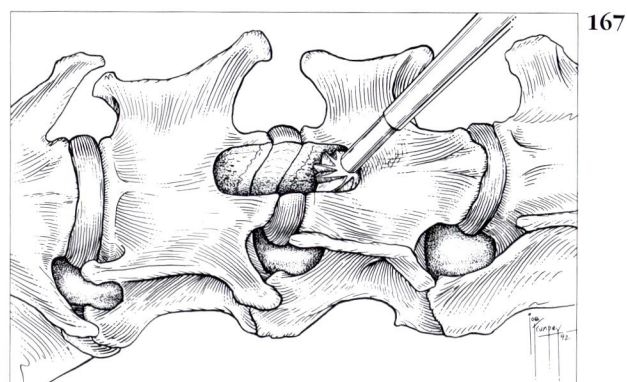

167 Partially completed slot. Somewhat more advanced than in the previous illustration.

168 The floor of the slot. This is the dorsal cortical bone of the vertebral body, the floor of the vertebral canal. It is important to judge the depth of the slot accurately. The cortical bone is white and hard (**a**), in contrast to the dark cancellous bone (**b**). The cancellous bone is removed over the whole slot area, using a small bur. The cortical bone is then thinned to allow easy removal; it is best to thin the whole area before entering the vertebral canal. The dorsal anulus fibrosus is visible (**c**). The shape of the opening into the vertebral canal must take into account the location of the venous plexus (see **169**). It is important that the slot is at most one third of the width of the vertebral body.

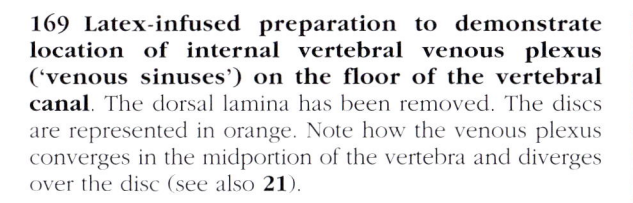

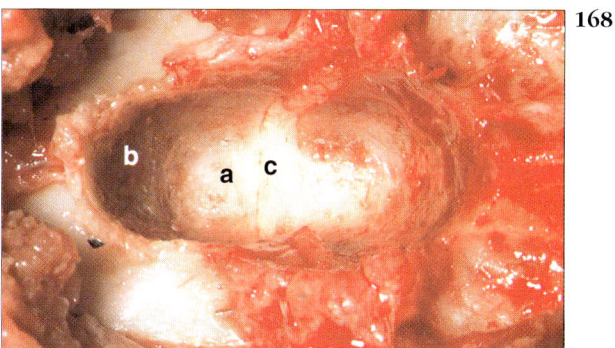

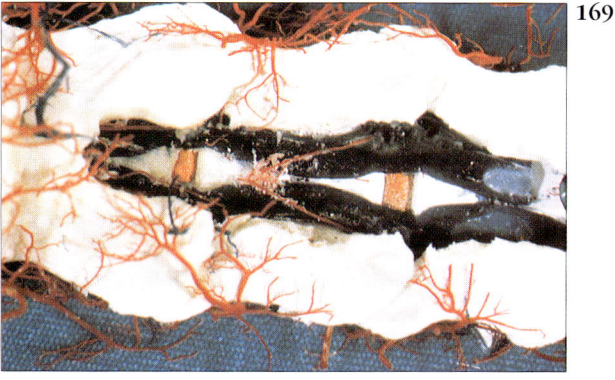

169 Latex-infused preparation to demonstrate location of internal vertebral venous plexus ('venous sinuses') on the floor of the vertebral canal. The dorsal lamina has been removed. The discs are represented in orange. Note how the venous plexus converges in the midportion of the vertebra and diverges over the disc (see also **21**).

79

DIAGNOSIS AND SURGERY OF SMALL ANIMAL SPINAL DISORDERS

170 The dorsal anulus fibrosus is incised on each side of the slot using a #11 blade. One incision can be seen uppermost in the picture. The nearside incision is being made.

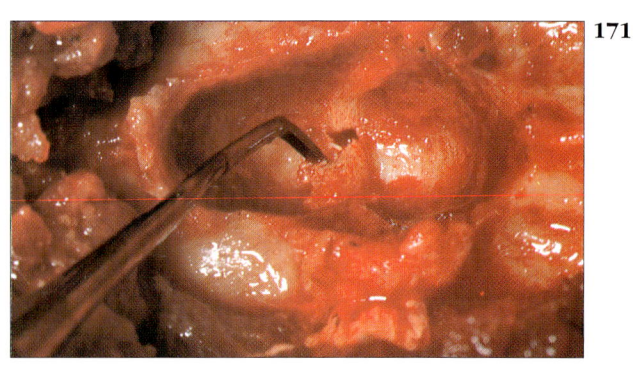

171 The anulus fibrosus is lifted with a suitable instrument (in this case, a pointed tartar scraper) and dissected free.

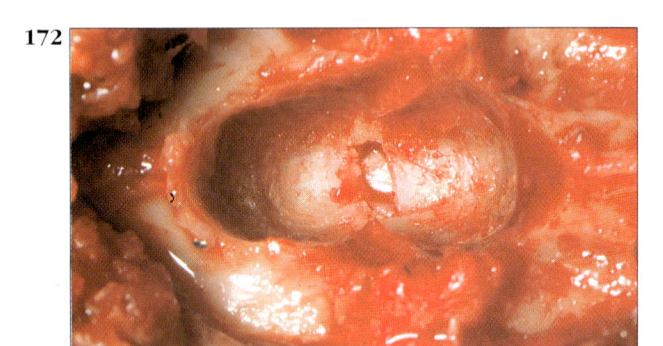

172 The dorsal anulus has been removed, allowing a view into the vertebral canal. This may reveal the dorsal longitudinal ligament, although this may be very thin or be damaged in dogs that have suffered disc extrusion. It is likely to be thicker in dogs with caudal cervical spondylomyelopathy. In this patient, the dura mater covering the spinal cord is in view. The identity of this tissue must be established before any manipulations or incisions are made. The ligament has longitudinal fibres. It may be necessary to complete bone removal before the tissue can be identified. When extruded disc material is present, it is wise to remove it from the midline first, thus avoiding damaging the venous plexus.

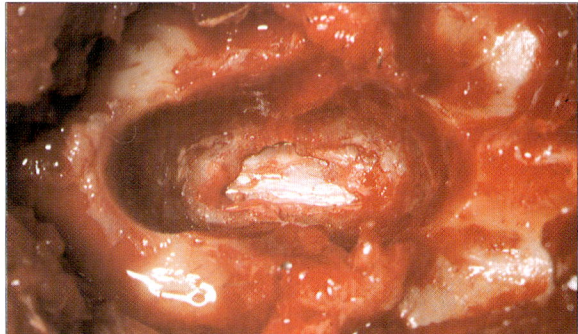

173 The slot is almost complete. The thin floor of the slot is elevated with a tartar scraper or small curette. This is most easily accomplished if the bone has been made very thin with the bur. The edges of the slot are removed with a curette, but bear in mind the position of the venous plexus. If haemorrhage from the plexus does occur, it may be possible to control it with Surgicell or a small piece of macerated muscle. Work should continue at the other end of the slot. Suction may be used continually while disc material is being removed, but this is not easy in the confined space and careful note must be taken of the amount of blood aspirated. If haemorrhage is severe, the slot is packed and time allowed for it to stop before the wound is closed. Any pressure on the jugular veins should be relieved. In a dog with a herniated disc, material is removed from the canal with a tartar scraper or curette. Pieces of anulus fibrosus are grasped with small haemostats. Great patience is required at this stage of the operation. Once all disc material is removed, the spinal cord will assume a normal position as shown here. This is often enough to stop bleeding. If the disc is asymmetrically positioned, it is possible to shape the base of the slot to allow more exposure on one side. However, the hazard of venous bleeding increases with this approach.

7 CERVICAL DISC DISEASE

174 Sagittal diagram showing access to disc material in the vertebral canal via the slot. Note again the starting position of the slot relative to the disc.

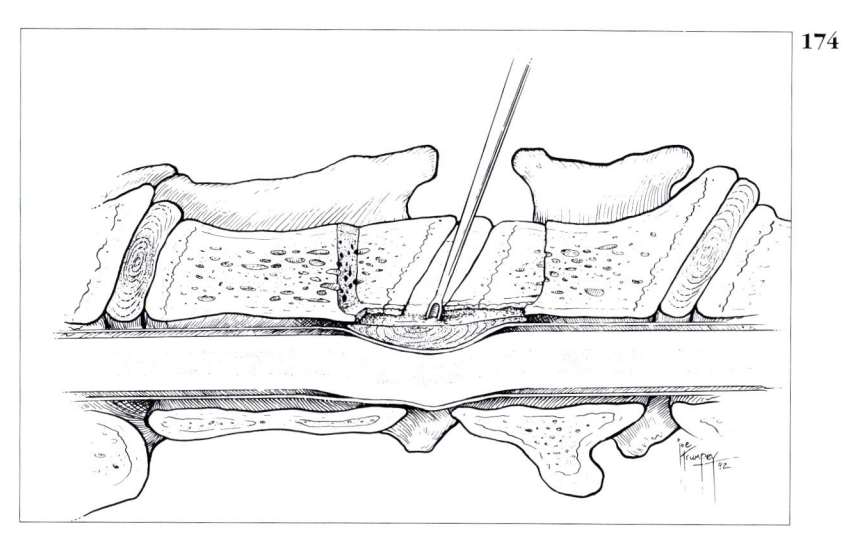

175 Wound closure. The slot may be filled with a fat graft or piece of surgical cellulose. The longus colli muscles are sutured with absorbable material.

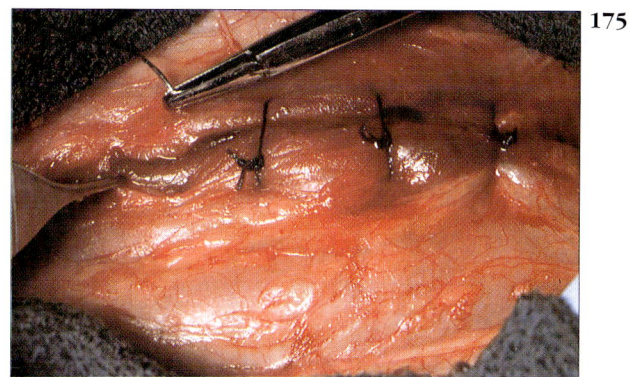

176 The sternohyoid muscles are loosely apposed with absorbable suture. The subcutis and skin are closed in a routine fashion.

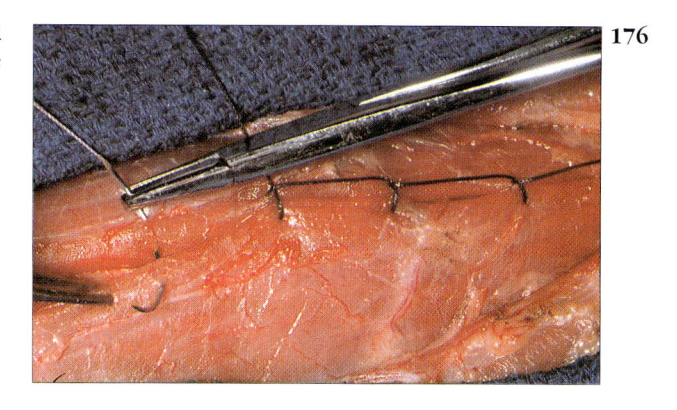

Accurate identification of the disc involved is necessary before performing a ventral slot. Removal of the disc material from the vertebral canal provides the most rapid resolution of clinical signs. Dogs that have longstanding pain and neurological deficits will usually respond well to decompression (see 'Prognosis,' page 83).

The best method of performing a ventral slot is by using powered instruments (Swaim, 1974). It is possible to perform the operation using a trephine and rongeurs, but this is a poor alternative.

Fenestration is a useful prophylactic procedure and can be performed on the other cervical discs at the time of the decompression (Russell and Griffiths, 1968).

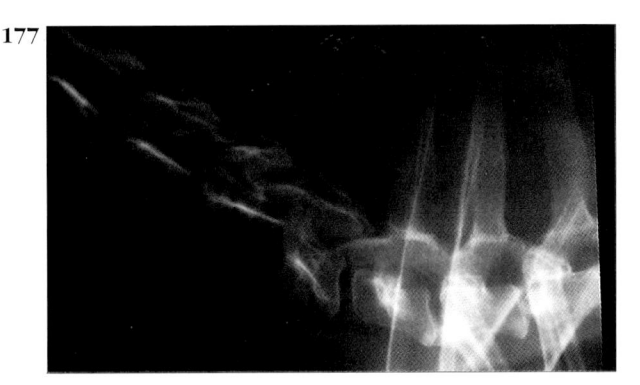

177, 178 Lateral (**177**) and ventrodorsal (**178**) radiograph of dog where subluxation had occurred following ventral slot. The slot had been made too wide, causing instability and allowing the vertebrae to collapse on themselves. The dog had severe neck pain for a week after surgery, prompting this further investigation.

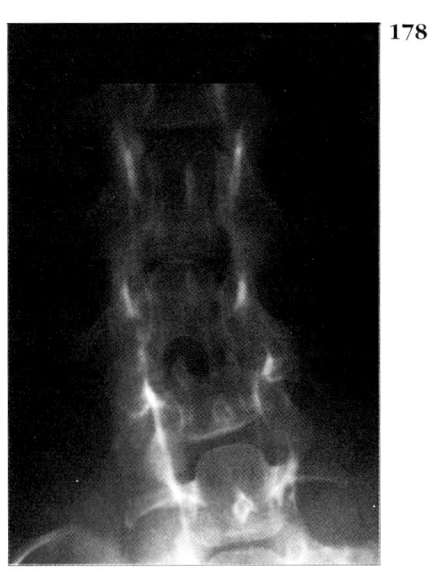

Hemilaminectomy

Hemilaminectomy via a dorsolateral approach is indicated in a few patients. If there is a markedly asymmetrical myelographic compression, as in the dog shown in **135**, there may be some doubt about the diagnosis. Intraforaminal extrusions occur occasionally, and these are best approached in this way (Felts and Prata, 1983; see **382–394**).

COMPLICATIONS

The ventral surgical approach should have few complications if proper care is exercised. It is possible to damage vital structures, particularly the recurrent laryngeal nerve.

Spinal cord damage during fenestration can occur if the intervertebral space is explored recklessly. Neurological deterioration after fenestration may occur, probably where incorrect fenestration technique leads to disc material being forced into the vertebral canal (Tomlinson, 1985).

Ventral decompression is more prone to complications than fenestration. Inaccurate identification of the disc involved, either on radiographs or at surgery, is a mistake.

Haemorrhage can be a problem at various stages. The longus colli muscles tend to bleed when removed from their insertion on the ventral process. Muscle removal away from the midline should be restricted as it may cause significant bleeding from the vertebral artery or its branches. Bleeding from the bone during burring can be controlled with bone wax. Severe haemorrhage can arise from the internal vertebral venous plexus (see **169**), and may be so severe that it is impossible to continue to explore the vertebral canal. Concurrent use of aspirin or the presence of coagulopathy (particularly VW disease in Dobermanns) increases the danger of severe haemorrhage (see Chapter 11).

One study reported death of three of 50 dogs undergoing ventral decompression for cervical disc herniation (Clark, 1986). One of the dogs died following uncontrollable haemorrhage from the venous plexus. The other two dogs experienced acute bradycardia and hypotension and died during the surgery. It is suggested that a syndrome of acute sympathetic blockade was responsible for these deaths. Anaesthetic complications are also seen following surgery for cervical disc disease (Stauffer *et al.*, 1988). Arrhythmias (bradycardia and ventricular premature contractions) were seen in 31% of dogs; these were 2.5 times more common in cervical disc surgery than thoracolumbar disc surgery. Two of 48 dogs died following cervical disc surgery in that study. Anaesthetic considerations are discussed in Chapter 6.

Removal of mineralized disc material is generally straightforward, but can be difficult if it is adherent to the dura mater. In dogs with CCSM, the compressive lesion is often a solid mass of hypertrophied anulus fibrosus and dorsal longitudinal ligament. This has to be removed by sharp dissection, which can damage the venous plexus or potentially even the spinal cord.

Neurological worsening occurs in some patients following ventral decompression. Extensive spinal cord manipulation may account for this, but it is not always clear why deterioration occurs, particularly in dogs with Type II disc protrusions. Fortunately, this situation is usually transient.

Vertebral instability may result if the slot is made too wide, leading to subluxation and possible nerve root compression (see **177, 178**). This will lead to marked deterioration in the condition of the patient. If this does occur, the lesion should be managed by distraction and fixation, as for a traumatic fracture or subluxation.

Infection of the intervertebral space (discospondylitis, see **467, 468**) can occur following either procedure if strict asepsis is not observed.

Swelling or oedema may be seen in the ventral neck. Care with hemostasis and wound closure helps to avoid this. Use of drains may occasionally be necessary (see Chapter 6).

The usual complications of long periods of recumbency occur in some patients (see Chapter 15).

Persistent neck pain occurs in a significant number of dogs that undergo fenestration, and may take up to a month to resolve. Following ventral decompression, neck pain usually resolves within a few days (see 'Prognosis,' below).

POSTOPERATIVE CARE (see Chapter 15)

Most patients are relatively pain free following surgery. Two weeks of restricted exercise should be enforced, even if improvement has been marked. Leash exercise for urination and defaecation is allowed, but a harness should be used rather than a collar.

If pain persists, anti-inflammatory drugs may be needed (**Table 35**, page 205). Diazepam or methocarbamol are beneficial in some patients.

Dogs with severe neurological deficits benefit from physiotherapy once the pain has subsided. Large breed dogs are prone to problems related to recumbency, and attention to bedding and cleanliness is required.

PROGNOSIS

The prognosis for dogs with cervical disc herniations is generally good. Non-surgically treated dogs may have a prolonged convalescent period (several weeks to months) and have an approximately 36% chance of recurrence of signs (Russell and Griffiths, 1968).

Fenestration

Following fenestration, recovery times vary. Denny (1978) reported that 11 of 12 dogs with neck pain recovered, although 30% of these took an average of two weeks for pain to subside. Of dogs with mild neurological deficits (thoracic limb paresis), 12 of 17 (70%) recovered in an average of 3.6 weeks (maximum 8 weeks). Of those with severe deficits (hemiparesis, tetraparesis, or tetraplegia), 6 of 10 (60%) recovered in an average of 6 weeks.

Decompression

The results of ventral decompression have also been analysed in a series of 54 patients (Seim and Prata, 1982). In dogs with neck pain and root signature (n=33), all dogs were normal or improved within 48 hours of surgery, and all were normal at 12 months after surgery. In dogs with moderate deficits, but still able to walk (n=14), 12 were improved at 48 hours and all were normal at 12 months. Interestingly, 2 of these dogs were worse (more severe pain or worse neurological status, or both) at 48 hours. Of dogs that were unable to walk before surgery (n=7), 6 were improved at 48 hours and 6 were normal at 12 months; the remaining dog had some residual deficits but was able to walk and was free of pain.

In a comparison of dogs with cervical disc disease that were able to walk before surgery, ventral decompression provided superior results to fenestration in all neurological parameters. Dogs recovered more rapidly and recovery rates were higher following ventral decompression. Surgical complications were fewer in fenestration (Fry et al., 1991).

Thus, ventral decompression carries a more favourable prognosis, both in terms of rate of recovery and time of convalescence. It is on this basis that we recommend ventral decompression for most dogs with cervical disc herniations.

CERVICAL DISC DISEASE IN CATS

Disc herniation is quite common in cats, particularly in the cervical region, but clinical signs related to these lesions are rare (Heavner, 1971; Littlewood et al., 1984; Wheeler et al., 1985). Type II protrusions are more frequent than Type I extrusions (King and Smith, 1960). Diagnosis and treatment are as discussed above.

REFERENCES

Clark, D.M. (1986) An analysis of intraoperative and early postoperative mortality associated with cervical spinal decompressive surgery in the dog. *Journal of the American Animal Hospital Association* **22**, 739–744.

Dallman, M.J., Pelattas, P. and Bojrab, M.J. (1992) Characteristics of dogs admitted for treatment of cervical intervertebral disk disease: 105 cases (1972–1982). *Journal of the American Veterinary Medical Association* **200**, 2009–2011.

Denny, H.R. (1978) The surgical treatment of cervical disc disease in the dog: a review of 40 cases. *Journal of Small Animal Practice* **19**, 251–297.

Felts, J.F. and Prata, R.G. (1983) Cervical disc disease in the dog: intraforaminal and lateral extrusions. *Journal of the American Animal Hospital Association* **19**, 755–760.

Fry, T.R., Johnson, A.L., Hungerford, L. and Toombs, J. (1991) Surgical treatment of cervical disc herniations in ambulatory dogs. *Progress in Veterinary Neurology* **2**, 165–173.

Griffiths, I.R. (1970) A syndrome produced by dorsolateral explosions of the cervical intervertebral discs. *Veterinary Record* **87**, 737–741.

Heavner, J.E. (1971) Intervertebral disc syndrome in the cat. *Journal of the American Veterinary Medical Association* **159**, 425–427.

King, A.S. and Smith, R.N. (1960) Disc protrusions in the cat: distribution of dorsal protrusions along the vertebral column. *Veterinary Record* **72**, 335–337.

Littlewood, J.D., Herrtage, M.E. and Palmer, A.C. (1984) Intervertebral disc protrusion in a cat. *Journal of Small Animal Practice* **25**, 119–127.

Russell. S.W. and Griffiths, R.C. (1968) Recurrence of cervical disc syndrome in surgically and conservatively treated dogs. *Journal of the American Veterinary Medical Association* **153**, 1412–1416.

Seim, H.B. and Prata, R.G. (1982) Ventral decompression for the treatment of cervical disk disease in the dog: a review of 54 cases. *Journal of the American Animal Hospital Association* **18**, 233–240.

Stauffer, J.L, Gleed, R.D., Short, C.E., Erb, H.N. and Schukken, Y.H. (1988) Cardiac dysrhythmias during anaesthesia for cervical decompression in the dog. *American Journal of Veterinary Research* **49**, 1143–1146.

Swaim, S.F. (1974) Ventral decompression of the cervical spinal cord in the dog. *Journal of the American Veterinary Medical Association* **164**, 491–495.

Tomlinson, J. (1985) Tetraparesis following cervical disk fenestration in two dogs. *Journal of the American Veterinary Medical Association* **187**, 76–77.

Wheeler, S.J., Clayton Jones, D.G. and Wright, J.A. (1985) Myelography in the cat. *Journal of Small Animal Practice* **26**, 143–152.

8. THORACOLUMBAR DISC DISEASE

Thoracolumbar disc disease is a common condition that predominantly affects chondrodystrophoid breeds of dog. Peak incidence is between three and six years of age. Non-chondrodystrophoid breeds are less frequently affected, and usually only after middle age. Disc lesions may be classified as Hansen Type I or Type II (see **15**, **16**). Hansen Type I disease is seen mainly in chondrodystrophoid dogs, whereas Type II is more typical for non-chondrodystrophoid breeds. Over 50% of all thoracolumbar disc lesions occur at the T_{12}/T_{13} and T_{13}/L_1 discs, and over 75% occur between T_{11}/T_{12} and L_1/L_2 inclusive. See **Table 16** for differential diagnosis.

CLINICAL SIGNS

Spinal hyperaesthesia and neurological deficits in the pelvic limbs are seen in dogs with thoracolumbar disc disease, and urinary dysfunction may be present in those with more severe lesions (**179**). The pain resulting from thoracolumbar disc disease is usually less dramatic than that associated with cervical disc disease. The dog may show kyphosis and a reluctance to run or jump, and discomfort can usually be elicited by deep palpation in the thoracolumbar region. Pain alone may be seen, and could be misinterpreted as being abdominal in origin. Neurological deficits range from mild ataxia and paresis to paraplegia, which may be accompanied by depressed or absent deep pain sensation caudal to the lesion. Pain arises because of combinations of anulus fibrosus and dorsal longitudinal ligament damage, and meningeal or nerve root irritation. The neurological deficits are caused by extradural spinal cord compression and injury.

Neurological deficits become more severe with greater spinal cord compression (see 'Spinal cord nerve fibres and the effect of compression,' page 12). In addition to the actual mass effect of the disc material, the rate at which spinal cord compression occurs is also important. If it is rapid, the spinal cord cannot compensate and more severe neurological deficits result. In the most extreme cases, there may be a combination of mass effect and a considerable impact injury to the spinal cord, resulting from explosive rupture of the disc.

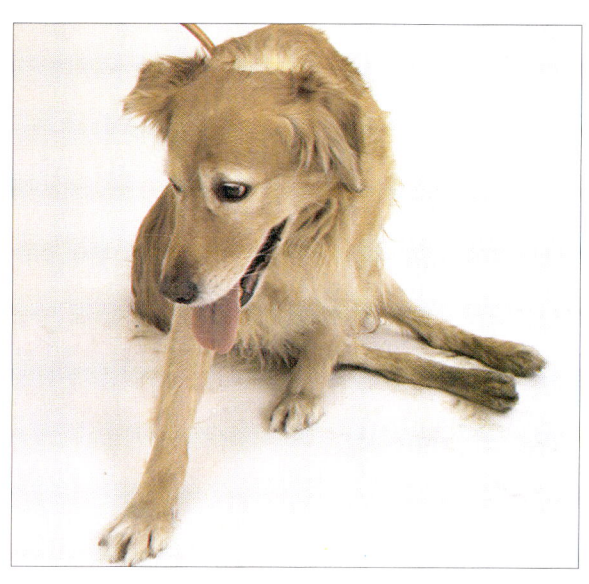

179 Paraplegic dog that had been treated one week previously with an injection of dexamethasone for thoracolumbar hyperaesthesia. The dog had not been confined to a cage at that stage, but it improved rapidly only to suffer from a sudden onset of paraplegia five days later. On presentation, the dog was also found to have urinary incontinence and to have depressed deep pain sensation caudal to the L_1 dermatome. The bladder was enormously distended with flocculent bloody urine, which had soaked the animal's hindquarters because of overflow. This case illustrates three important points in the management of thoracolumbar disc disease.
- Corticosteroids often improve the animal's demeanour causing it to over exert itself if not confined to a cage. This can precipitate further extrusion of material from the weakened disc, with disastrous results.
- The bladder of a paraplegic animal should be regularly palpated for the development of distension, and should be expressed at least three times daily if the animal is found to be incontinent (any urine soaked areas should also be bathed and dried).
- When deep pain sensation is depressed, definitive treatment should be started within the first 48 hours.

Table 16 Differential diagnosis for thoracolumbar disc disease

Discospondylitis
Inflammatory CNS disease
Trauma
Neoplasia
Congenital disorders
Ischaemic myelopathy

The majority of dogs with thoracolumbar disc herniations demonstrate UMN neurological deficits. In many patients this is combined with a panniculus reflex cut-off (see **35**). Approximately 10–15% of dogs show LMN deficits because of lesions affecting L_3/L_4, L_4/L_5, L_5/L_6, or L_6/L_7 discs (see Chapter 1).

Progressive myelomalacia

Progressive myelomalacia (the ascending syndrome) affects up to 3–6% of dogs with severe neurological deficits related to thoracolumbar disc disease (Denny, 1978; Davies and Sharp, 1983). It usually has a delay in onset of several days after the dog becomes paralysed, and may only become evident during the postoperative period.

In affected dogs, the onset of paralysis will usually have occurred over less than 12 hours, and most have grade 4 or 5 deficits. Profound hyperaesthesia and toxaemia are the hallmarks of the condition (**180**). The clinician should be suspicious of this problem if a paralysed dog becomes depressed, there is progressive loss of pelvic limb reflexes, and the level of panniculus cut-off moves cranially.

Extensive epidural and subarachnoid haemorrhage occurs, together with epidural fat necrosis and both arterial and venous thrombosis (**181**). The disc material in most dogs with progressive myelomalacia spreads along the epidural space for some distance, often completely encircling the dura mater but causing little spinal cord deformation. This type of disc herniation has been called Type III (Funkquist, 1962; Griffiths, 1972). Total or subtotal necrosis of the spinal cord in progressive myelomalacia can extend from the cranial thoracic to the sacral spinal cord segments. As soon as this condition is recognized, euthanasia should be performed on humane grounds as patients will die within a few days, usually of respiratory failure.

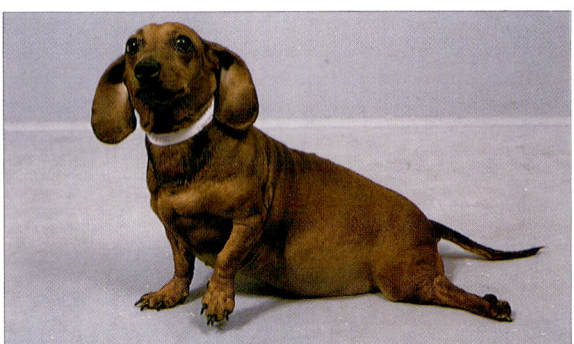

180 Extensive myelomalacia of the spinal cord. This dog presented with a grade 5 lesion and then developed depression, anorexia, vomiting, toxaemia and profound hyperaesthesia two days later. The panniculus cut-off point had moved cranially from the T_{13} to the T_9 dermatome, and there was progressive loss of the patellar and withdrawal reflexes, combined with marked hypotonicity of both pelvic limbs. A necropsy confirmed extensive myelomalacia of the spinal cord.

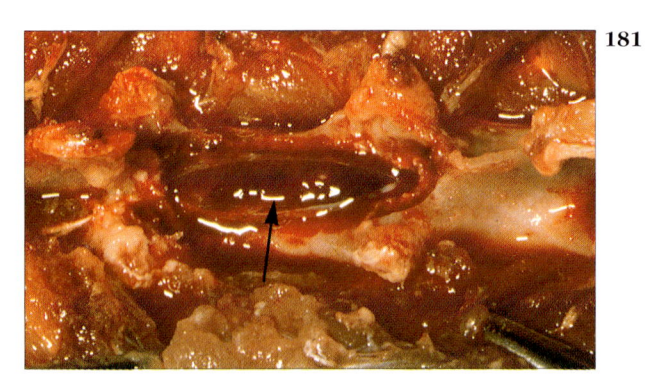

181 Progressive myelomalacia. A dorsal laminectomy and durotomy performed in a dog with progressive myelomalacia shows a swollen and grossly haemorrhagic spinal cord (arrow).

8 THORACOLUMBAR DISC DISEASE

DIAGNOSIS

Radiography

Survey radiographs indicate whether disc disease is present, but are only accurate in identifying the exact location in two thirds of disc herniations (Kirberger *et al.*, 1992). A tentative diagnosis of disc disease can be made from survey radiographs, if this correlates with the results of the neurological localisation (**182**), but survey radiographs should not be used as the sole means of confirming the diagnosis if decompressive surgery is planned.

Myelography

For a more definitive diagnosis, especially if decompressive surgery is contemplated, a myelogram should be performed. Lumbar injection is preferred as there is often considerable spinal cord swelling and cervical myelograms tend to stop cranial to the disc lesion. In lumbar myelography, contrast medium can be injected with some force, thus outlining the lesion (see Chapter 4). Lateral and ventrodorsal radiographs should be taken (**183, 184**). It is often possible to determine the side of the vertebral canal the disc material lies from clinical signs and the ventrodorsal myelogram. If in doubt, oblique views should be taken.

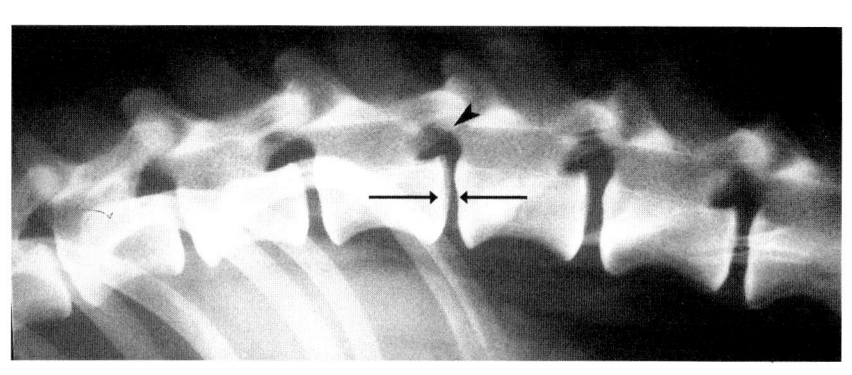

182 Survey lateral radiograph from a dog with a disc extrusion at L_1/L_2. There is narrowing of both the intervertebral space (**a**) and foramen (arrow). Note that the thoracic intervertebral spaces are normally narrower than the lumbar spaces.

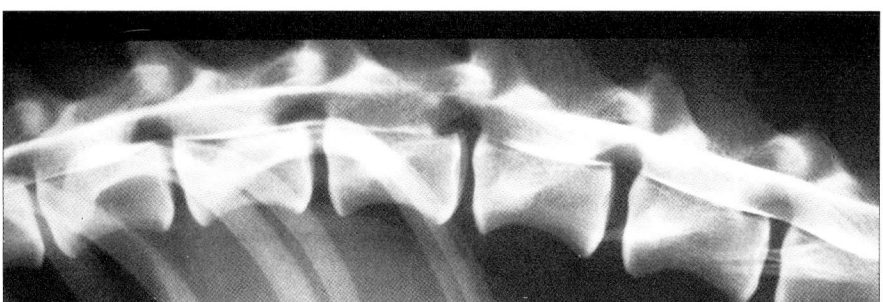

183 Lateral myelogram on the same dog as 182. There is poor filling of the subarachnoid space over the L_1/L_2 intervertebral space, with an indistinct ventral contrast column over the L_2/L_3 disc.

184 The ventrodorsal view of 183. This reveals tremendous compression of the spinal cord, due to a massive epidural lesion located on the left side of the vertebral canal (right side of the radiograph), centred over the L_2 vertebra. The left-sided contrast column can be clearly seen to deviate towards the midline just caudal to the L_2/L_3 disc (arrow). The left-sided column is barely discernible over the T_{13}/L_1 disc, and the right-sided column is absent between T_{13}/L_1 and L_2/L_3 disc spaces.

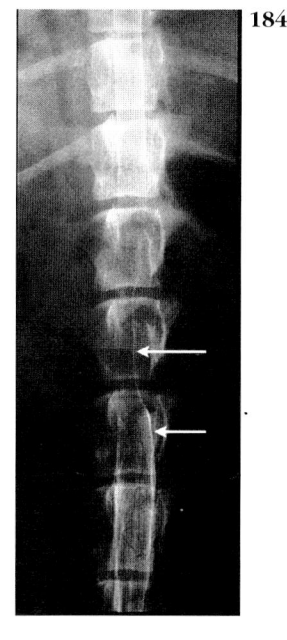

CSF analysis

Analysis of CSF may show mild abnormalities in dogs with disc disease (Thomson *et al.*, 1989). It should be analysed to help rule out other conditions (see **Table 16**), particularly in dogs less than one year or older than seven years of age.

TREATMENT

Many dogs will recover from moderate neurological deficits following either nonsurgical or surgical treatment. Patients with severe neurological deficits (grades 3–5) (see Assessing the severity of the lesion, page 30) who are seen within eight hours of the time of spinal cord injury may benefit from high dose methylprednisolone therapy (Chapter 6). Certain generalizations can be made regarding the advantages of each type of therapy.

Nonsurgical treatment

Strict cage rest is the overriding principle behind this therapy, although judicious use of anti-inflammatory medication can be helpful. The animal must rest quietly in a confined space (travelling cage size) for at least two weeks, during which time it should only be removed to allow it to urinate and defaecate. A satisfactory response to treatment should be followed by a further two weeks rest, and then by a gradual increase in exercise between the fifth and eighth weeks.

Animals that will not rest, those that are allowed out of confinement for even half an hour a day, or that are kept in too large a cage, may not respond or may even get worse. It is important that the patient be evaluated regularly for any signs of deterioration in the neurological status, which indicates treatment failure, as does a lack of improvement within two weeks.

Advantages of nonsurgical treatment are that it is inexpensive, requires no equipment other than a suitable cage, and can be continued at home, if necessary, after an initial few days of direct observation. It gives an overall recovery rate of about 90% for dogs with grade 1–3 deficits (**Table 17**). About half the dogs with grade 4 lesions will recover with cage rest, but it is ineffective for the vast majority of dogs with grade 5 lesions. However, occasional dogs with grade 5 lesions will respond, and one or two weeks of cage rest is reasonable when there is no alternative other than euthanasia.

Although a useful treatment option, nonsurgical therapy is rarely the treatment of choice for paraparetic or paraplegic dogs where there are no financial constraints. The major long term problem is that over one third of dogs will suffer a recurrence (**Table 18**). Another disadvantage is that the dog can deteriorate during treatment, possibly as far as grade 5. In addition, there is a natural tendency to underemphasize the diagnostic evaluation of a dog to be treated by cage rest, with the possibility that other causes for the neurological deficits can be overlooked. Physiotherapy must also be delayed until the latter part of the treatment period, and recovery of the neurological deficits may be slow or incomplete.

Table 17 Results of treatment for thoracolumbar disc disease

Neurological grade	Percent successful treatment (number of dogs)		
	Conservative[1]	Hemilaminectomy[2]	Fenestration[3]
1	100 (8)	100 (8)	95 (19)
2	84 (38)	100 (33)	95 (60)
3	100 (10)	95 (20)	85 (47)
4	50 (6)	90 (37)	94 (18)
5	7 (14)	50 (21)* 6 (15)**	33 (6)

* Dogs operated on within 48 hours of the onset of paraplegia.
** Dogs operated on more than 48 hours after the onset of paraplegia.
[1] Davies and Sharp, 1983.
[2] Lineberger and Kornegay (Unpublished).
[3] Denny, 1978; Davies and Sharp, 1983; Butterworth and Denny, 1991.

Table 18 Recovery times and recurrence rates after treatment for thoracolumbar disc disease

Neurological grade	Mean recovery time in weeks		
	Conservative[1]	Hemilaminectomy[2]	Fenestration[3]
1	3	N/A	2.5
2	6	N/A	4
3	9	1	5.5
4	12	2.5	8
5	N/A	2*	N/A
Recurrence rate (%)	34[1], 40[4]	H, 27[4] H/F, 16[4]	0[1], 2[3], 16[4]

* Dogs operated on within 48 hours of the onset of paraplegia.
H, hemilaminectomy without fenestration; H/F, hemilaminectomy with fenestration of at least T_{11}/T_{12} to L_1/L_2.
N/A, data not available.
[1] Davies and Sharp, 1983.
[2] Lineberger and Kornegay (Unpublished).
[3] Butterworth and Denny, 1991.
[4] Levine and Caywood, 1984.

A short course of corticosteroids without cage rest does *not* constitute effective nonsurgical treatment. A high proportion of dogs referred for emergency decompressive surgery have been treated in the preceding days or weeks with corticosteroids but with no cage confinement (see **179**). The corticosteroids relieve the dog's discomfort but often make it more active. This renders the dog very susceptible to further herniation of disc material and subsequent development of severe neurological deficits. For this reason, we may withold anti-inflammatory medication during the initial period of nonsurgical treatment in order to encourage the animal to rest.

SURGERY

Dorsolateral hemilaminectomy (185–214)

The usual way to perform a hemilaminectomy is to use power instruments, but it can be performed with rongeurs (see **200**). Ideally, it should be performed on the same side as the disc herniation.

The results of the neurological examination (asymmetry in the degree of paresis and the level of the panniculus reflex cut-off) and the myelogram usually agree on the side of maximum compression. When the side of the lesion is not obvious by these means, the history may reveal that the neurological deficit was initially apparent or worse in one pelvic limb, and this is then taken to be the side of the lesion. In the absence of any evidence to lateralize the lesion, the hemilaminectomy may have to be extended dorsally to allow access to the opposite side of the spinal cord (see **209**).

Hemilaminectomy is the treatment of choice for most dogs with neurological deficits of grade 2 or more. Decompression should be performed as soon as possible after the onset of neurological signs, especially for dogs with severe deficits. This is crucial in animals with depressed or absent deep pain sensation. Those with grade 5 neurological deficits should be regarded as emergencies, requiring surgery within 24 hours to have the best chance for a successful outcome. Reasonable results can still be obtained if surgery is performed within 48 hours, but after three days the results are dismal (Knecht, 1972; Henry, 1975; Lineberger and Kornegay, unpublished data) (see **Table 17**). The rate of recovery is also faster after hemilaminectomy than after the other two methods of treatment (see **Table 18**), and there is less likelihood of any residual neurological deficits after surgical decompression of the spinal cord.

Disadvantages relate mainly to the need for myelography and for special equipment and surgical expertise. Specific recommendations for hemilaminectomy include the following.

- Grade 5 lesions of less than 48 hours duration.
- Neurological deterioration or lack of response to other types of therapy.
- Recurrence after previous treatment.
- Myelographic evidence of significant spinal cord compression.
- Presence of LMN deficits.

Hemilaminectomy without fenestration can result in a recurrence rate as high as 27% (Levine and Caywood, 1984), so we recommend concomitant disc fenestration. The ideal treatment for disc herniation is spinal cord decompression with fenestration of all high risk discs (T_{11}/T_{12}–L_4/L_5 inclusive). This requires considerable dissection if undertaken from a dorsolateral approach. A compromise is usually reached entailing fenestration of at least the affected disc and the one on either side (if possible also including T_{12}/T_{13} and T_{13}/L_1).

We do not recommend dorsal laminectomy for thoracolumbar disc disease: it has no advantages over hemilaminectomy, and yet causes considerably more biomechanical instability (see Chapter 13). Access to extruded disc material is better from a hemilaminectomy and fenestration is also easier.

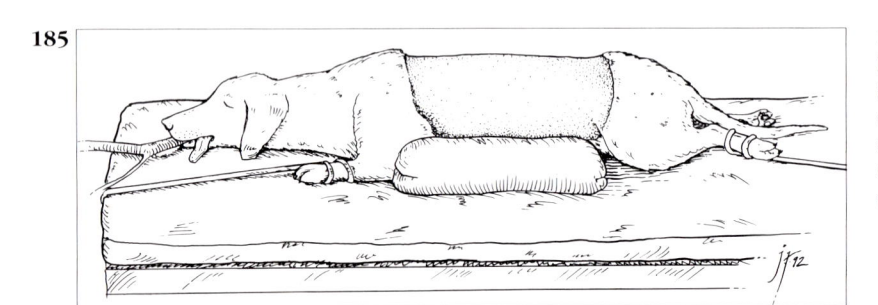

185 Positioning for thoracolumbar hemilaminectomy. The trunk is supported by sandbags on each side of the abdomen. Some surgeons prefer to have the patient rotated slightly, with the side to be approached positioned uppermost.

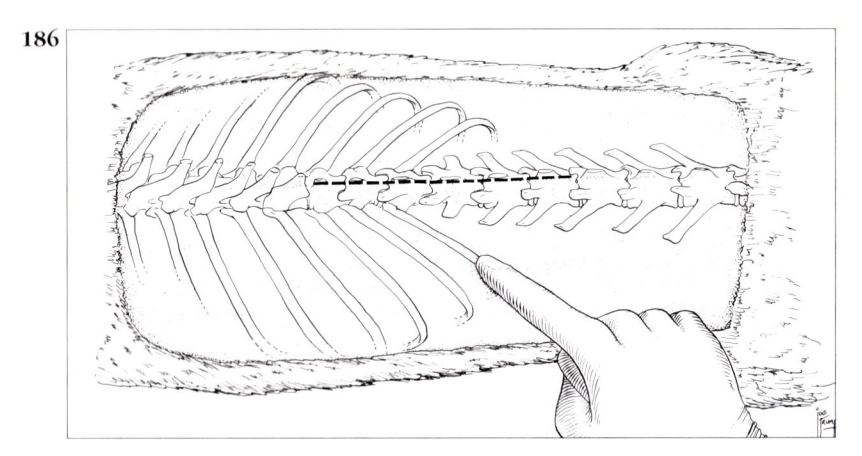

186 Incision site. Most hemilaminectomies are performed near the thoracolumbar junction. It is important to identify the last rib (shown by finger) and the transverse process of L_1. The incision is made just off the midline, again on the side of the spine to be approached.

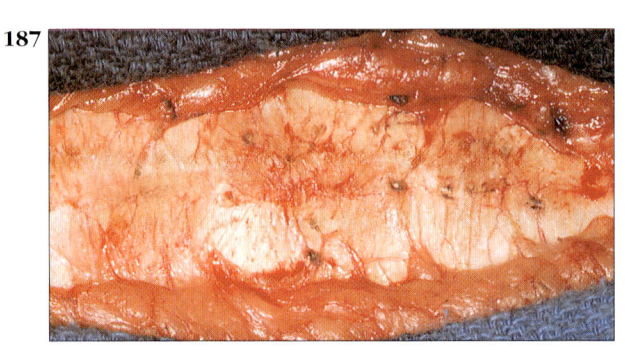

187 The patient's head is to the left throughout the procedure. The skin and superficial muscles have been generously incised a few millimetres away from the spinous processes, and the subcutaneous fat has been reflected for 1–2 cm on either side of the midline. This has revealed the thick lumbodorsal fascia, which covers the spinous processes. Although creating additional dead space, this exposure considerably facilitates subsequent repair of this important fascial plane.

8 THORACOLUMBAR DISC DISEASE

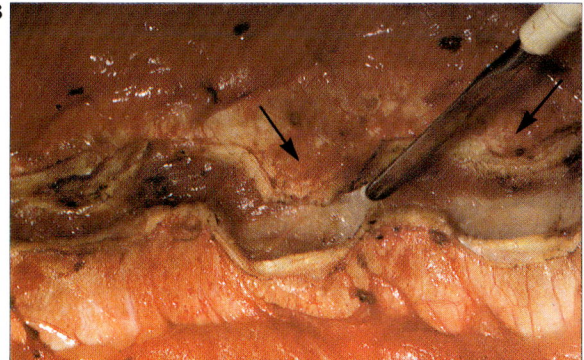

188 The lumbodorsal fascia is incised on the midline, extending around the near side of the spinous processes, over at least five vertebrae. Use of the electroscalpel tends to reduce minor haemorrhage during this and ensuing stages of the exposure of the vertebral bodies. Here two spinous processes (arrows) have already been exposed to show the relationship of the fascial incision to the spinous processes.

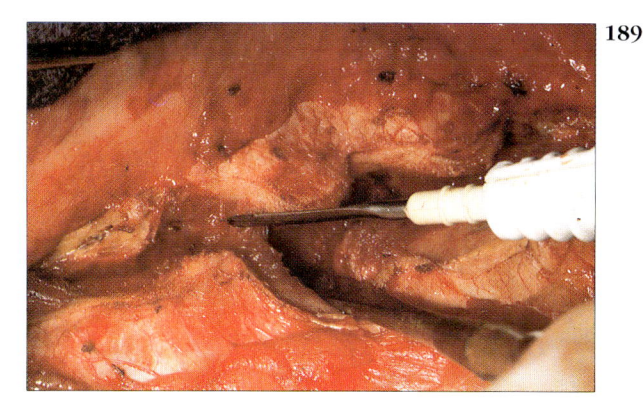

189 A periosteal elevator or similar instrument is used to lever muscle away from the nearside of each spinous process. Muscular insertions on the cranial and caudal ends of each spinous process are cut close to the bone, here using the electroscalpel.

190 A handheld (Langenbeck/Senn) retractor is placed adjacent to the spinous process, and pulled laterally and slightly cranially to expose the dorsal surface of the articular processes of this and the adjacent cranial vertebral body. Here the lateral retraction shows an articular process with muscles still attached (arrow). While maintaining this traction, the muscular attachments onto the articular processes are cut as close as possible to the joint capsule.

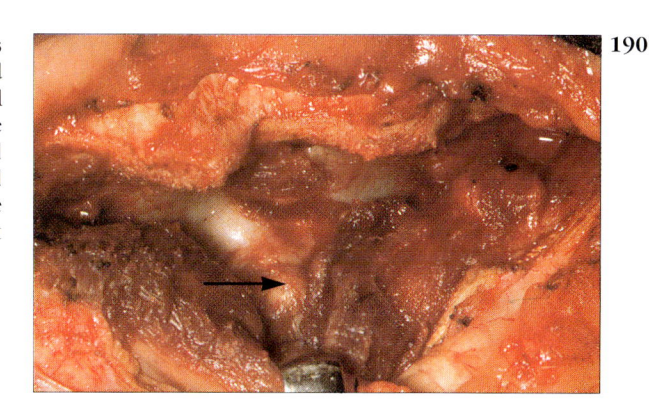

191 Diagram to show craniolateral traction applied to muscles with a handheld retractor. The incision of the muscles from the articular processes is shown (dotted lines). The incision should be made as close as possible to the bone; this reduces haemorrhage.

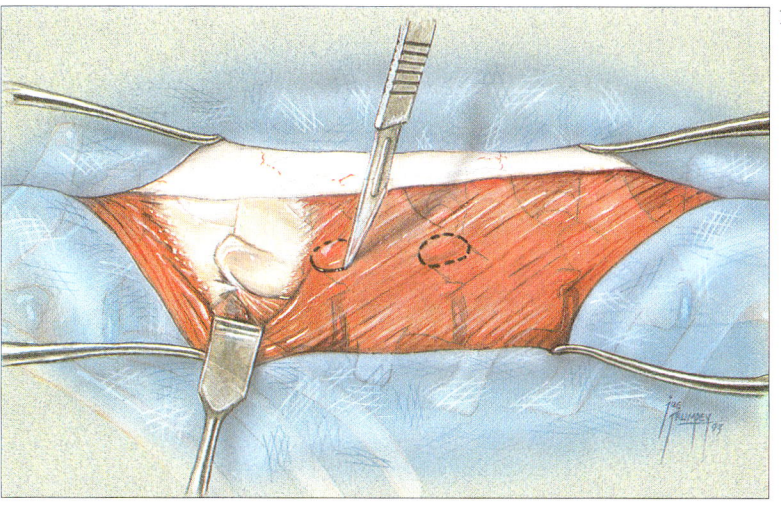

DIAGNOSIS AND SURGERY OF SMALL ANIMAL SPINAL DISORDERS

192 The muscular attachments have been severed, and the isolated articular processes are clearly visible (arrow). Bipolar electrocautery is helpful to retard bleeding from the proximity of the articular processes. It is useful to separate any remaining tags of muscle away from the joint and the base of each process, by using a blunt elevator covered with a gauze sponge (see **193**). The procedure outlined in **189–192** is repeated for two articulations on either side of the one overlying the target intervertebral space.

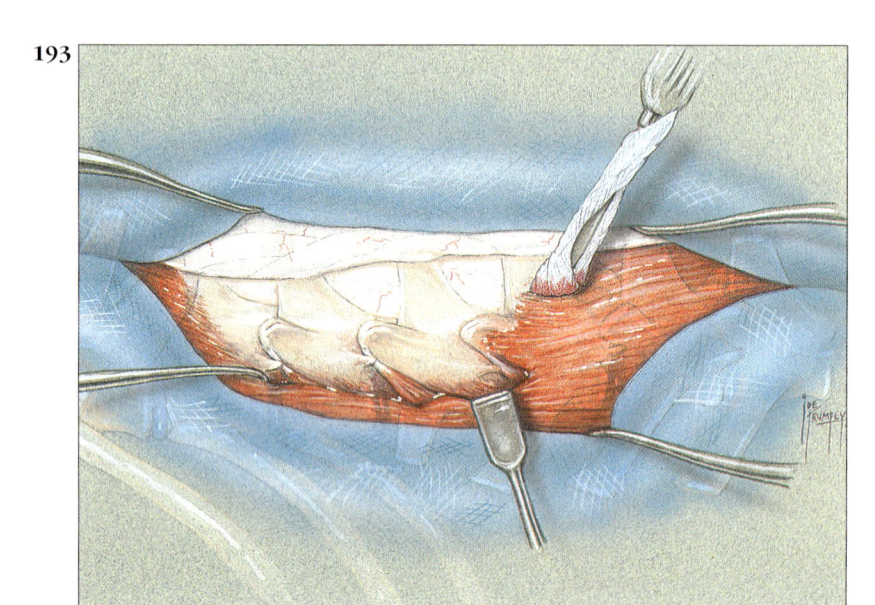

193 Diagram to illustrate cleaning away of muscle tags from the lamina and articular processes, using a periosteal elevator and gauze sponge. Gelpi retractors have been inserted to maintain the exposure.

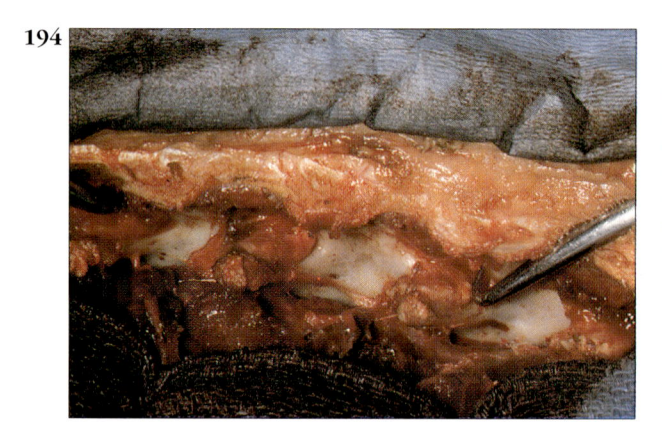

194 Gelpi retractors are placed between the interspinous space and the laterally dissected epaxial muscle mass, at a site one intervertebral space cranial and one space caudal to the target intervertebral space. Before maximally distracting the retractors, a moistened towel drape is placed over the muscle to protect it and prevent desiccation. An impervious paper drape, which has been sutured to the skin, is seen on the far side of the surgical site.

8 THORACOLUMBAR DISC DISEASE

195 Diagram to illustrate aspects of anatomy referred to previously. Muscles are being elevated from the lamina with a periosteal elevator. The exposed articular processes are visible, beneath which are seen muscular insertions on the accessory processes.

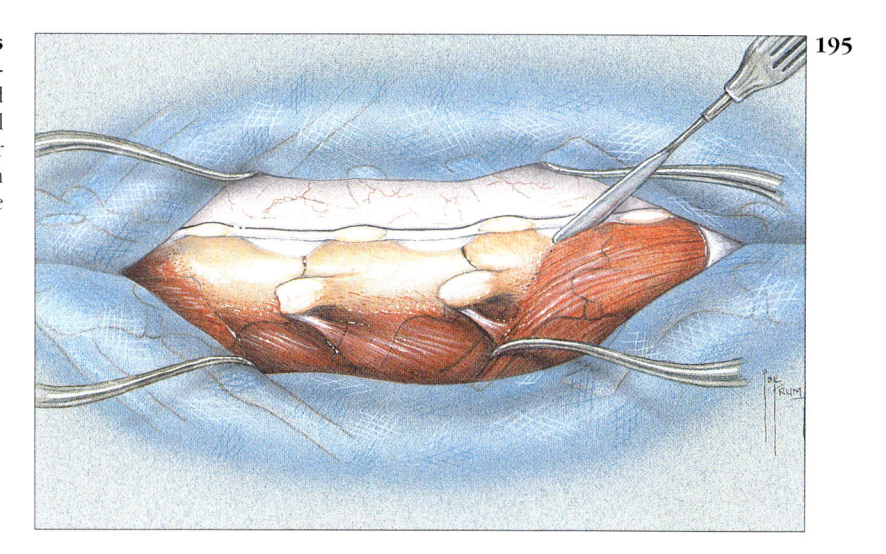

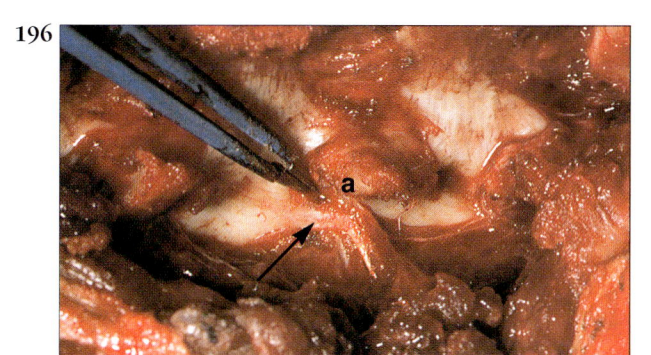

196 Maximal lateral retraction of the muscles reveals almost the entire lateral aspect of the two adjacent vertebrae. The thin, tendinous attachment can be seen on the accessory process (arrow) of the most cranial of the two vertebrae. There is frequently a small branch of the spinal artery that runs dorsal to this accessory process, which requires use of bipolar cautery as shown.
(**a**) articular process.

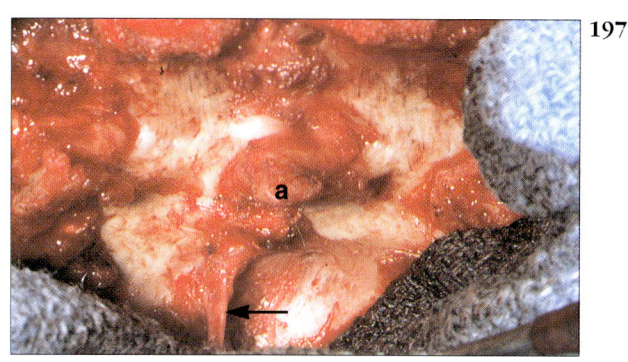

197 The tendinous attachment to the accessory process has been cut, and the main branches of the spinal artery, vein and the spinal nerve appear as a common neurovascular bundle (arrow).
(**a**) articular process.

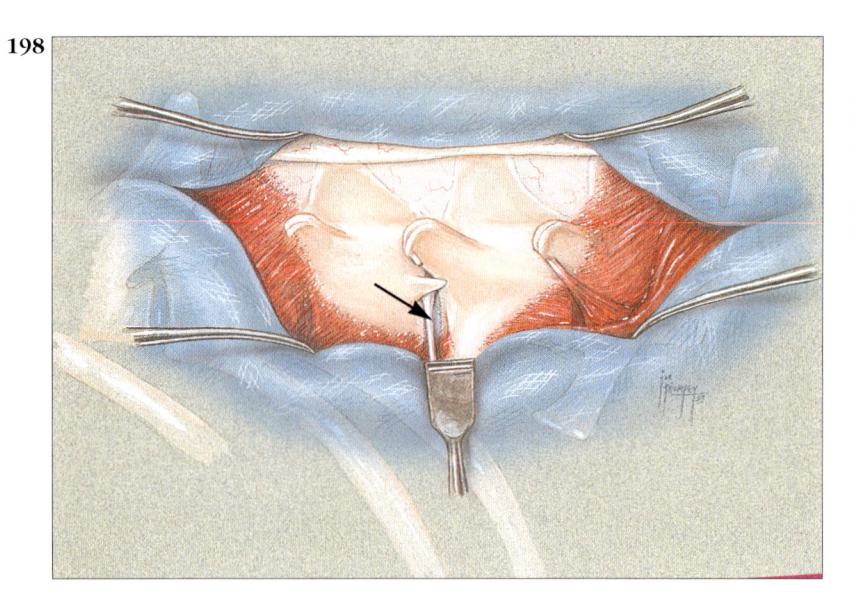

DIAGNOSIS AND SURGERY OF SMALL ANIMAL SPINAL DISORDERS

198 Diagram to show the approach for fenestration at the site of the hemilaminectomy, before entry into the vertebral canal. Lateral retraction is provided by a handheld retractor. This exposes the spinal nerve (arrow), behind which lies the lateral anulus fibrosus.

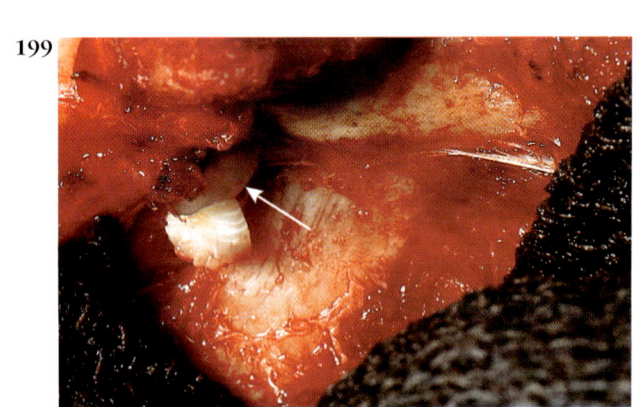

199 A window of anulus has been removed (see also 229). The concentric layers of anulus can be seen, and the jelly-like nucleus of this 'normal' disc is extruding laterally (arrow). The transverse process (**a**) is seen caudal to the incised anulus.

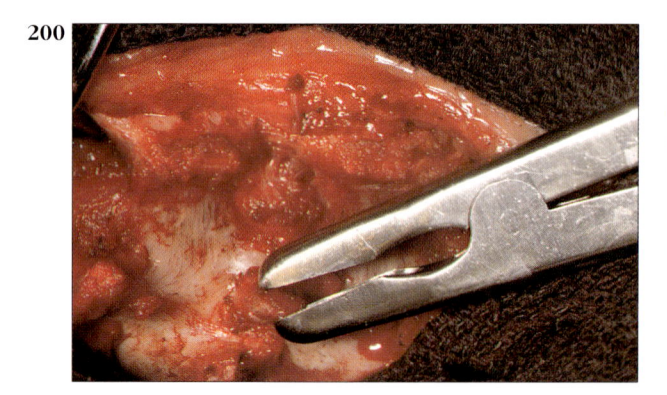

200 Rongeurs are used to remove the articular processes at the site of entry into the vertebral canal. Fine rongeurs can be used to perform the entire hemilaminectomy if desired, although most surgeons prefer to use power instruments. To start the procedure using rongeurs, the adjacent spinous processes are grasped with clamps, which are then used to lever the two vertebrae apart. The rongeurs can then be carefully introduced into the intervertebral foramen to start the bone removal.

8 THORACOLUMBAR DISC DISEASE

201 The extent of the proposed hemilaminectomy window has been drilled. It is oval or kidney-shaped over the intervertebral foramen.

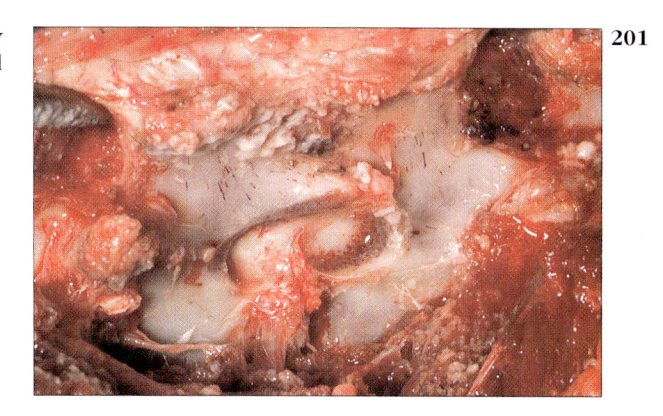

202 Surgical site with towel drapes removed to show the relationship of the suction tip (arrow) in the 'gutter' formed between the vertebral body and the epaxial muscle mass, the tip of the irrigator over the hemilaminectomy site, and the drill itself. Also note the manner in which the surgeon is holding the drill, steadying the bur guard with the left hand resisting any downward movement.

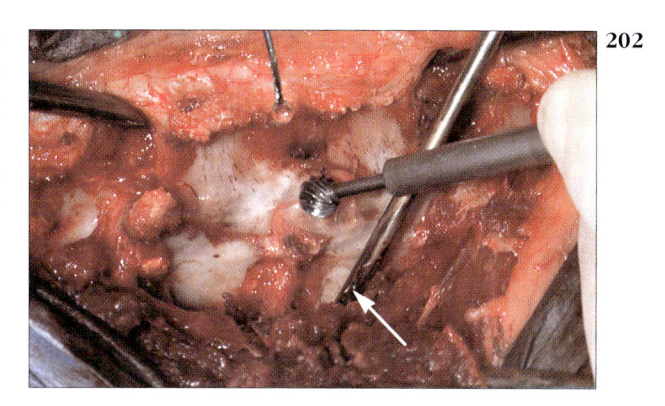

203 The bur has been used to remove bone from the base of the articular processes, exposing the underlying grey/pink, coarse cancellous bone (arrow) of the most caudal vertebral body. Bone removal is a little further advanced over the cranial-most vertebral body, where the inner cortical bone plate is revealed (white arrow).

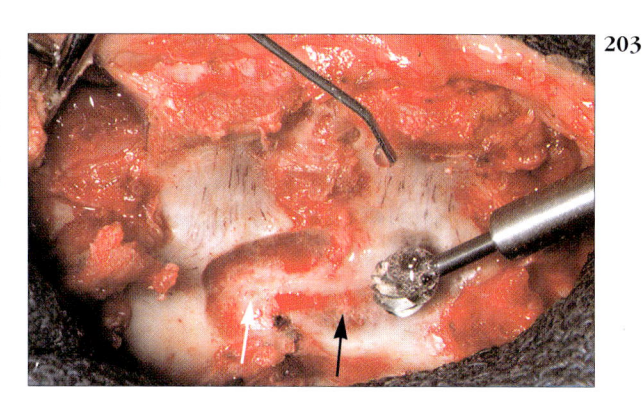

204 The inner cortical bone plate of each vertebral body has been exposed here (arrow). When the bone is eggshell thickness, it is removed with a probe, curette, or small rongeur (see **304, 305**).

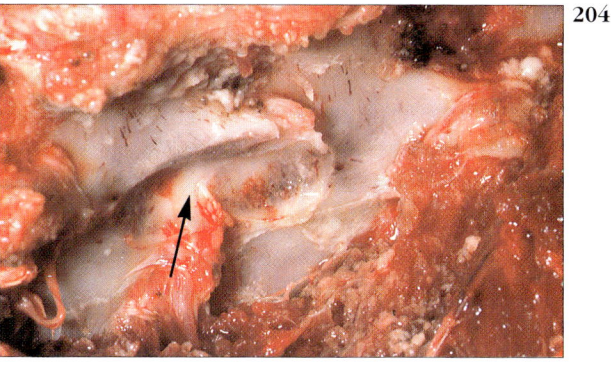

95

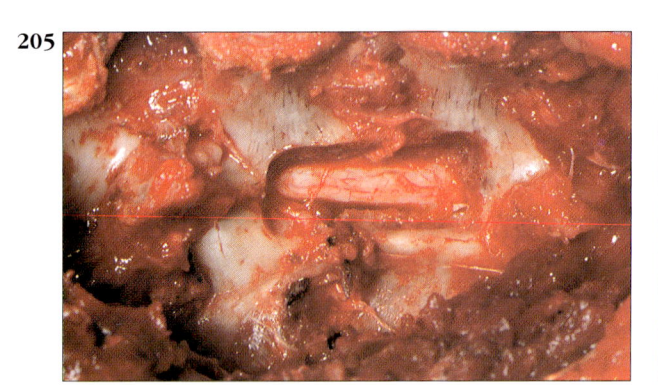

DIAGNOSIS AND SURGERY OF SMALL ANIMAL SPINAL DISORDERS

205 All bone has been removed over the laminectomy site. This exposes the spinal cord covered by pial blood vessels and the transparent dura mater.

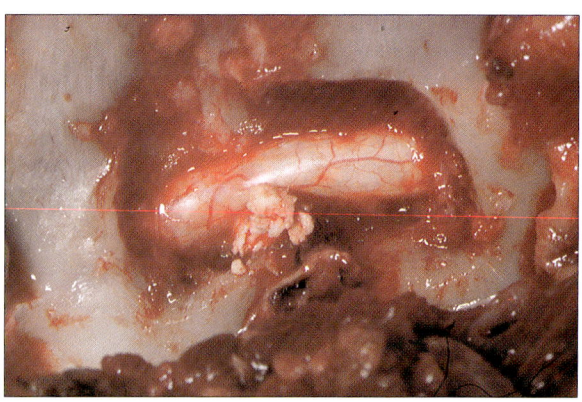

206 Extruded disc *in situ*, compressing the spinal cord. The disc is removed by a combination of gentle suction and use of a thin tartar scraper to scoop material from beneath the spinal cord.

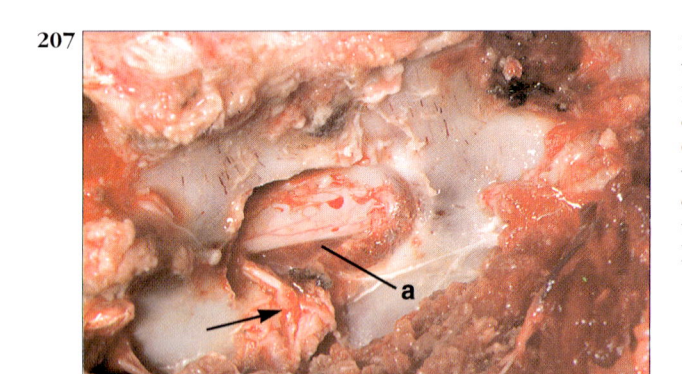

207 This laminectomy has been extended ventrally to expose the spinal nerve and ganglion (arrow). Bleeding from the spinal artery at this stage must be controlled, using bipolar cautery. The venous plexus (venous sinuses) is just visible on the floor of the vertebral canal (**a**). Great care should be taken to avoid damaging the venous structures, although it is not uncommon for them to bleed during removal of herniated disc material.

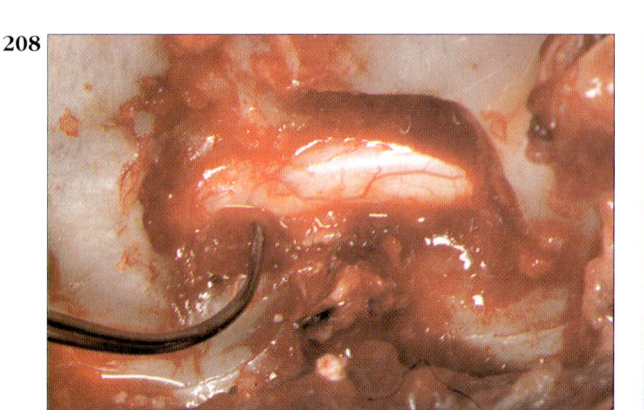

208 Control of venous haemorrhage may be achieved by using a small piece of muscle. This is first macerated, then placed on the surgical site. It is then gently pressed over the defect in the wall of the vein.

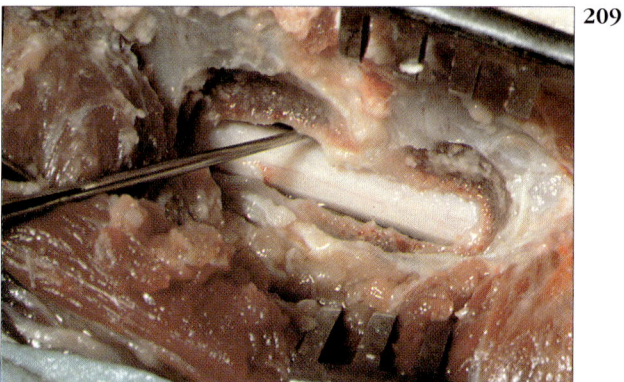

209 The hemilaminectomy can be extended dorsally to allow access to the opposite side of the vertebral canal. This is sometimes necessary if the disc material lies on the opposite side of the vertebral canal.

8. THORACOLUMBAR DISC DISEASE

210 A durotomy has been performed using a 26-gauge hypodermic needle to reveal the spinal cord covered by small pial blood vessels and by thin dorsal nerve rootlets (a). Collapse of the subarachnoid space has caused the dura mater to become opaque. The venous plexus is clearly visible at the floor of the vertebral canal (**b**). This should not be performed routinely (see page 106).

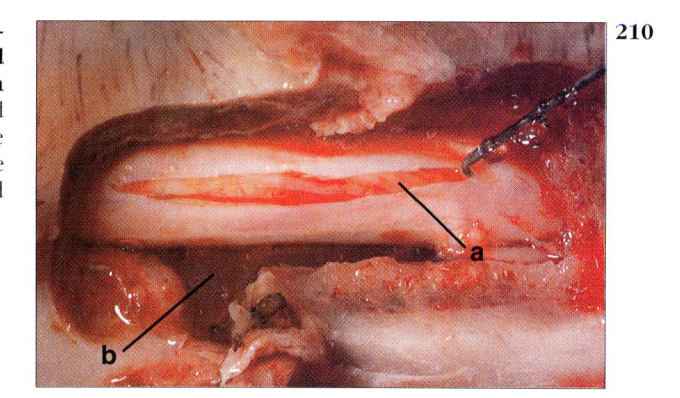

211 The fenestration may be performed after the hemilaminectomy. Here the spinal nerve is seen retracted cranially to reveal the lateral anulus fibrosus. The site of the incision in the anulus is shown. Subsequent disc fenestrations are performed in a similar manner, using the original dorsolateral approach to the spine. Alternatively, a new lateral approach can be made after the fascial incision is closed, as described for lateral fenestration below.

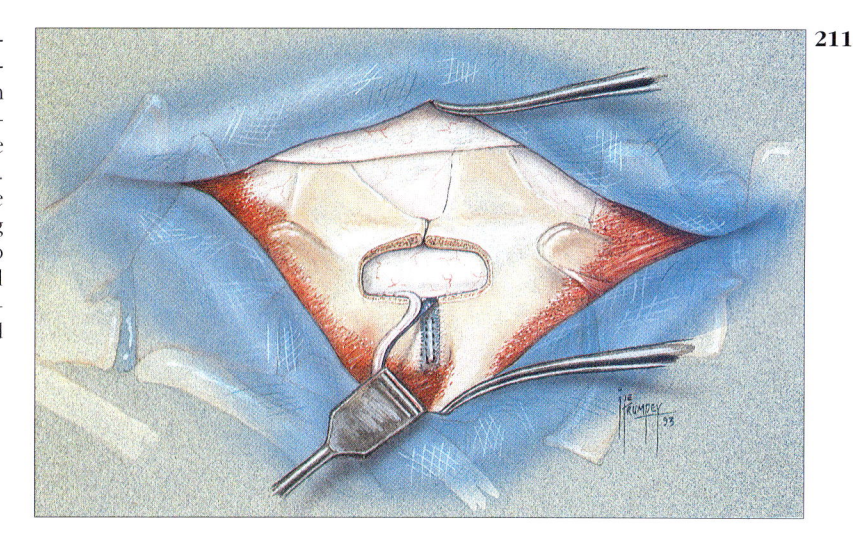

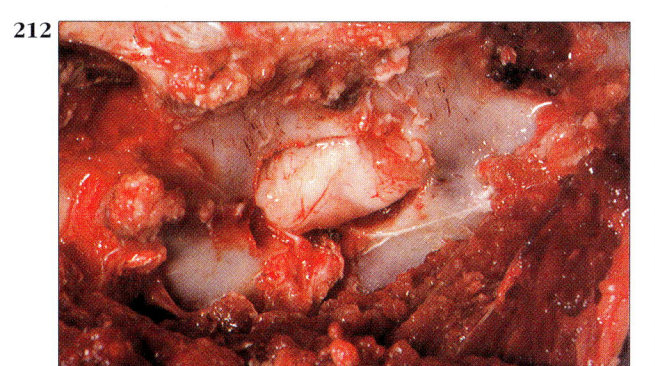

212 The hemilaminectomy site is covered by a piece of subcutaneous fat. This should be only 3–5mm thick, and is held in place by the epaxial musculature after the retractors have been removed.

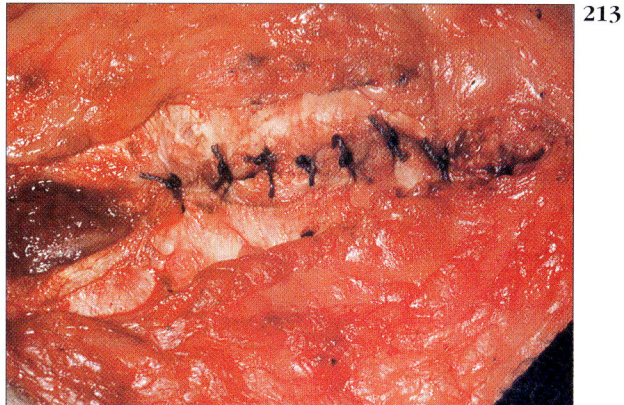

213 Repair of the fascial layer using absorbable sutures in a simple interrupted pattern. Although multifilament absorbable material has been used here, there is evidence that this may be associated with a higher rate of postoperative wound infection (Hosgood, 1992). Monofilament nylon or polydioxanone (PDS, Ethicon) may be better.

214

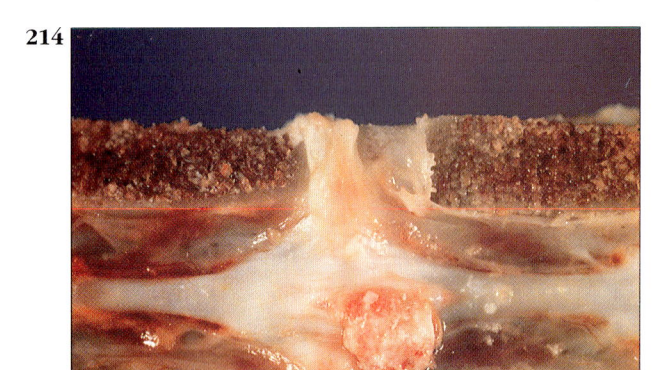

214 Dorsal view of the floor of the vertebral canal, with the spinal cord removed, to show a Type I disc extrusion. The calcified nuclear material lies at the level of the intervertebral foramen, to one side of the dorsal longitudinal ligament. Note how this ligament fans out over, and then merges with, the dorsal surface of the anulus fibrosis.

Minihemilaminectomy (215–218)

The main value of minihemilaminectomy is that it preserves the articular processes (Braund *et al.*, 1976; Black, 1988) and so results in less instability. Because the approach is lateral rather than dorsolateral, disc fenestration is easier.

Minihemilaminectomy is simplest to perform in small, thin dogs and is more difficult in larger animals. It is possible to preserve the articular facets as is done in minihemilaminectomy while performing the standard dorsolateral approach for hemilaminectomy.

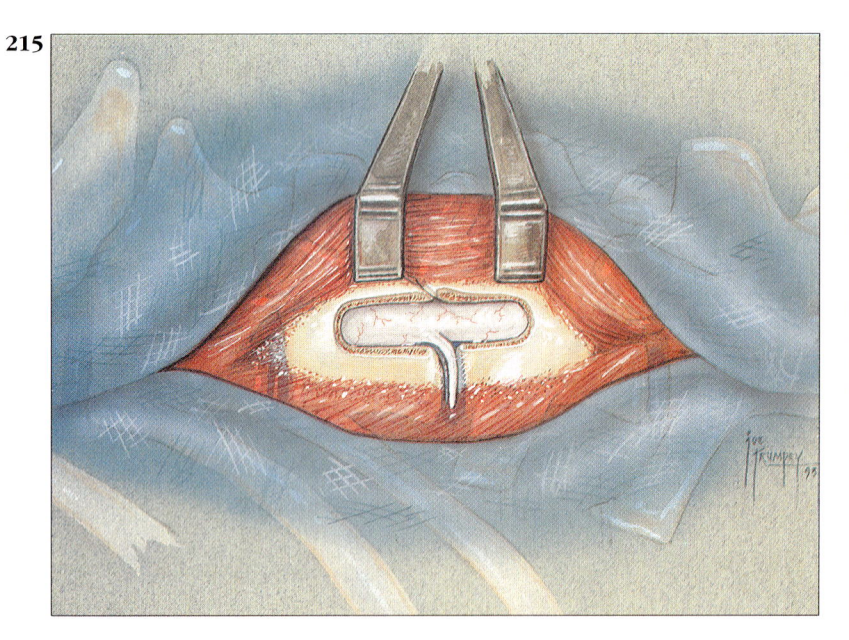

215

215 Minihemilaminectomy. A lateral approach to the spine is made as for fenestration (see below). The epaxial muscles are elevated dorsally to reveal the lateral aspect of the vertebrae, including the transverse process and accessory processes. A hemilaminectomy is performed as described below, but from a more ventral position over the intervertebral foramen, thus preserving the articular processes. Fenestration of this and other discs is as described below.

8. THORACOLUMBAR DISC DISEASE

216 Gelpi retractors and two pairs of army navy retractors have been used to elevate the epaxial muscle mass. This provides good exposure of the lateral aspect of the vertebral body. A hemilaminectomy has been performed, which gives good access to the vertebral canal but preserves the articular processes (not visible here, as they are obscured by the muscle and retractors).

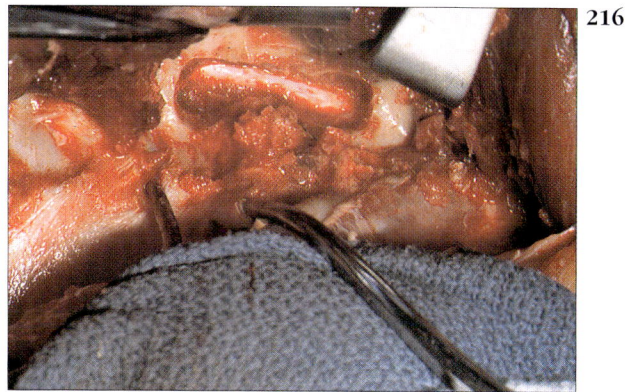

217 Close-up of the minihemilaminectomy site. The dorsal aspect of the spinal cord is visible, while the floor of the vertebral canal is largely obscured by a massive disc extrusion (arrow), which is extending both dorsally and laterally. This is a good example of a chronic disc herniation. Chronic disc herniations frequently adhere to the dura mater. Attempts to free these adhesions to remove the disc often result in a worsening of the neurological status. It is often better to decompress the site, and if the disc material cannot be easily removed, it should be left. Extra decompression of the spinal cord can be provided dorsally (see **209**), if there is significant spinal cord deformity.

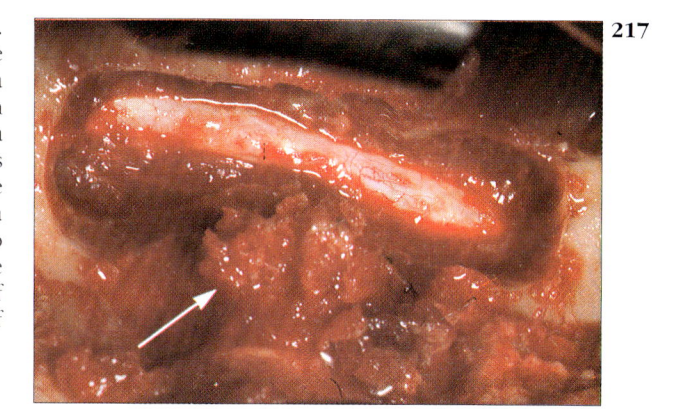

218 Diagram of transverse section through the lumbar region of a dog to show the approach for minihemilaminectomy. The lateral approach allows access to disc material within the vertebral canal while leaving the articular processes intact. The lateral aspect of the vertebral arch has been removed, and here the curette is removing the extruded nucleus pulposus.

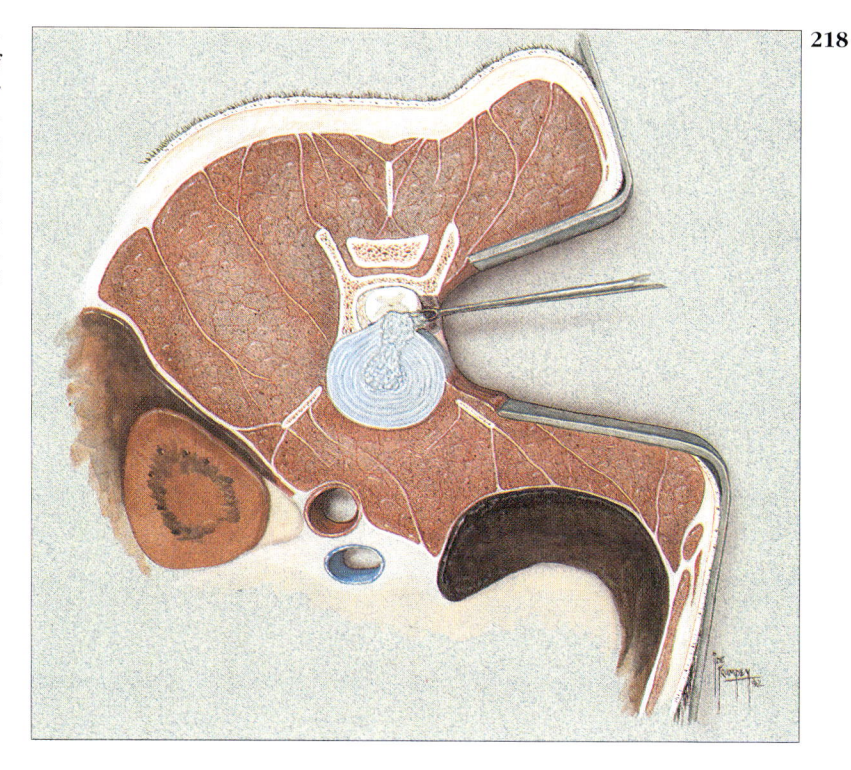

Lateral fenestration (219–239)

The approach can be made from either side, but is normally undertaken from the left with the dog in right lateral recumbency. Although relatively straightforward in principle, fenestration requires a thorough understanding of anatomy and should be undertaken only after careful preparation and practice on cadavers. It is usual to fenestrate the discs from T_{11}/T_{12} to L_3/L_4 inclusive. The more caudal lumbar discs should be fenestrated if there is evidence of LMN disease, taking particular care not to damage the large ventral branches of spinal nerves at this level. Some surgeons believe fenestration has no merit as the sole surgical procedure. We maintain that in certain properly selected patients fenestration is appropriate. Suggested specific recommendations for fenestration include the following.
- Recurrent episodes of pain.
- Recurrent mild (grade 2) neurological deficits.
- If decompression cannot be performed for technical reasons.

Overall recovery rates after fenestration in dogs with lesions of grade 1–3, and possibly grade 4 lesions, appear to be equivalent to those after decompression (see **Table 17**, page 88). It has been suggested in one study that dogs with grade 5 lesions undergoing fenestration may have a 65% chance of recovery (Denny, 1978), but our experience is much less favourable.

The major advantage of fenestration is the low recurrence rate (see **Table 18**). There is also no need for special instrumentation. It can be used in circumstances where myelography is not available. In comparison to nonsurgical therapy, fenestration has the added advantage that physiotherapy can be instituted immediately.

The main disadvantages of fenestration are that recovery periods are longer and residual neurological deficits are more common than after hemilaminectomy, probably because the spinal cord is not decompressed (see **Table 18**). Fenestration cannot be regarded as the treatment of choice for dogs with grade 5 lesions.

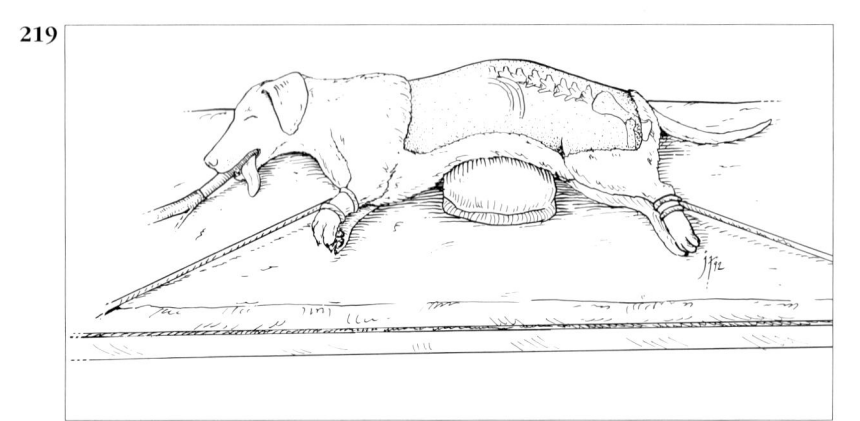

219 Positioning for lateral fenestration. The patient is in right lateral recumbency with the thoracic limbs tied extended and the pelvic limbs extended backwards. A thin sandbag is placed under the dog at the level of the thoracolumbar junction to open up the disc spaces of interest; this may be moved as required to approach the lumbar discs.

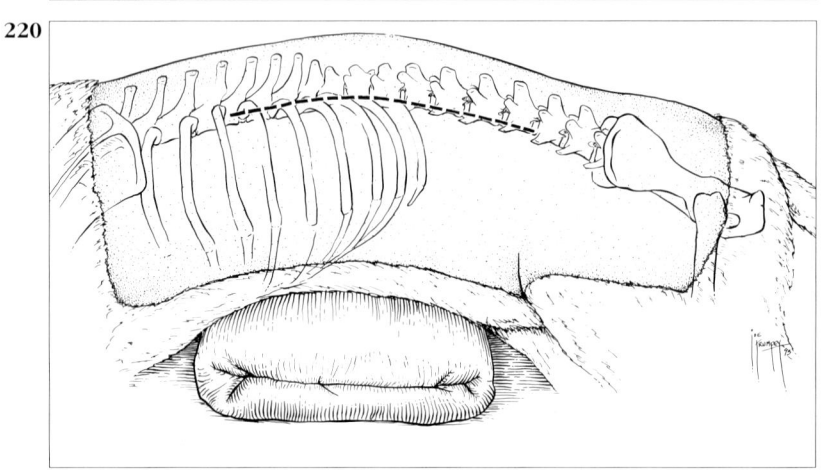

220 Skin incision. The skin incision is made over the lateral aspect of the spine, at the level of the lumbar transverse processes. The incision extends from approximately T_8–L_5.

8. THORACOLUMBAR DISC DISEASE

221 The dog's head is to the left in all illustrations. The skin and superficial fascia have been incised to show the lumbodorsal fascia. At the cranial edge of the incision, the fascia can be seen to have a more muscular appearance.

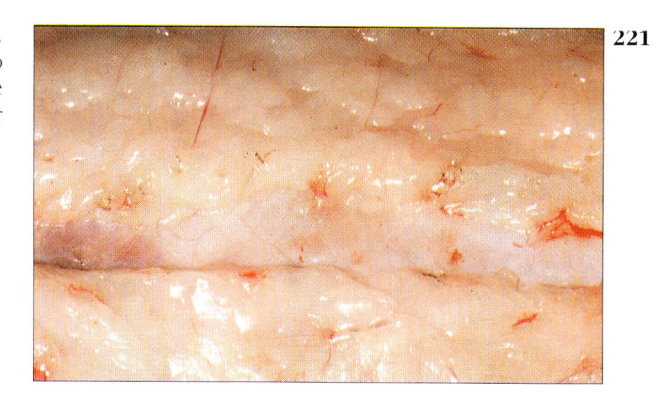

222 A small incision has been made in the lumbodorsal fascia to show the layer of fat beneath. This can be very substantial, even in apparently lean dogs. The incision is in the centre of the exposed portion of fascia, to facilitate finding the fascial edges when undertaking the repair.

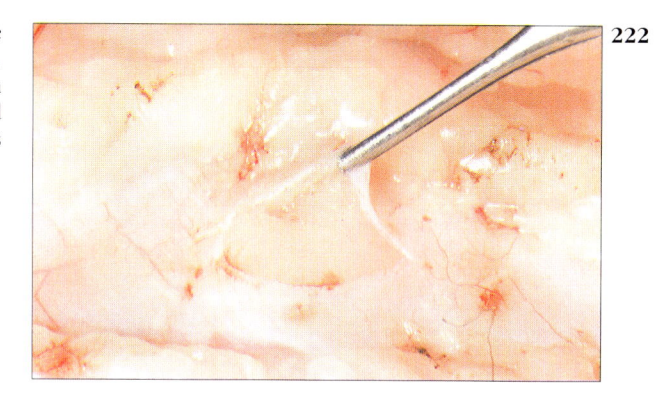

223 The fascia is incised over the full length of the approach.

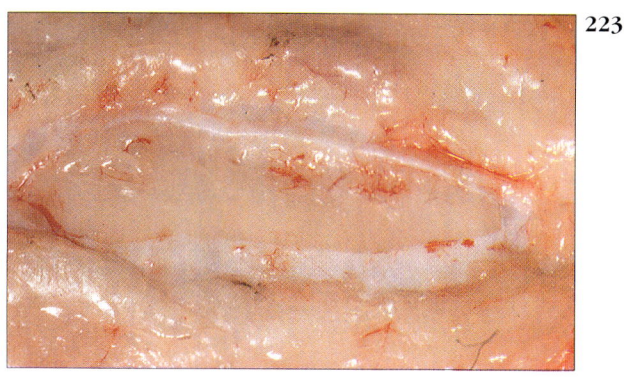

224 The deep layer of fat has been incised to reveal the iliocostalis lumborum muscle and the thirteenth rib (arrow). The longissimus dorsi muscle is covered by a fascial sheath that is just visible under the layer of fat (**a**). The degree of exposure shown in this figure is a little more excessive than required, but has been made here for illustrative purposes.

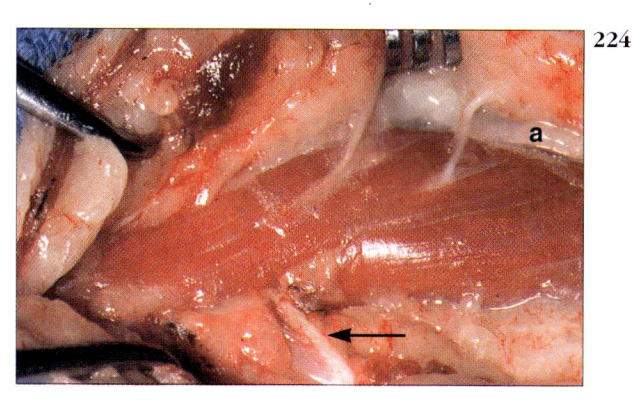

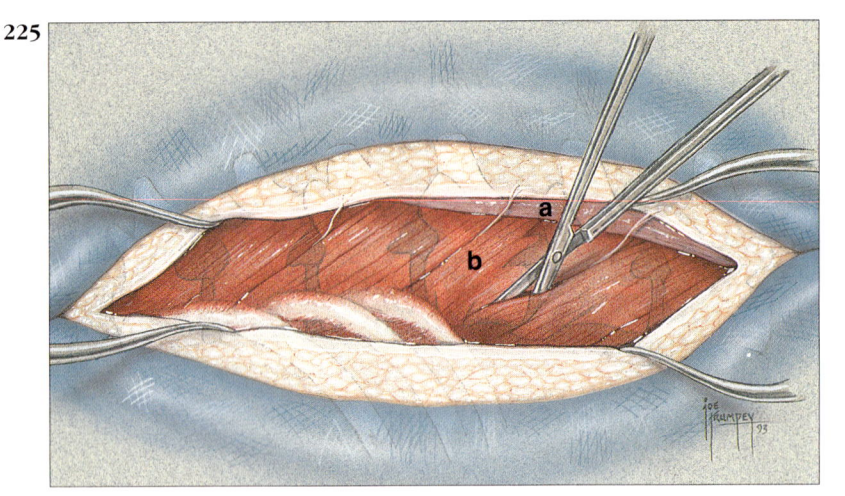

DIAGNOSIS AND SURGERY OF SMALL ANIMAL SPINAL DISORDERS

225 Diagram to show the deep anatomy and muscle separation through the iliocostalis lumborum muscle, in this case over the L₁/L₂ intervertebral space. The longissimus dorsi muscle is in the dorsocaudal part of the surgical field (**a**). The iliocostalis lumborum muscle fibres are seen running obliquely to insert on the ribs (**b**).

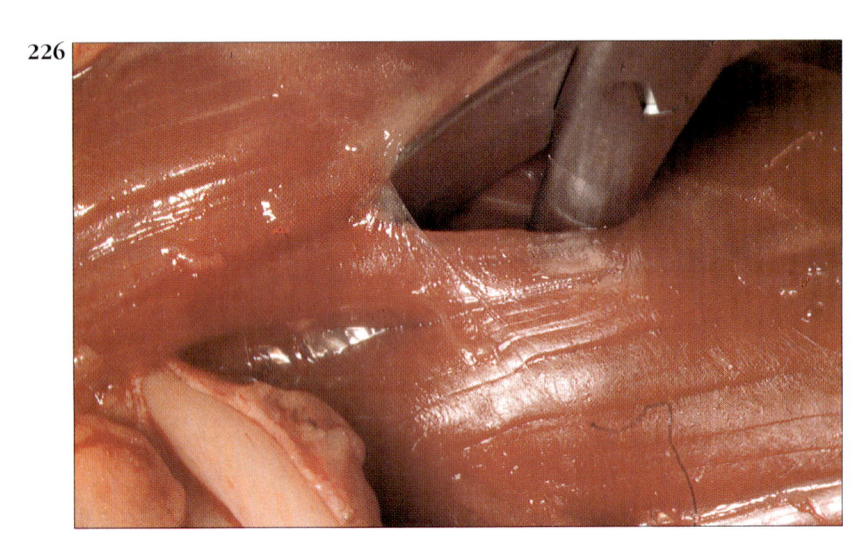

226 Close-up to show separation of the iliocostalis lumborum muscle over the T₁₃/L₁ disc. This is performed by opening a pair of Metzenbaum scissors in the same direction as the muscle fibres. The thirteenth rib (with the periosteum reflected for clarity of illustration) is clearly evident in the lower left hand side of the picture.

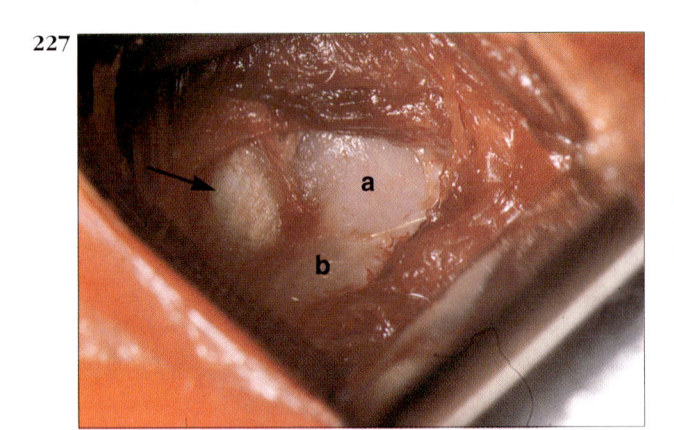

227 Retraction of the iliocostalis muscle. This reveals the body (**a**) and transverse process of the L₁ vertebral body (**b**) and the T₁₃/L₁ disc (arrow). Note the fibres of the anulus fibrosus (over which lies a fine layer of connective tissue). This is best removed by using an elevator covered with a surgical swab (see **193** for technique), pushing the tissue in a craniodorsal direction (to the top left corner of the disc when approaching from the left side of the dog).

102

8. THORACOLUMBAR DISC DISEASE

228 Close-up diagram of the site approached in 227. The muscle separation has revealed the lateral aspect of the anulus fibrosus, which lies just cranial to the transverse process of the lumbar vertebra. Note the small vessel that lies over the disc; this is pushed off the disc with the connective tissue as described in **227**. The incision in the anulus fibrosus is shown by the dotted line. Note the accessory process, which marks the dorsal margin of the intervertebral foramen (arrow).

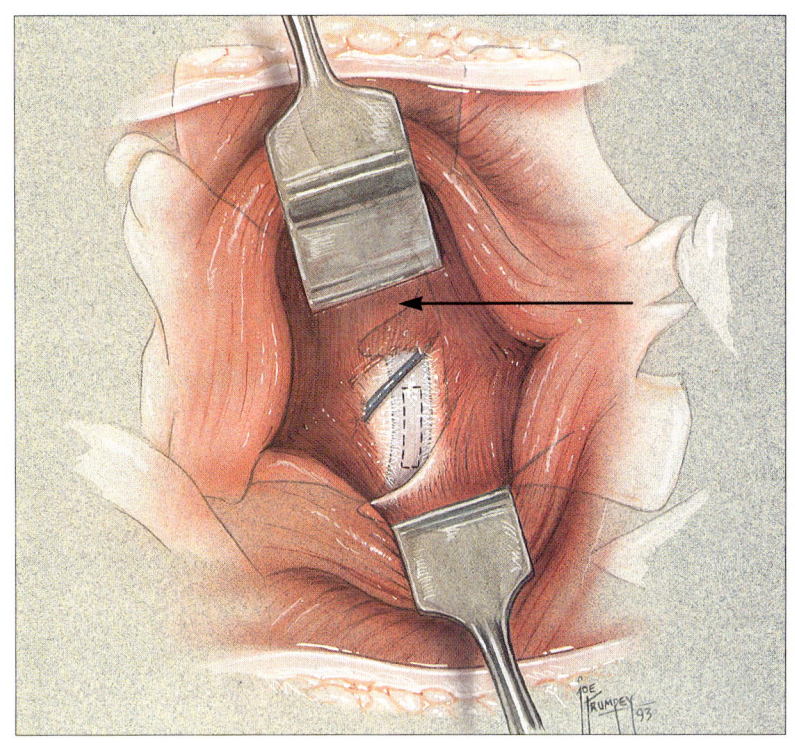

229 Incising the disc with a # 11 scalpel blade reveals the window of anulus and the jelly-like nucleus pulposus (arrow). This view is from the same angle as **227**. The window is initially made by four separate stab incisions, which are then joined at the corners. The hole in the anulus fibrosus must be made larger than any instrument that is going to be used for removal of nucleus pulposus. Disc removal is done with a small curette, a Rosen mobilizer or the # 11 blade itself. It is important to remove as much nuclear material as possible, as any left will remain in the intervertebral space and could cause a clinical problem later. The adjacent discs may be approached from the same muscle separation, but it is usually preferable to make a new approach.

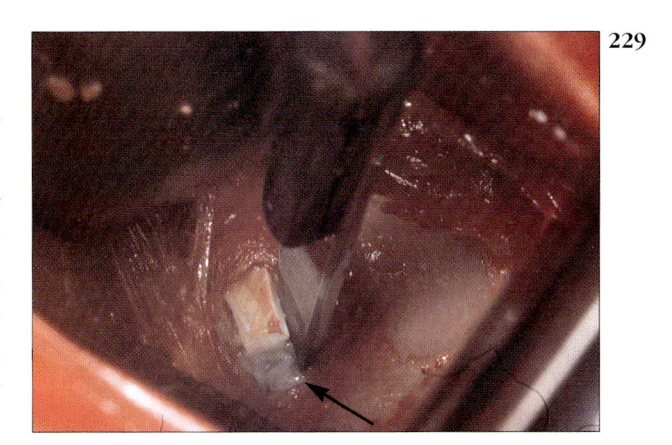

230 The approach to thoracic discs is different. They may be approached by separating the iliocostalis lumborum muscle as for lumbar discs. Alternatively, the muscle can be cut close to the insertion on the twelfth and thirteenth ribs.

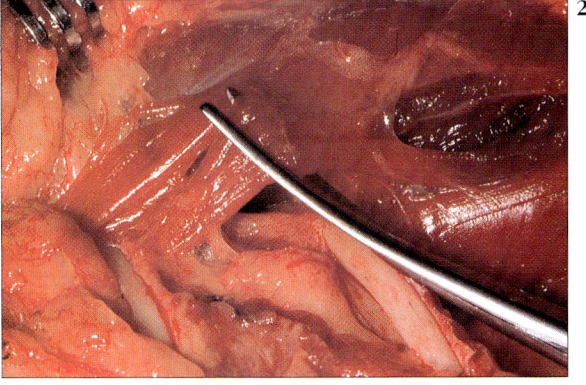

103

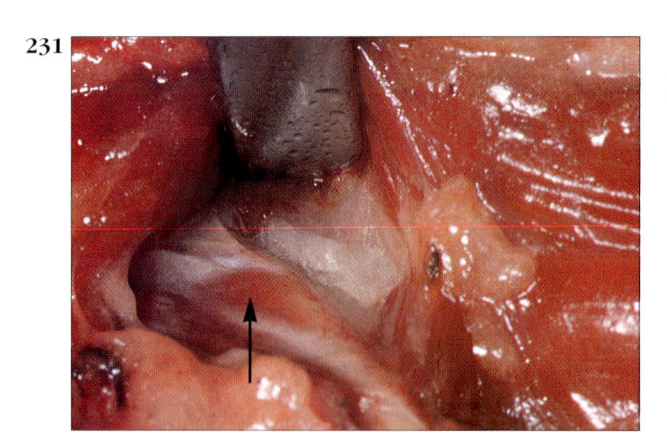

DIAGNOSIS AND SURGERY OF SMALL ANIMAL SPINAL DISORDERS

231 Retraction of the iliocostalis lumborum muscle dorsally reveals the levator costarum muscle (arrow). This will be separated from the rib and retracted in a cranial direction.

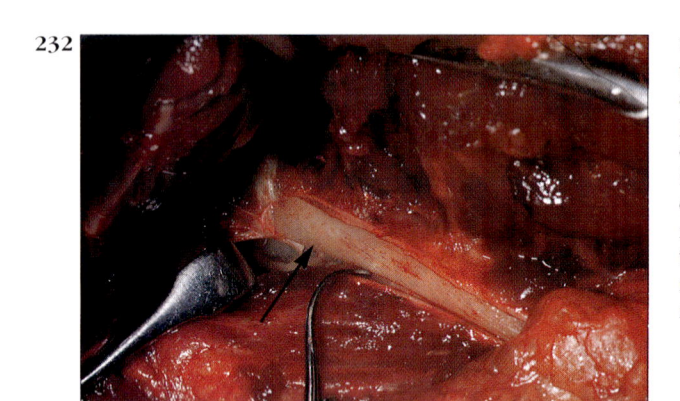

232 The periosteum of the rib has been incised at the caudal border of the levator costarum muscle, and then undermined by a tartar scraper used as a periosteal elevator. The periosteum has been elevated close to the neck of the rib, and a Langenbeck retractor is being used to retract the levator costarum muscle in a cranial direction. At this level, the plane of dissection is medial and dorsal to the pleural reflection. Dissection of the deep fascia that attaches to the cranial margin of the rib (arrow) is then continued proximally, towards the neck and head of the rib.

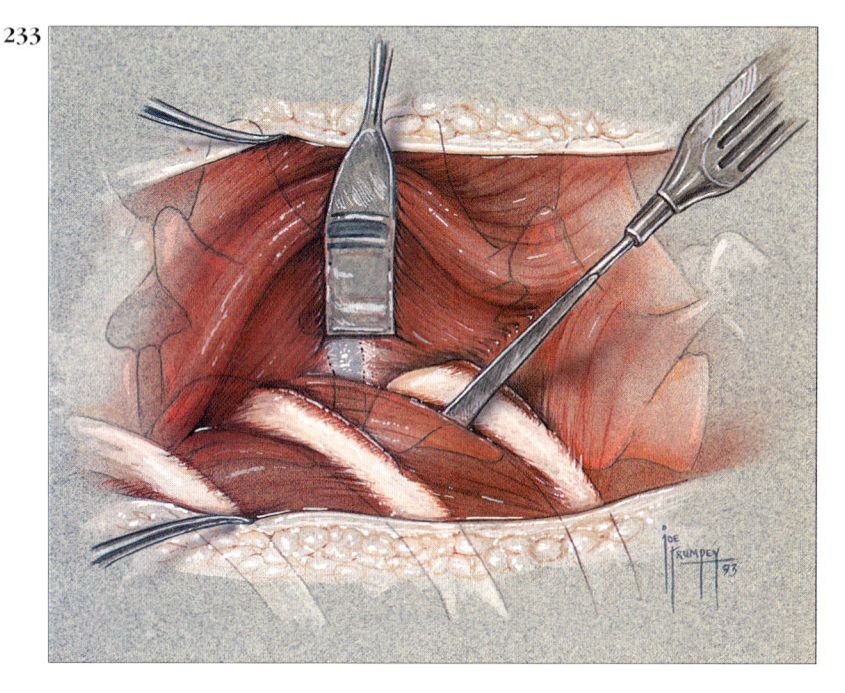

233 Diagram to show the features described in 231. Here the levator costarum muscle is being elevated from the rib with a periosteal elevator. A handheld retractor is positioned to keep the iliocostalis lumborum muscle retracted dorsally. Gelpi retractors can be used here, but must be positioned with care to avoid tearing the pleura.

8. THORACOLUMBAR DISC DISEASE

234 Close-up of the region deep to the cranially reflected levator costarum (a). Blunt dissection (which is most easily accomplished using a narrow, blunt periosteal elevator covered by a piece of gauze sponge, used to gently 'wipe' away loose connective tissue in this area) has begun to expose the intervertebral disc (**b**) just cranial to the rib. The ligament of the tubercle of the rib (**c**) is particularly prominent from this angle; (**d**) shows rib.

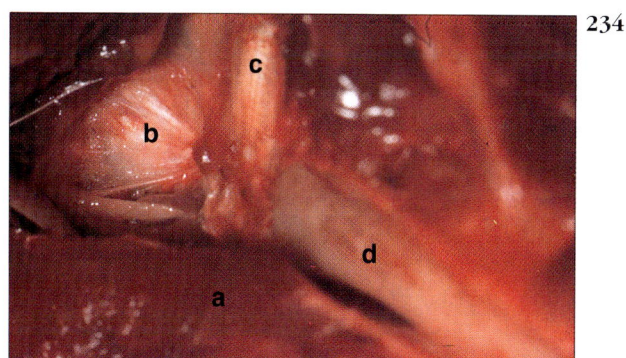

235 Diagram to show the lateral aspect of the disc exposed, with the levator costarum muscle retracted cranioventrally, and the epaxial muscles retracted dorsally. The site of the fenestration is shown.

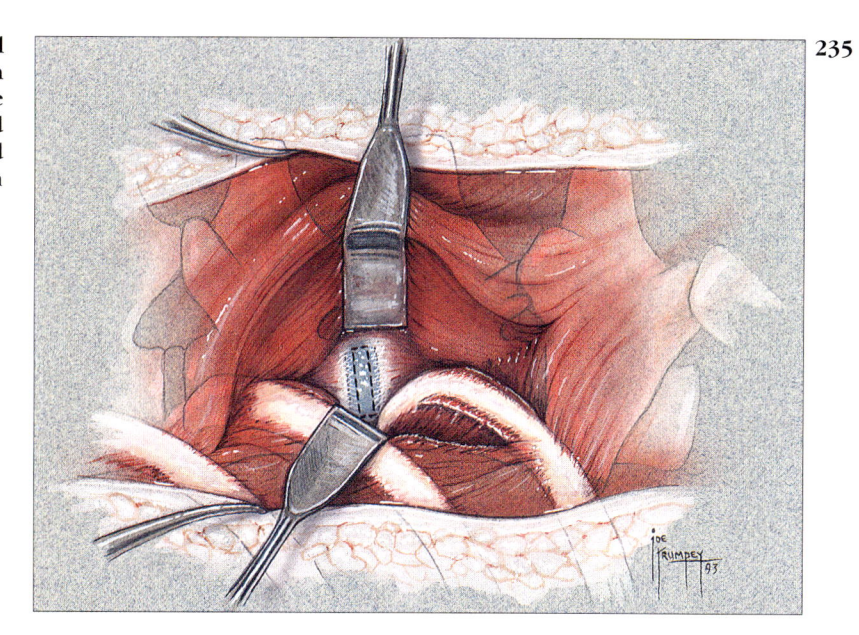

236 Blunt dissection has been completed, and the disc is now clearly visible (a). Handheld retractors are being used to elevate the epaxial muscle away from the last two ribs. Joint capsule overlies the rib head and tubercle (**b**).

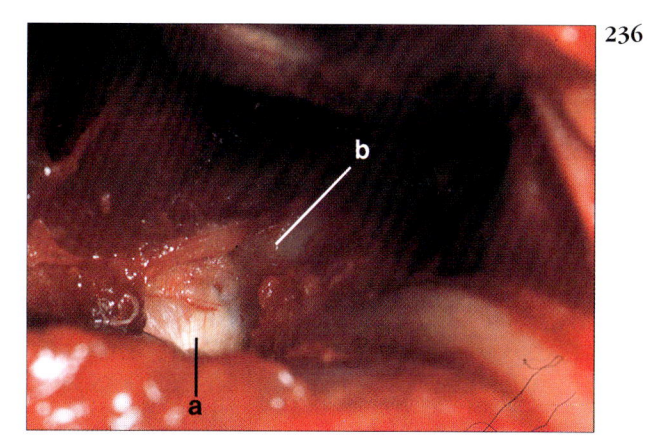

DIAGNOSIS AND SURGERY OF SMALL ANIMAL SPINAL DISORDERS

237 A # 11 scalpel blade can be seen cutting deeply into the anulus. The fenestration is then completed in the manner described in **229** and in Chapter 7. The surgeon should ensure that the window in the anulus fibrosus is slightly larger than the instrument to be used for curettage of nuclear material (see 'Complications,' below). A 4mm drill bit can be used instead of a #11 blade, and may allow more complete evacuation of nuclear material (Holmberg et al., 1990).

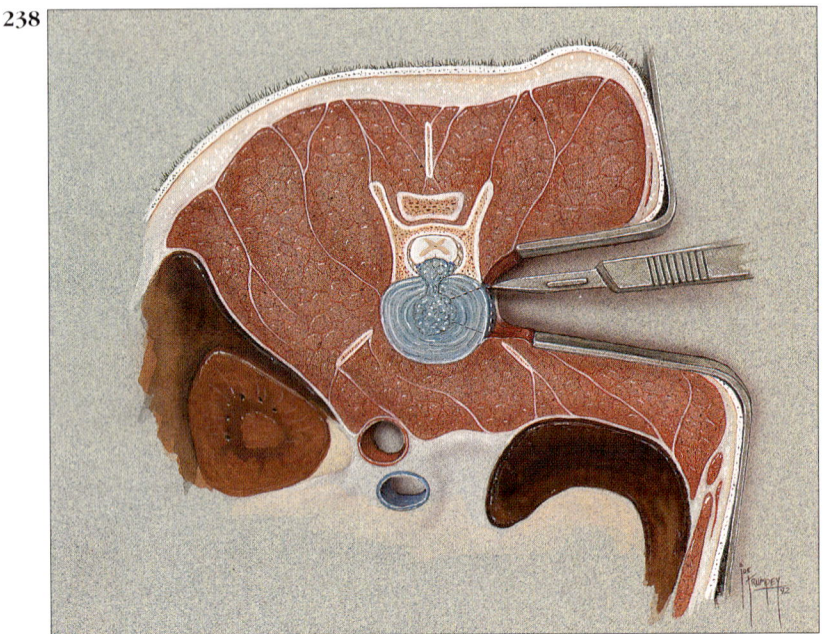

238 Diagram of a transverse section through a dog in the lumbar region to show the approach used in fenestration. The approach allows access to the lateral anulus fibrosus and to disc material in the intervertebral space. However, there is no access to disc material in the vertebral canal.

239 The iliocostalis muscle is repaired using absorbable suture material. The muscle separations in the lumbar area do not need to be sutured if they are small. Repair of the lumbodorsal fascia is best performed using monofilament absorbable suture material in a simple continuous pattern. The advantage of incising the lumbodorsal fascia in a region that has been cleared of subcutaneous fat can be appreciated from this figure.

Other surgical considerations

During hemilaminectomy, decompression of spinal cord swelling, as opposed to removal of the disc material, is only required if the spinal cord bulges against the sides of the hemilaminectomy defect. In this case, removal of additional bone should be performed until the bulging is no longer visible, or until epidural fat or pulsation of the dura mater can be seen.

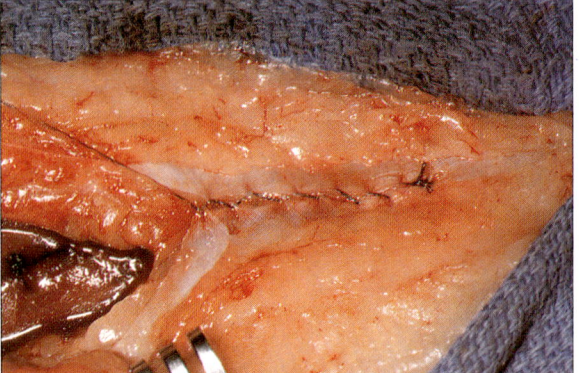

Performance of a durotomy may be considered in dogs with discoloured or very swollen spinal cords (see **210**). If there is widespread malacia of the cord, this indicates a hopeless prognosis and suggests that euthanasia should be performed (see **181**). Although durotomy may provide additional decompression of the spinal cord, the relative risks and benefits of this technique are not clear. In experimental situations durotomy was of value when performed immediately after trauma, but was of no benefit two hours after the injury (Parker and Smith, 1972, 1974).

COMPLICATIONS

Damage to the spinal cord during fenestration is unlikely but could occur if the surgeon mistakes important landmarks. Neurological deterioration following fenestration could occur if curettage of the disc is performed through too small a window in the anulus fibrosus, which can force nuclear material into the vertebral canal. Thus the window must always be made larger than the instrument to be used for disc removal. If neurological deterioration does occur, the dog will usually improve within a few days. If the dog has deteriorated by more than one neurological grade, and certainly if it has lost deep pain sensation, myelography and decompression should be performed promptly.

In dogs with chronic, fibrotic disc lesions, removal of disc material adherent to the dura mater should not be performed too aggressively, as the spinal cord is easily damaged. Here it is preferable just to decompress the spinal cord and not to make prolonged attempts to remove all disc material (see **217**).

One problem that can occur during hemilaminectomy is inaccurate identification of the correct site of the lesion, either at radiography or at surgery. If disc material is not found on exploration of the vertebral canal, the surgeon should reassess whether the correct intervertebral space has been approached. Misleading landmarks should be looked for, such as fusion of the last rib to the vertebral body (which can be mistaken for the first lumbar transverse process) or sacralization of L_7 (which will suggest that there are only six lumbar vertebrae). Identification of the site can be assisted by injecting 0.1 ml of methylene blue and radiographing the patient before surgery with the needle *in situ*, thus identifying the location of the injection.

If the correct site has been approached, but there is no disc material, then the hemilaminectomy must be extended. This is performed in whichever direction the spinal cord appears most compressed or swollen, often indicated by a local absence of epidural fat or failure of the dura mater to pulse. It may sometimes be necessary to extend the hemilaminectomy over three or four intervertebral spaces. Preservation of the articular processes by performing multiple 'exploratory' minihemilaminectomies is recommended before expanding the decompression over the affected area. If no disc material can be found, the original diagnosis should be reassessed.

Marked haemorrhage can occasionally arise from the internal vertebral venous plexus, or from branches of the spinal artery or vein. A small piece of muscle or surgical cellulose usually controls plexus bleeding (see **208**).

POSTOPERATIVE CARE (see Chapter 15)

Analgesia should be provided on a routine basis for the first 12 hours after surgery. If required beyond 24 hours, low doses of non-steroidal anti-inflammatory drugs such as carprofen can be used, or a muscle relaxant such as methocarbamol to relieve muscle spasm (see **Table 35**, page 205). Postoperative physiotherapy and restricted exercise on a leash is strongly recommended following decompressive surgery.

The most important aspect of postoperative care is to ensure that the bladder is regularly emptied of all urine. Urinary retention is the most common postoperative problem in thoracolumbar disc disease. Pharmacological management of urination should be used whenever urinary function is impaired (see 'Control of urinary function,' page 210).

Persistence of back pain is sometimes encountered after fenestration, and this can take up to a month to resolve. Time is sometimes necessary for disc material within the vertebral canal to be rendered non-irritant to the meninges or nerve roots.

A minor potential complication of both hemilaminectomy and fenestration relates to flaccidity of the body wall, caused by stretching or section of the segmental spinal nerves. This usually resolves within one or two weeks of the surgery.

Iatrogenic infection of an intervertebral space (see 'Discospondylitis,' page 194), or of the surgical wound itself, can occasionally occur following surgery (see Chapter 15).

PROGNOSIS

The prognosis for a functional recovery is good for dogs with grade 1, 2, and 3 lesions, almost irrespective of the treatment used (see **Table 17**, page 88). Dogs with grade 4 lesions show a similar overall response after either hemilaminectomy or fenestration.

When hemilaminectomy is performed within 24 or at the most 48 hours of the onset of a grade 5 lesion, the animal has an approximately 50% chance of making a functional recovery. The preoperative use of methylprednisolone may increase the recovery rate in this category to about 70% (Seimering and Vroman, 1992). The three most important points relating to prognosis are as follows.

- The clinician assesses the dog's neurological status accurately, and assigns it to the correct category.
- Any dog that presents with, or that subsequently develops, a grade 5 neurological status, must undergo hemilaminectomy within 24 or at the most 48 hours, in order to have the optimum chance of a functional recovery.
- One of the three treatments discussed here should be used in patients with disc disease. Use of methylprednisolone may be an advance in the management of human spinal cord injury, but currently it cannot be considered to be the definitive treatment for dogs with intervertebral disc disease (see also Chapter 6).

THORACOLUMBAR DISC DISEASE IN CATS

Disc disease and vertebral canal encroachment is quite common in cats, but clinical signs are rare (Gilmore, 1983). Other causes of such signs are much more common, particularly trauma, neoplasia, inflammatory CNS disease, and ischaemic neuromyopathy (aortic embolism). Thus, a diagnosis of disc disease in a cat should only be made after thorough patient evaluation, including myelography.

REFERENCES

Black, A.P. (1988) Lateral spinal decompression in the dog: A review of 39 cases. *Journal of Small Animal Practice* **29**, 581–588.

Braund, K.G., Taylor, T.K.F., Ghosh, P. and Sherwood, A.A. (1976) Lateral spinal decompression in the dog. *Journal of Small Animal Practice* **17**, 583–592.

Butterworth, S.J. and Denny, H.R. (1991) Follow-up study of 100 cases with thoracolumbar disc protrusions treated by lateral fenestration. *Journal of Small Animal Practice* **32**, 443–447.

Davies, J.V. and Sharp, N.J.H. (1983) A comparison of conservative treatment and fenestration for thoracolumbar disc disease in the dog. *Journal of Small Animal Practice* **24**, 721–729.

Denny, H.R. (1978) The lateral fenestration of thoracolumbar disc protrusions: a review of 30 cases. *Journal of Small Animal Practice* **19**, 259–266.

Funkquist, B. (1962) Thoracolumbar disc protrusion with severe cord compression in the dog. I: Clinical and pathoanatomical observations with special reference to the role of development of the symptoms of motor loss. *Acta Veterinaria Scandinavia* **3**, 256–274.

Gilmore, D.R (1983) Extrusion of a feline intervertebral disc. *Veterinary Medicine/Small Animal Clinician* **78**, 207–209.

Griffiths, I.R. (1972) The extensive myelopathy of intervertebral disc protrusion in dogs ('the ascending syndrome'). *Journal of Small Animal Practice* **13**, 425–437.

Henry, W.B. (1975) Dorsal decompressive laminectomy in the treatment of thoracolumbar disc disease. *Journal of the American Animal Hospital Association* **11**, 627–635.

Holmberg, D.L., Palmer, N.C., Vanpelt, D. and Willan, A.R. (1990) A comparison of manual and power assisted thoracolumbar disc fenestration in dogs. *Veterinary Surgery* **19**, 323–327.

Hosgood, G. (1992) Wound complications following thoracolumbar laminectomy in the dog: A retrospective study of 264 procedures. *Journal of the American Animal Hospital Association* **28**, 47–52.

Knecht, C.D. (1972) Results of surgical treatment for thoracolumbar disc protrusion. *Journal of Small Animal Practice* **13**, 449–453.

Kirberger, R.M., Roos, C.J., and Lubbe, A.M. (1992) The radiological diagnosis of thoracolumbar disc disease in the dachshund. *Veterinary Radiology* **33**, 255–261.

Levine, S.H. and Caywood, D.D. (1984) Recurrence of neurological deficits in dogs treated for thoracolumbar disc disease. *Journal of the American Animal Hospital Association* **20**, 889–894.

Lineberger, E. and Kornegay, J.N. (Unpublished observations).

Parker, A.J. and Smith, C.W. (1972) Functional recovery from spinal cord trauma following incision of spinal meninges in dogs. *Research in Veterinary Science* **16**, 276–279.

Parker, A.J. and Smith, C.W. (1974) Functional recovery from spinal cord trauma following delayed incision of spinal meninges in dogs. *Research in Veterinary Science* **18**, 110–112.

Siemering, G.B. and Vroman, M.L. (1992). High dose methylprednisolone sodium succinate: An adjunct to surgery for canine intervertebral disc herniation. *Veterinary Surgery* **21**, 406.

Thomson, C.E., Kornegay, J.N. and Stevens, J.E. (1989). Canine intervertebral disc disease: Changes in cerebrospinal fluid. *Journal of Small Animal Practice* **30**, 685–688.

9. ATLANTOAXIAL SUBLUXATION

Atlantoaxial subluxation causes neck pain and neurological deficits related to cervical spinal cord compression. The neurological deficits range from mild ataxia and proprioceptive deficits to severe tetraparesis (Geary *et al.*, 1967; Cook and Oliver, 1981).

The anatomical relationships between the atlas (first cervical vertebra–C_1) and the axis (second cervical vertebra–C_2) are shown in **240** (see also **8** and **20**). Note there is no intervertebral disc between C_1 and C_2. The atlantoaxial joint allows rotation of the head; C_1 pivots around the dens of C_2, but there is little flexion. The relationship between C_1 and C_2 is largely maintained by ligaments (see **20**).

A number of pathological processes may lead to atlantoaxial subluxation.
- Absence of the dens (**241**).
- Fracture or separation of the dens (**242**).
- Failure of the ligaments (absence or rupture, **243**).

Most patients have an underlying congenital abnormality.

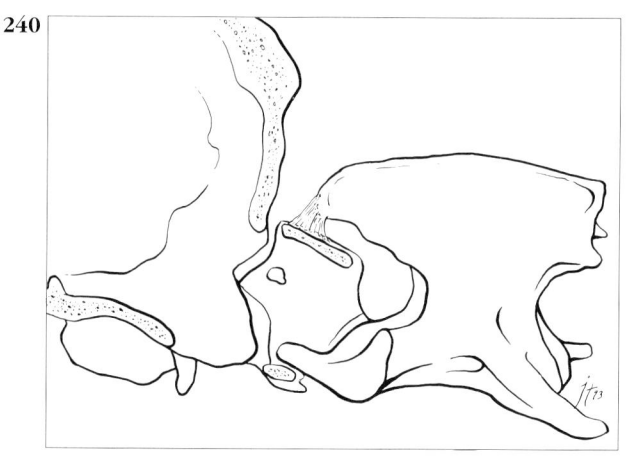

240 Diagram to show the normal relationship between C_1 and C_2 (see also **8** and **20**).

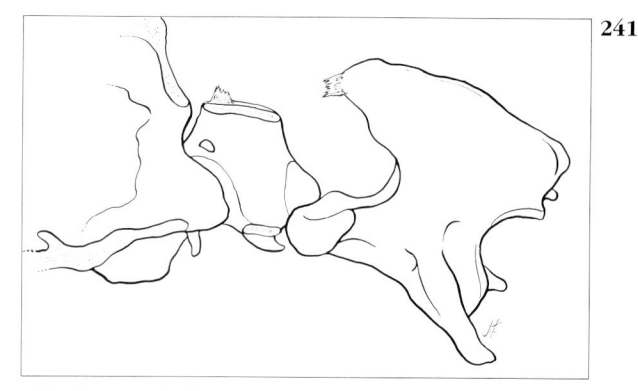

241 Congenital absence or hypoplasia of the dens. This is the most common abnormality and is most often seen in small breed dogs, particularly Yorkshire terriers, Miniature poodles, Pomeranians, and Pekingese. As this is a congenital abnormality, clinical signs are usually seen in immature patients. Rare cases have been seen in cats and large breed dogs (Shelton *et al.*, 1991; Wheeler, 1992).

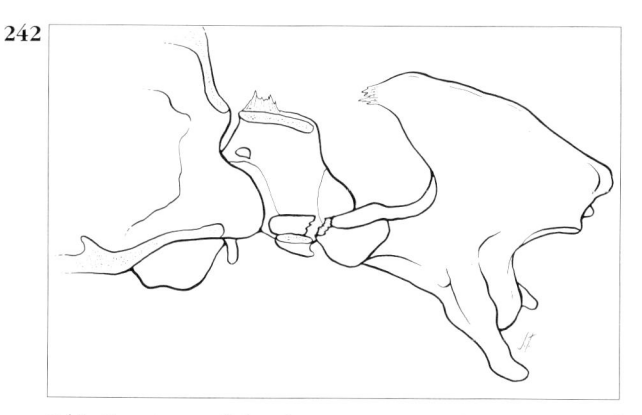

242 Fracture of the dens can occur in any type of dog or cat. There is an ossification centre between the dens and the body of C_2, predisposing to fracture or separation.

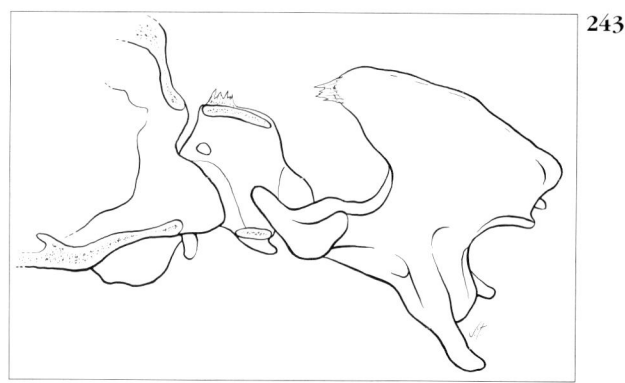

243 Rupture or absence of the ligaments, particularly the transverse ligament of the atlas and the dorsal atlantoaxial ligament can lead to subluxation (Watson and DeLahunta, 1989). This is a serious type of subluxation, as the dens protrudes dorsally into the spinal cord.

CLINICAL SIGNS

Neck pain is seen in most patients and can be severe, particularly following trauma.

Neurological signs reflect cervical spinal cord compression and are variable. In mild cases, conscious proprioceptive deficits alone may be seen. Weakness or severe paresis indicate more significant spinal cord compression. Asymmetry of signs, or preferential involvement of either the thoracic limbs or pelvic limbs may occur. Tetraplegia is rarely encountered, as spinal cord damage of this severity usually leads to respiratory failure.

A history of trauma usually indicates a fracture. However, trauma will occasionally precipitate a crisis in a dog that has a congenital abnormality but has previously shown no clinical signs.

DIAGNOSIS

Examination
Atlantoaxial subluxation should be considered in any young, small breed dog with the clinical signs described, or any dog with signs of a cranial cervical myelopathy after trauma. The neurological examination indicates a cranial cervical lesion, and palpation of the neck often locates the origin of pain to the C_1/C_2 region. It is very unwise to flex the neck where atlantoaxial subluxation is suspected as this may considerably worsen the situation.

Differential diagnosis
The differential diagnosis for an immature, small breed dog with cranial cervical signs is given in **Table 19**. Cervical disc disease is the most likely differential diagnosis. It is prevalent in small breeds, but is rare in dogs less than two years old, where inflammatory CNS disease is the most likely differential diagnosis. In older dogs, cervical disc disease must be considered, and in larger dogs, discospondylitis could be present. Following trauma, fracture of other cervical vertebrae should be considered.

Table 19 Differential diagnosis of atlantoaxial subluxation

Clinical picture	Diagnoses
Immature, small breed dog	Inflammatory CNS disease Trauma
Mature dogs	Cervical disc extrusion Inflammatory CNS disease Discospondylitis Neoplasia Trauma

Radiography

Survey radiography
Survey radiographs provide the diagnosis in most cases. General anaesthesia is required for taking the radiographs, with the possible exception of dogs with fractures. Accurate positioning is essential in evaluating the cranial cervical region, and this is not possible in the conscious patient, particularly if neck pain is present (Chapter 4). It is a common error to diagnose atlantoaxial subluxation on radiographs of conscious dogs, where the positioning is inadequate and the region of interest is far from the centre of the film.

The lateral projection will reveal the presence of subluxation. Mild flexion of the cranial cervical region may be required to demonstrate the malalignment of the vertebra, but this must not be excessive. The ventrodorsal view will highlight the dens and show whether it is normal (**244, 245**).

It is safe to position the dog in dorsal recumbency with the neck extended for the ventrodorsal projection. This is preferable to the open-mouth view.

Myelography
Myelography is unlikely to be required. Cerebellomedullary cistern puncture either for myelography or CSF sampling should not be performed in dogs with atlantoaxial subluxation; lumbar puncture is preferable if either are deemed necessary.

9 ATLANTOAXIAL SUBLUXATION

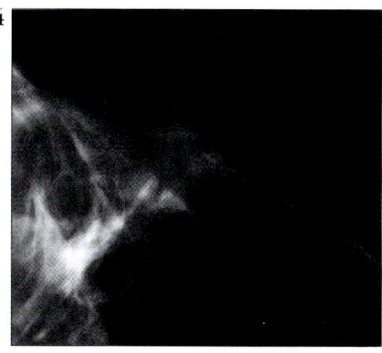

244 Lateral radiograph of a dog with atlantoaxial subluxation. Compare the angulation of the articulation with the normal cervical spine in **71**.

245 Ventrodorsal radiograph of dog in 244. Compare with normal radiograph in **72**; note the small dens in this radiograph (arrow).

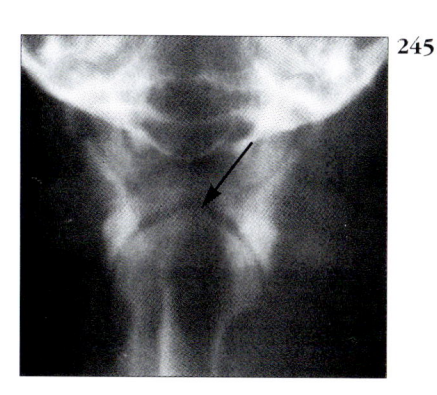

TREATMENT

Nonsurgical treatment
Nonsurgical treatment by cage rest, application of a neck brace and use of anti-inflammatory medications may lead to improvement (see **416**). However, in patients with congenital lesions, improvement is usually transient and deterioration often occurs upon return to normal activity. With the advent of the safer ventral surgical approach, nonsurgical treatment is rarely indicated in dogs with congenital disorders, although successful cases have been reported. Animals with traumatic injuries may respond well to nonsurgical treatment (Denny, 1983).

Surgical treatment
Surgery is indicated for most patients with congenital lesions. Even dogs with profound neurological deficits are likely to benefit from stabilization. One of two procedures is most often used: ventral fusion or dorsal wiring. Dorsal wiring is more hazardous and has a high morbidity. It has largely been supplanted by ventral fusion, which is recommended.

SURGERY

Ventral fusion (246–265)
Ventral fusion by lag screw fixation is the preferred method of treatment.

246 Positioning of a dog for surgery. The patient is placed with the neck in extension; this reduces the subluxation. The approach is essentially the same as for the ventral approach to the neck for cervical disc surgery (see Chapter 7 for details). The area is prepared and draped, including the proximal humerus to allow bone graft collection (see **327** and **328**).

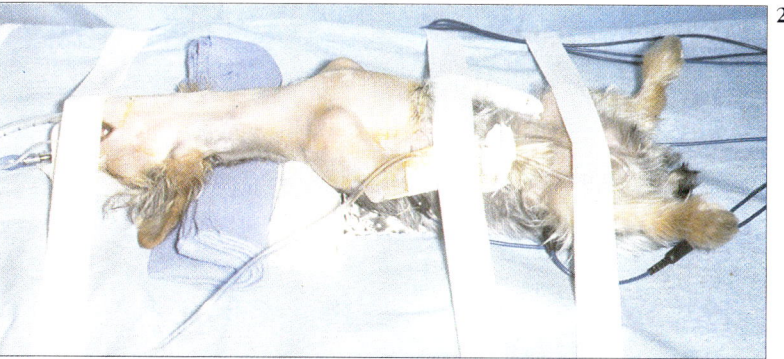

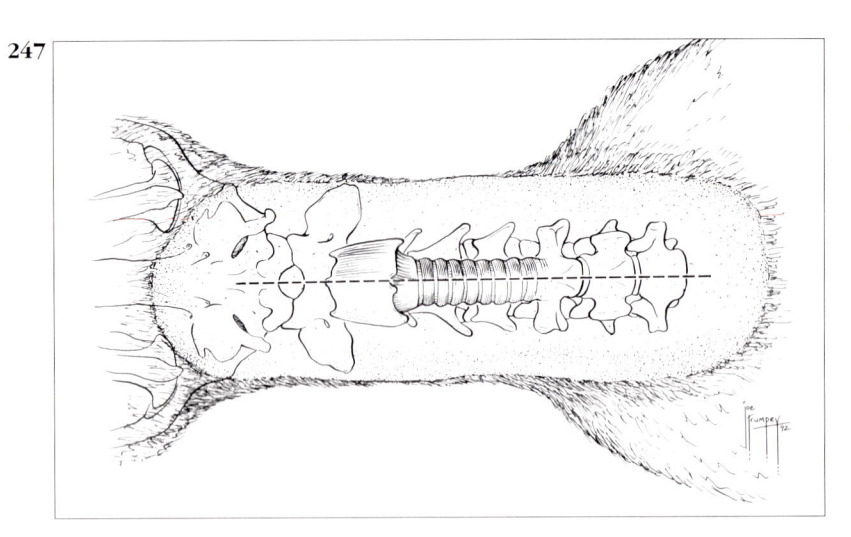

DIAGNOSIS AND SURGERY OF SMALL ANIMAL SPINAL DISORDERS

247 Site of incision. Note that the incision extends cranial to the larynx. The dog's head is to the left in all illustrations.

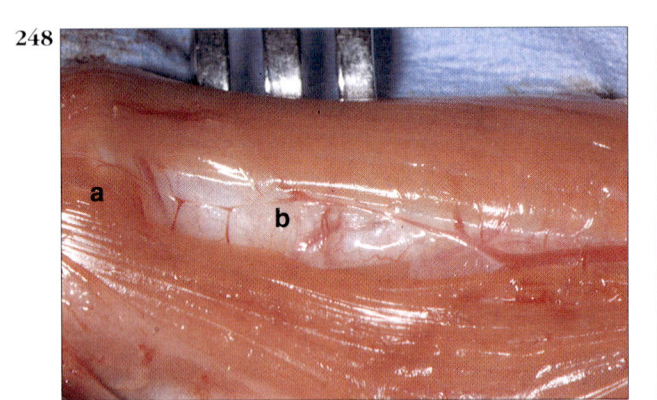

248 Incision through the superficial fascia reveals the sternohyoid muscles (see **140** and **141**). The larynx (**a**) is at the cranial end of the incision, and the trachea is visible (**b**).

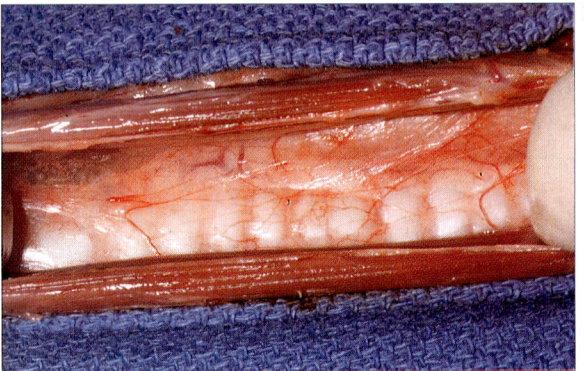

249 The sternohyoid muscles are separated and retracted to expose the trachea. At the cranial edge of the incision, the sternothyroid muscle becomes apparent, lying immediately ventral and lateral to the sternohyoid muscle.

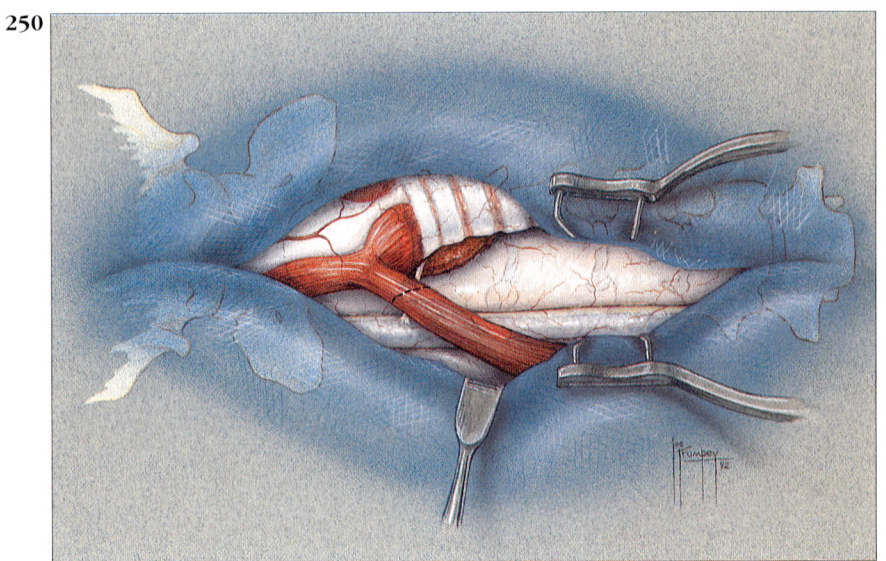

250 The sternothyroid muscle inserts on the thyroid cartilage. It is helpful to section the muscle as shown by the dotted line. The vascular bundle visible in **252** can be seen under the muscle insertion.

9 ATLANTOAXIAL SUBLUXATION

251 The sternothyroid muscle is mobilized and divided close to the larynx. Leave an adequate portion near the thyroid cartilage to allow repair. The thyroid gland is visible (**a**).

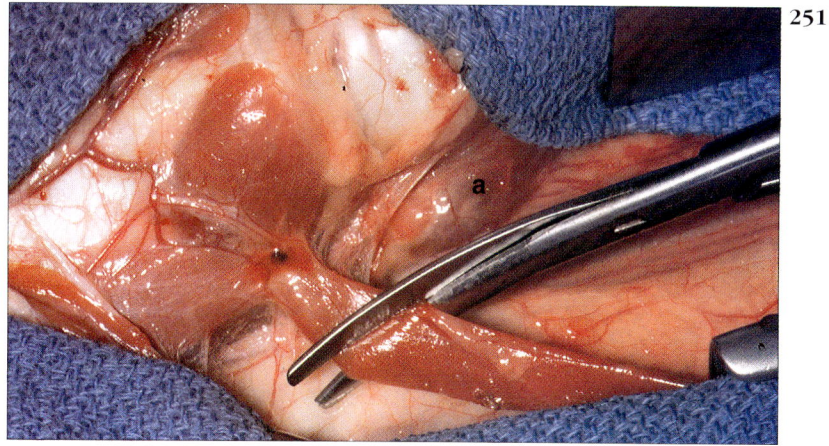

252 A vascular bundle supplies the thyroid gland; this must be preserved.

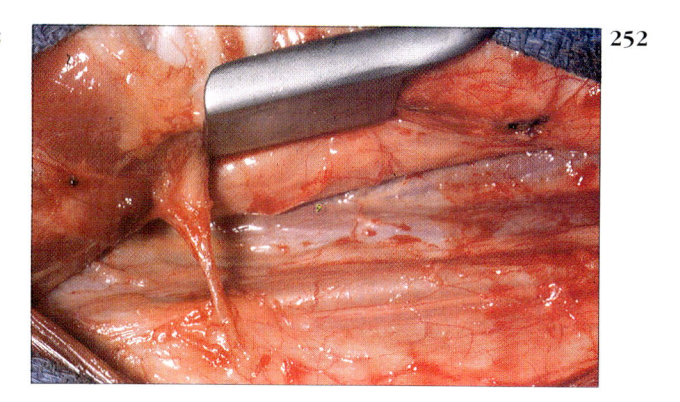

253 The vital structures are retracted laterally and maintained with self-retaining retractors. Adequate padding with moist towels or sponges must be provided for the trachea. The deep fascia is divided, and the longus colli muscles can clearly be seen inserting on the ventral process of C_1. The surgeon's finger is on the ventral process of C_1 in this photograph.

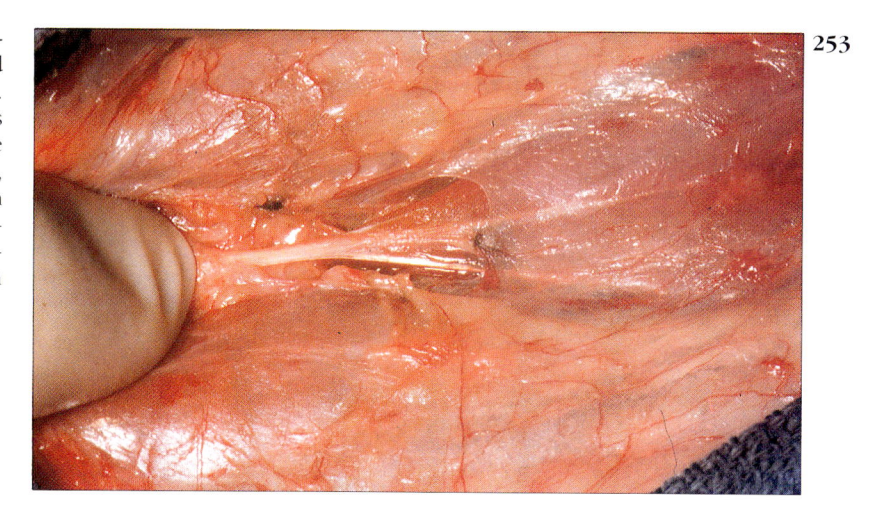

113

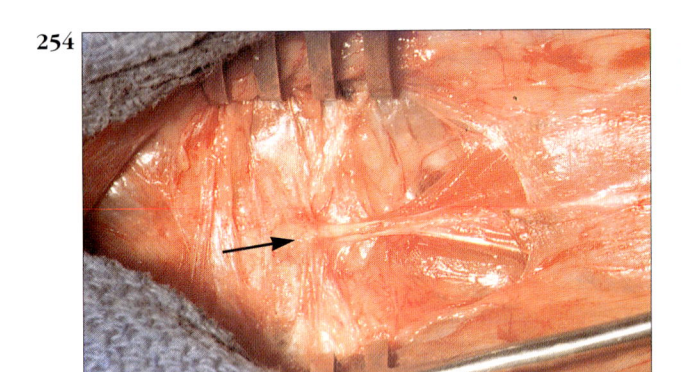

DIAGNOSIS AND SURGERY OF SMALL ANIMAL SPINAL DISORDERS

254 Deep fascia further dissected to show the tendons of the longus colli muscles inserting on the ventral process of C_1 (arrow).

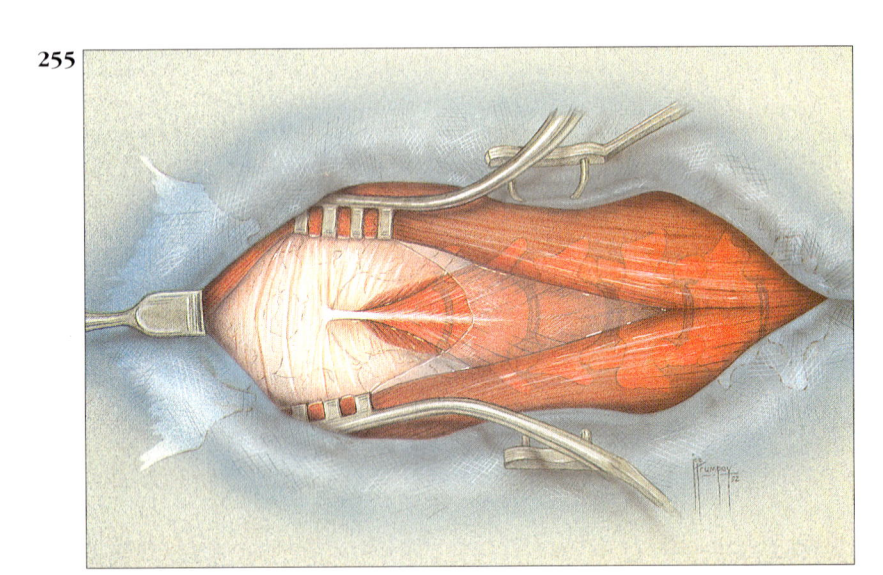

255 Diagram of deep anatomy as shown in 254. Note the relationship of the soft tissues to the underlying skeletal structures.

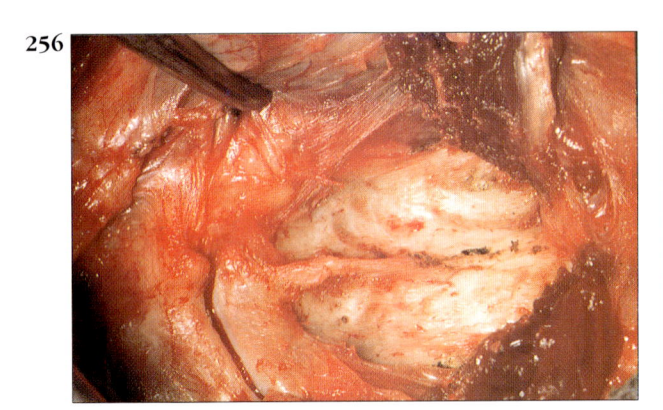

256 The tendons of the longus colli muscles are elevated from the ventral process of C_1. The muscles are elevated caudolaterally from the body of C_2 (exposed here). Dissection of the fascia reveals the synovial joint capsule of the C_1/C_2 joints. Here the capsule has been incised and partially removed on the dog's right side – bottom of picture.

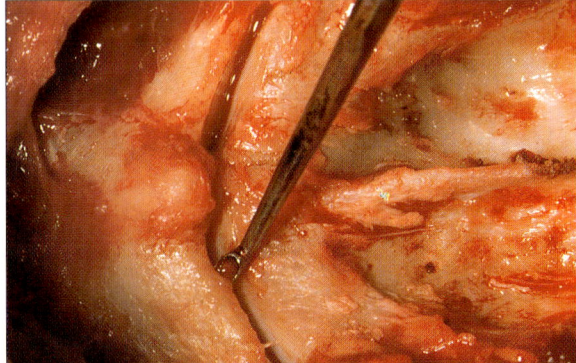

257 The joint spaces can be clearly seen. The articular cartilage is removed with a curette, #11 blade, or a small bur.

9 ATLANTOAXIAL SUBLUXATION

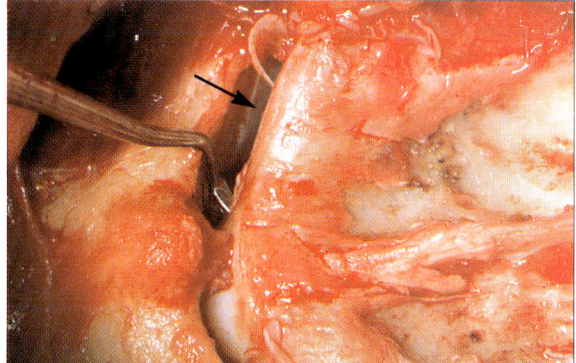

258 The joint space can be opened using a dental tartar scraper or small Hohmann retractor. This is a useful manoeuvre in order to support C_2 during drilling. Here the caudal articular cartilage has been removed revealing the subchondral bone (arrow).

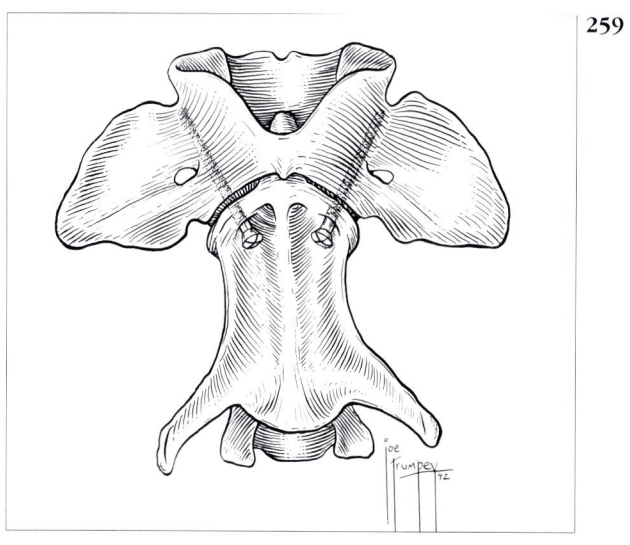

259 Position of screws. The screws are angled away from the midline at an angle of approximately 30°, and downward (dorsally) at approximately 20° from the horizontal (Sorjonen and Shires, 1981).

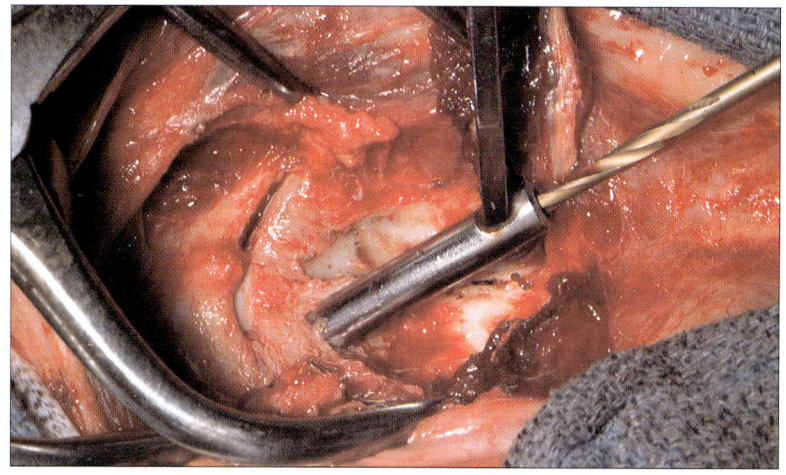

260 Placement of screws. In most miniature dogs, 1.5 mm cortical bone screws are used. A 1.1 mm hole is drilled in C_2 and across the articulation. The body of C_2 tends to move down, away from the surgeon; use of the stabilization technique shown in **258** can help prevent this. Once the hole has been drilled in one side of C_2, a tartar scraper may be inserted in the hole to stabilize the vertebra while the other hole in C_2 is drilled. The following order for drilling, tapping, and screw placement is preferred.
1. Drill both 1.1 mm holes in C_2.
2. Drill 1.1 mm hole through one of these holes into C_1 on one side only. Ensure far cortex is penetrated.
3. Drill 1.5 mm glide hole on the same side in C_2.
4. Measure depth of the hole through C_2 into C_1.
5. Tap this hole with 1.5 mm tap.
6. Place screw through C_2 into C_1. Do not fully tighten.
7. Repeat steps **2** to **6** on the other side.

Performing the operations in this order avoids the problem of drilling holes and not being able to locate the deep hole after the other screw has been tightened.

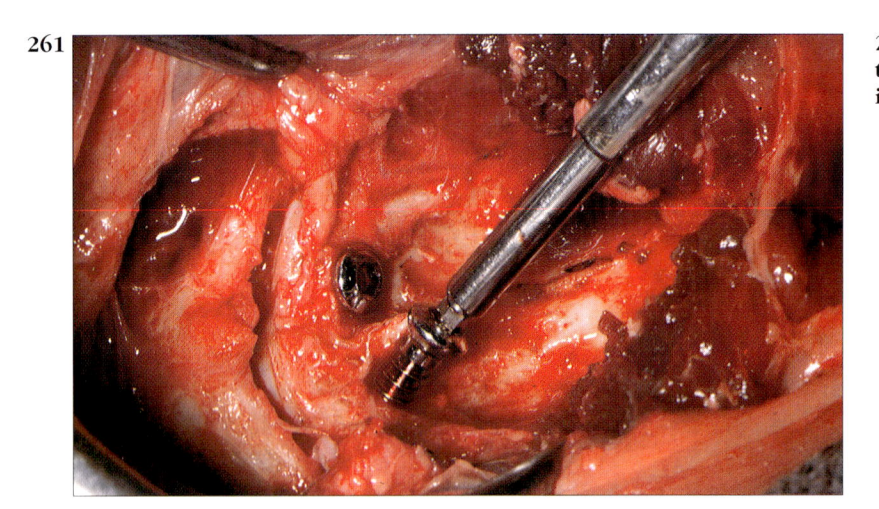

DIAGNOSIS AND SURGERY OF SMALL ANIMAL SPINAL DISORDERS

261 Here one screw is in position, and the other is being inserted before final tightening.

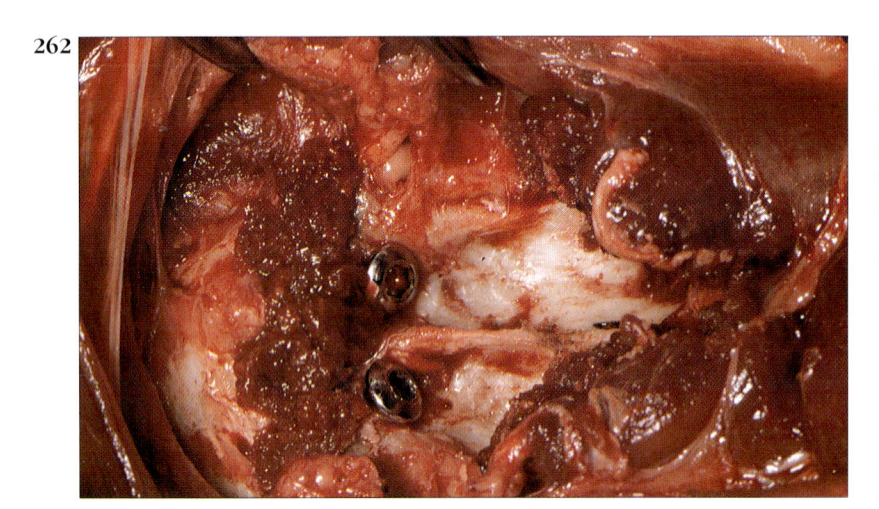

262 Cancellous bone is harvested from the proximal humerus and placed in and around the joint space before tightening the screws. The longus colli is apposed with absorbable sutures. If possible, the sternothyroid muscle is repaired. Thereafter closure is routine (see Chapter 7).

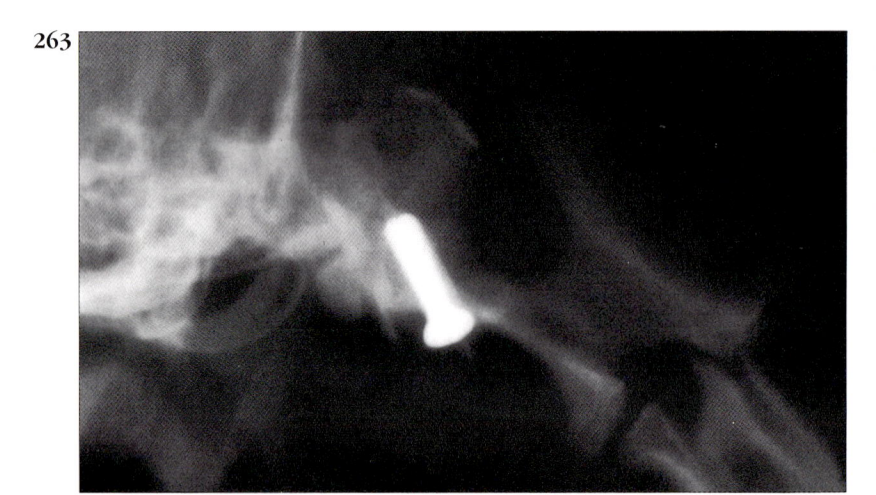

263 Postoperative lateral radiograph showing well-positioned screws. The subluxation has been reduced, and the vertebrae are in a relatively normal position. The screws are of an appropriate length and are angled correctly.

9 ATLANTOAXIAL SUBLUXATION

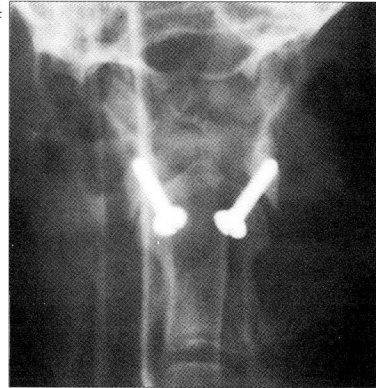

264 Postoperative ventrodorsal radiograph. The screw position is acceptable here.

265 Postoperative ventrodorsal radiograph. Here the screws are not correctly positioned. The screw on the right of the radiograph (left of the dog) is not adequately angled away from the midline and was probably not crossing the joint. It snapped soon after surgery and the dog had a partial recurrence of signs. The dog was managed by addition of an external support and made a good recovery.

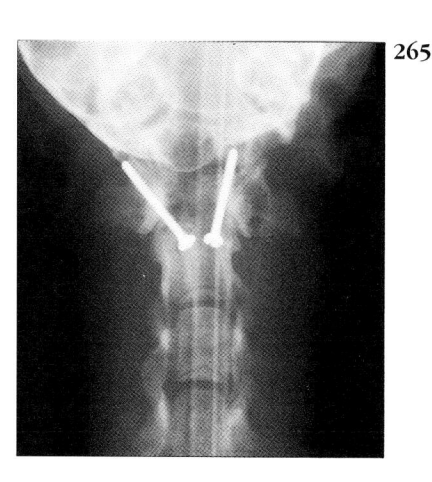

The ventral approach can be accompanied by odontoidectomy via a ventral slot in C_1 if the dens is compressing the spinal cord. This can be performed either before or after screw placement.

Pins may be used as an alternative to lag screws. Kirschner wires may be inserted by hand or with a pneumatic driver. Stability of the pins is increased by placing methylmethacrylate bone cement over the exposed ends.

Dorsal wiring (266–276)

This was the first described method of surgical treatment. The approach is straightforward, but the manipulations required for wire placement are difficult. The complications associated with it do not make it the treatment of first choice (see below).

266 Incision site relative to the skeleton. The finger is on the occipital protuberance; the incision is made just off the midline.

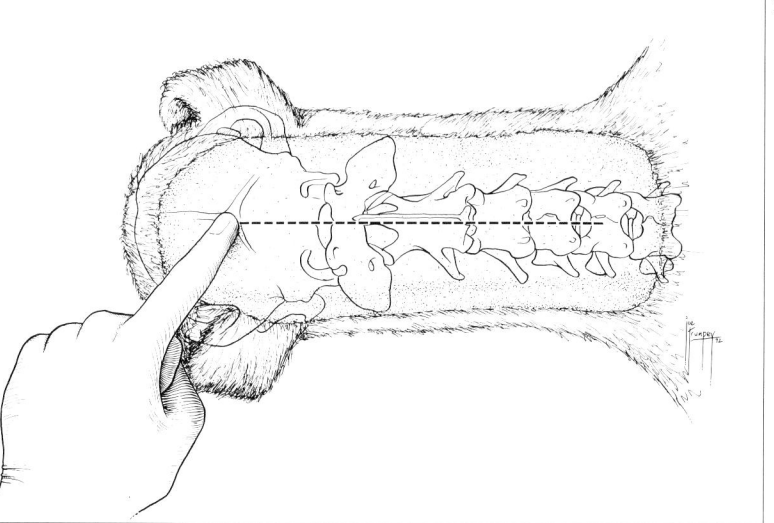

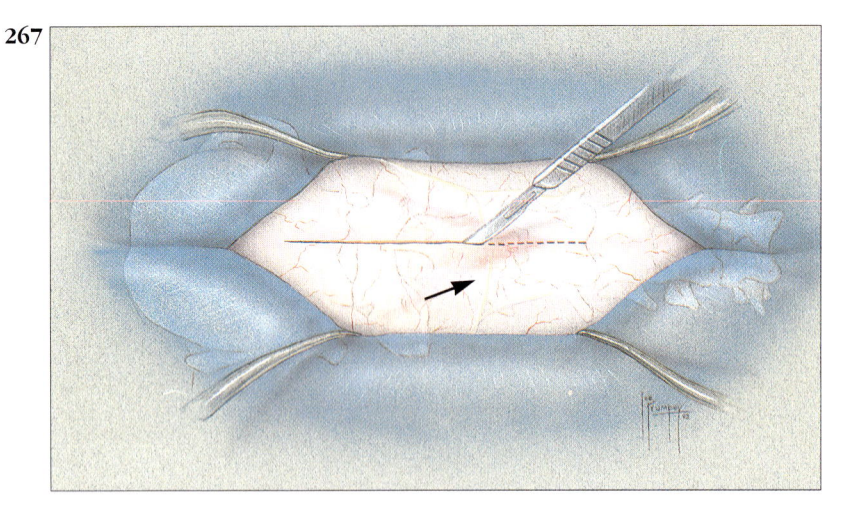

DIAGNOSIS AND SURGERY OF SMALL ANIMAL SPINAL DISORDERS

267 Diagram of the incision site showing position of the skeletal structures. The skin and superficial fascia have been incised from the occipital protuberance to the spinous process of C_4. Note the subcutaneous segmental nerves diverging from the midline (arrow).

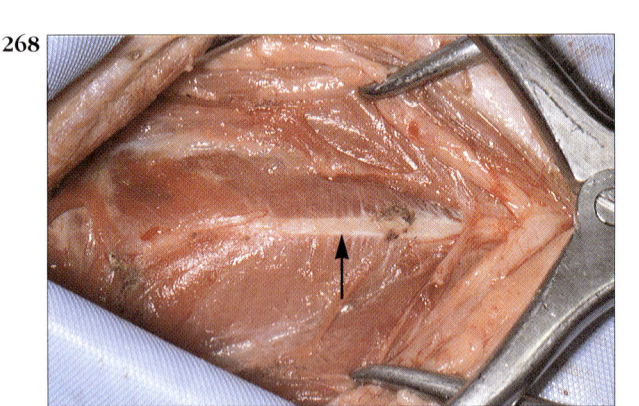

268 The dissection is continued on the midline to the dorsal arch of C_1 and the spinous process of C_2 (arrow).

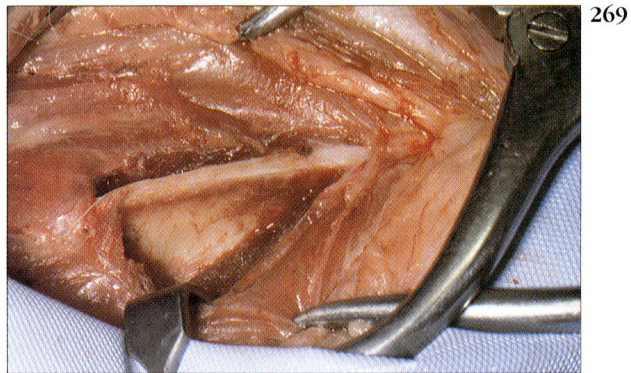

269 Exposure of the spinous process of C_2. Manipulation and movement of the vertebrae must be kept to a minimum; for this reason, it is preferable to use sharp dissection.

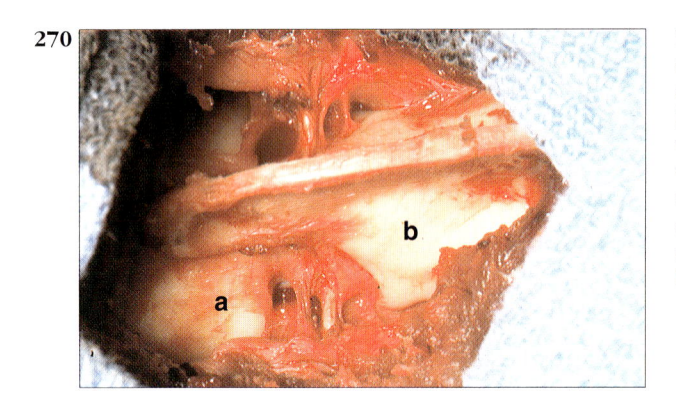

270 Muscles removed from C_1(a) and C_2(b). Lateral retraction is maintained by Weitlander or Adson–Baby self-retaining retractors. This reveals the neurovascular bundle, containing the C_2 nerve root (which leaves the vertebral canal between C_1 and C_2) and a branch of the vertebral artery. It is vital that these structures are not disrupted; severe haemorrhage can result if they are damaged. There are also significant branches of the vertebral artery close to the transverse processes of C_2, which must be avoided (see **21**).

9 ATLANTOAXIAL SUBLUXATION

271 Diagram to show the relationship between skeletal structures, vascular and nervous tissues.
(**a**) Dorsal notch of the foramen magnum.
(**b**) Dorsal arch of C$_1$.
(**c**) Spinous process of C$_2$.
(**d**) C$_2$ nerve root and vessels. Note the branches of the vertebral artery close to the transverse processes of C$_2$.

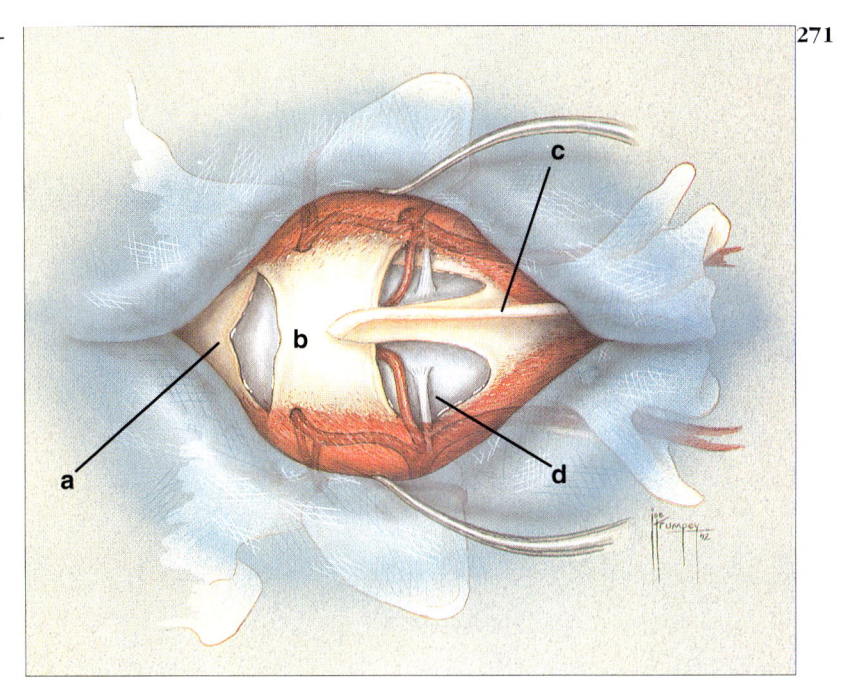

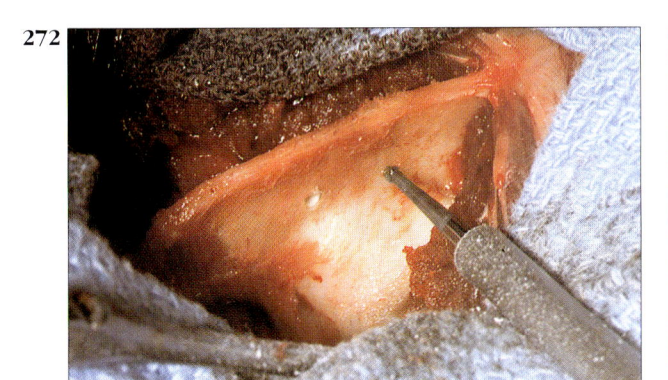

272 Two holes are drilled in the spinous process of C$_2$.

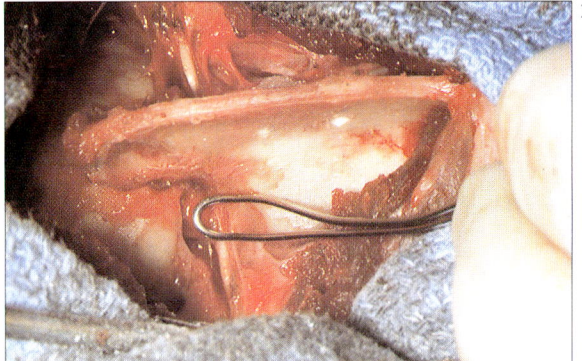

273 The dorsal atlantoaxial ligament between C$_1$ arch and C$_2$ spinous process is disrupted in atlantoaxial subluxation. The periosteum and soft tissues are removed to allow access to the vertebral canal between C$_1$ and C$_2$. A double loop of wire is passed under the arch of C$_1$ in a cranial direction. Pressure on the spinal cord must be avoided. The internal periosteum of the vertebral canal may be continuous with the dura mater, and gentle dissection is required to allow passage of the wire.

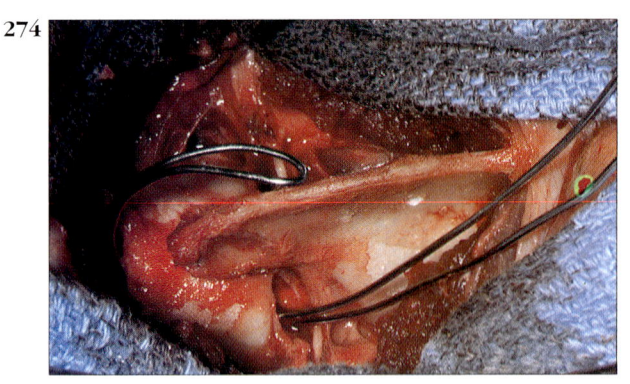

274 The loop of wire is retrieved from the atlanto-occipital space. This space may need to be enlarged in order to grasp the wire. This is best achieved by removing bone from the occiput, thus preserving the dorsal arch of C_1, which is required for the fixation.

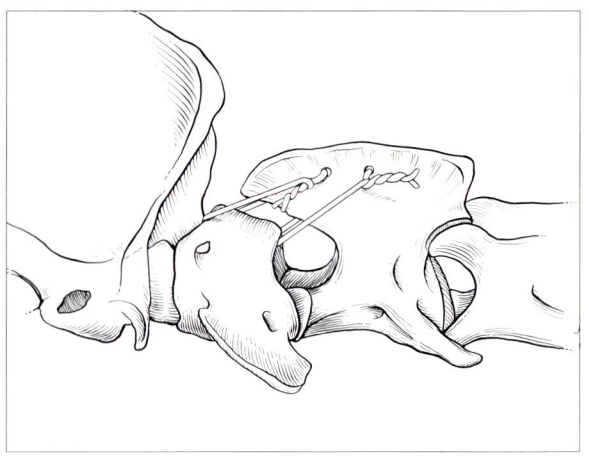

275 Arrangement of wires after tightening and cutting the ends.

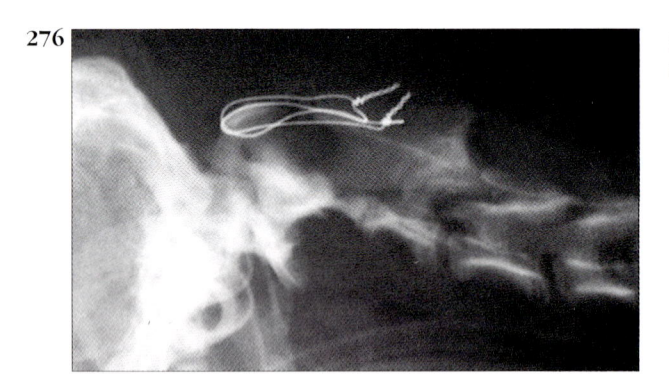

276 Postoperative radiograph showing some reduction of the subluxation.

COMPLICATIONS

Ventral fusion

The ventral approach to the neck is straightforward and should not lead to any untoward complications. Care must be taken to avoid damage to the vital structures, particularly the recurrent laryngeal nerve and the vascular supply to the thyroid gland. Ischaemia and subsequent necrosis of the thyroid gland could result from interruption to the blood supply.

Implant failure—either migration or breakage—can occur (see **265**). If this occurs early in the postoperative period, repeat surgery is often required. However, if it occurs later (4–6 weeks), the atlantoaxial joint generally remains aligned and stable. Use of a cancellous bone graft makes successful fusion more likely.

Worsening of the neurological status could occur, with increased locomotor disability or respiratory depression. Careful patient handling during radiography and positioning, and gentle manipulation of the vertebrae at surgery should reduce this likelihood. Inaccurate placement of screws or pins into the vertebral canal may result in neurological deterioration; proper technique should avoid this.

Thomas *et al.*, (1991) reported that 6 of 18 dogs that underwent ventral stabilization (using a variety of methods, including pins, screws and T-plates) died or were euthanatized within seven days of surgery. Two had tracheal problems (probably a result of excessive tracheal retraction) and two died suddenly for no obvious reason while apparently recovering well.

In our experience, complications are infrequent in ventral fixation and are certainly less common than in dorsal approaches.

Dorsal fixation

Marked neurological deterioration can occur following this procedure. Another serious consequence is respiratory failure due to interference with respiratory centres in the brain stem and their descending pathways, which may be irreversible. Denny et al., (1988) reported respiratory problems in 4 of 13 dogs treated by dorsal methods; only one of these 4 dogs recovered.

Failure of the implant is also possible, either by breakage of the wire or a 'cheesewire' effect cutting through the dorsal arch of C_1 or the spinous process of C_2. As there is no other support for the implant (as provided by the bone graft and joint fusion in the ventral approach) the tendency is for failure and recurrence of the subluxation.

POSTOPERATIVE CARE (see Chapter 15)

External support may be useful following surgery, by use of a light casting material. This may be left in place for a month, but should be removed periodically to allow inspection of the wound.

Postoperative pain is common and adequate analgesia should be provided, avoiding drugs that may depress respiration.

Strict rest is enforced for 3–4 weeks following surgery, after which restricted exercise is allowed.

PROGNOSIS

The prognosis in dogs with congenital lesions depends largely on the neurological status at presentation; more severe deficits have less favourable outlooks. Dogs with neck pain and mild deficits have a good prognosis. Those with tetraparesis have a guarded outlook, although in one report, four of seven dogs that were unable to walk before surgery had a good outcome (Thomas et al., 1991).

Reported results of surgical treatment vary. Geary et al., (1967) reported good results in 3 of 4 dogs in which dorsal wire technique was used, but one dog required two operations. Denny et al., (1988) compared both techniques, finding that 8 of 13 dogs treated by the dorsal method recovered, compared with 9 of 10 that were treated by ventral lag screw. Thomas et al., (1991) had successful results in only 2 of 11 dogs treated by dorsal methods, and 8 of 18 treated by ventral decompression and fusion.

In our experience, the ventral fixation method described here is very successful and our results are similar to those described by Denny et al., (1988).

ATLANTOAXIAL SUBLUXATION IN CATS

There are several reports of this condition in cats, two of which had hypoplasia of the dens, which was treated successfully by ventral cross pinning. The clinical signs were similar to those seen in dogs, and the considerations discussed above apply (Jaggy et al., 1991; Shelton et al., 1991).

REFERENCES

Cook, J.R. and Oliver, J.E. (1981) Atlantoaxial subluxation in the dog. *Compendium on Continuing Education for the Practicing Veterinarian* **3**, 242–250.

Denny, H.R. (1983). Fractures of the cervical vertebrae in the dog. *Veterinary Annual* **23**, 236–240.

Denny, H.R., Gibbs, C. and Waterman, A. (1988) Atlantoaxial subluxation in the dog: a review of thirty cases and an evaluation of treatment by lag screw fixation. *Journal of Small Animal Practice* **29**, 37–47.

Geary, J.C., Oliver, J.E. and Hoerlein, B.F. (1967) Atlantoaxial subluxation in the canine. *Journal of Small Animal Practice* **8**, 577–582.

Jaggy, A., Hutto, V.L., Roberts, R.E. and Oliver, J.E. (1992) Occipitoatlantoaxial malformation with atlantoaxial subluxation in a cat. *Journal of Small Animal Practice* **32**, 366–372.

Shelton, S. B., Bellah, J., Chrisman, C. and McMullen, D. (1991) Hypoplasia of the odontoid process and secondary atlantoaxial luxation in a Siamese cat. *Progress in Veterinary Neurology* **2**, 209–211.

Sorjonen, D.C. and Shires, P.K. (1981) Atlantoaxial instability: a ventral surgical technique for decompression, fixation, and fusion. *Veterinary Surgery* **10**, 22–29.

Thomas, W.B., Sorjonen, D.C. and Simpson, S.T. (1991) Surgical management of atlantoaxial subluxation in 23 dogs. *Veterinary Surgery* **20**, 409–412.

Watson, A.G. and DeLahunta, A. (1992) Atlantoaxial subluxation and absence of transverse ligament of the atlas in a dog. *Journal of the American Veterinary Medical Association* **195**, 235–237.

Wheeler, S.J. (1992) Atlantoaxial subluxation with absence of the dens in a rottweiler. *Journal of Small Animal Practice* **33**, 90–93.

10. LUMBOSACRAL DISEASE

The clinical signs of lumbosacral lesions differ from those seen at other locations of the spine, because of the unique anatomical structure of the region. The vertebral canal of the caudal lumbar spine contains not spinal cord but the cauda equina. This is the collection of peripheral nerves that course caudally from the terminal spinal cord. The spinal cord ends in the L_6 vertebra in most dogs and in L_7 in cats (see **3**, **4**).

The lumbosacral joint is a site of considerable transfer of forces and is susceptible to degenerative changes. Flexion is the main movement, but some rotational movement also occurs. Motion is limited by the various ligamentous structures and the intervertebral disc. Degenerative changes in these structures, particularly Hansen Type II degeneration of the disc, may alter the mobility. Abnormal motion often leads to compensatory skeletal changes, for example, development of spondylosis deformans, osteophyte proliferation, and soft tissue overgrowth of the joint capsules. These changes in themselves can lead to clinical problems by compression of neural structures in the vertebral canal and intervertebral foramina.

Lumbosacral lesions can cause pelvic limb gait abnormalities, lameness, or LMN neurological deficits. The femoral and obturator outflow is spared, so limb signs are restricted to sciatic dysfunction. The lower urinary tract, tail, and anus may be affected. Pain is common (**277**).

Various diseases affect the lumbosacral spine and neurological structures in this region. Degenerative and congenital conditions are focussed on here.

Larger breeds of dogs, particularly German shepherds, are most often involved, but occasionally small dogs are affected. The condition is seen in a wide range of ages of dogs but is rare in cats. Young, working dogs that have been heavily trained are particularly prone to this disorder (Oliver *et al.*, 1978; Denny *et al.*, 1982; Hurov, 1985; Chambers, 1989; Wheeler, 1990, 1992).

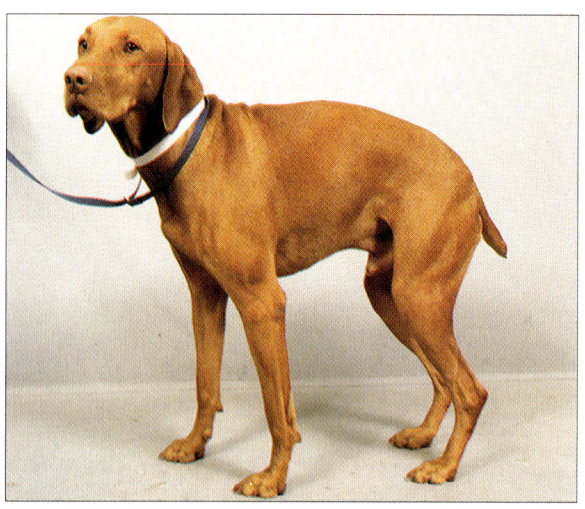

277 Dog in a typical posture of low back pain. There was lameness in one pelvic limb and marked pain on palpation over the lumbosacral junction.

A number of abnormalities may combine to cause compression of the cauda equina or L_7 nerve roots (**278–280**), including the following.
- Stenosis of the vertebral canal.
- Hansen Type II disc protrusion at the L_7/S_1 intervertebral space.
- Spondylosis deformans may impinge on the L_7 spinal nerve as it traverses the intervertebral foramen.
- Instability and malalignment between L_7 and S_1.
- Soft tissue proliferation, usually of the joint capsule or ligamentous structures.
- Vascular compromise.
- Osteochondrosis of the sacrum (Lang *et al.*, 1992).

Tumours (see Chapter 12) and fractures (see Chapter 13) occur and should be considered in the differential diagnosis. Discospondylitis occurs at the lumbosacral junction (see **281, 282**); management is discussed in Chapter 14.

Cats with sacrocaudal injuries often have urinary and faecal incontinence, and possibly pelvic limb paresis. The signs mainly result from traction injury to the cauda equina and may indicate a lumbosacral lesion, but the physical findings of a damaged sacrum or tail provide the diagnosis (see Chapter 13).

10 LUMBOSACRAL DISEASE

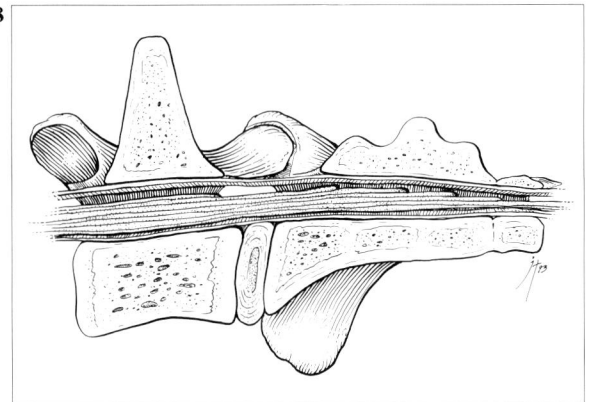

278 Sagittal section to show the normal relationship between L_7 and the sacrum.

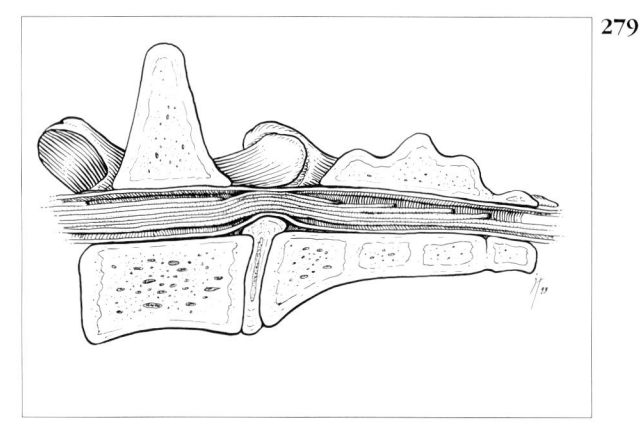

279 Hansen type II disc protrusion compressing the cauda equina.

280 **Instability leading to ventral subluxation of the sacrum relative to L_7.** This type of abnormality is often associated with marked spondylosis, which may narrow the intervertebral foraminae and compress the L_7 spinal nerves (see **283**).

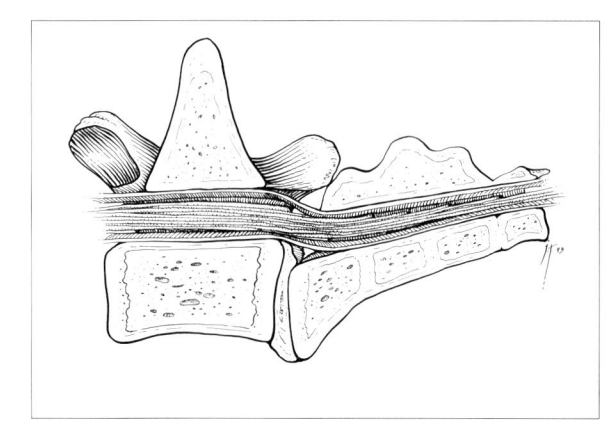

CLINICAL SIGNS

The signs reflect damage to the skeletal structures and interference with neurological function. Pain, lameness, and reluctance to exercise are seen in lumbosacral disc lesions and nerve root irritation. Acute injuries may be associated with severe pain.

Compressive cauda equina lesions can cause a variety of clinical signs, depending on the nature and severity of the neurological impairment. They range from no deficits, through mild paresis with conscious proprioceptive deficits, to severe paraparesis, tail paralysis, and urinary and faecal incontinence. Limb deficits are restricted to interference with sciatic nerve function, causing LMN signs in the muscles of the caudal thigh and those distal to the stifle.

Urinary dysfunction results from interference with pelvic and pudendal nerve function. Urinary incontinence is LMN in nature, with urine dribbling and a bladder that is easily expressed by manual pressure. Rarely, urinary dysfunction may be the only clinical sign of lumbosacral disease. Faecal incontinence is related to poor anal tone, which may be present even when the anal reflex is intact.

Dogs with degenerative lumbosacral lesions may present with nonspecific clinical signs, but low back pain is quite different from that seen in thoracolumbar lesions.

Diagnosis of lumbosacral disease depends on recognising the clinical signs described here and a careful physical examination, which will pinpoint the focus of pain. Owners often report some or all

Table 20 Clinical signs of lumbosacral disease

Severity	Sign
Mild	Low back pain
	Hyperaesthesia, pruritus, or self-mutilation over lumbosacral area
	Difficulty sitting
	Difficulty jumping
	Difficulty climbing
	Pelvic limb lameness, worsening with exercise
Severe	Pelvic limb paresis
	Pelvic limb muscle atrophy
	Tail paresis
	Faecal incontinence
	Anal areflexia
	Urinary incontinence

of the signs listed in **Table 20**, and the disability has frequently been present for a lengthy period.

DIAGNOSIS

Examination

The vague signs may make accurate diagnosis difficult in some patients, as many other diseases could be causing or complicating the clinical picture. Thus, a thorough physical, orthopaedic, and neurological examination is essential, including a rectal examination. In view of the difficulty in interpreting some of the ancillary diagnostic tests, the clinical signs may be the main basis for reaching a diagnosis.

Conscious proprioception testing, hopping, and the withdrawal and patellar reflexes are important. Note the degree of hock flexion when the withdrawal reflex is tested; lack of hock flexion is a sensitive indicator of LMN dysfunction in the sciatic nerve. The patellar reflex may appear exaggerated if sciatic nerve function is depressed. This phenomenon of pseudohyperreflexia must be differentiated from the increased reflex that occurs with UMN-type deficits seen with lesions cranial to the L_4 segment. Pseudohyperreflexia results from decreased tone in muscles innervated by the sciatic nerve, which normally counteract the extension of the stifle induced by the patellar reflex. The anal reflex and sphincter tone should also be evaluated.

Hyperaesthesia is a frequent finding, and the hindquarters should be palpated carefully to locate the focus of pain. Manipulation of the limbs and spine may provoke a pain response, but it may be difficult to distinguish pain associated with spinal disease from that caused by orthopaedic problems. Direct pressure over the lumbosacral joint may pinpoint a specific focus of pain, especially with the spine extended.

The owner should be carefully questioned regarding the patient's urinary function. Urinary incontinence with a LMN bladder may be seen with lumbosacral lesions (see 'Control of urinary function,' page 210).

Differential diagnosis

The differential diagnosis of lumbosacral disease includes neurological disorders and several other conditions. If a patient clearly has neurological deficits, other causes of spinal or peripheral nerve disease must be considered (see Chapter 3).

The considerations are somewhat different in a dog with the rather nonspecific syndrome seen in many cases of lumbosacral disease (**Table 21**). Dogs with the orthopaedic diseases listed have a normal neurological examination. Dogs with de-

10 LUMBOSACRAL DISEASE

Table 21 Differential diagnosis of lumbosacral disease

Clinical picture	Diagnoses
Large breed dog; mild clinical signs	Neurological disease (discospondylitis, neoplasia, congenital anomaly, degenerative myelopathy, cauda equina neuritis)
	Orthopaedic disease (coxofemoral arthritis, cruciate rupture, gracilis contracture, other conditions causing pelvic limb lameness)
	Other (prostatic disease)
Severe neurological deficits	Degenerative myelopathy
	Ischaemic myelopathy
	Neoplasia
	Discospondylitis
	Trauma

generative myelopathy are pain free; the withdrawal reflex is normal, but the patellar reflex may be depressed due to dorsal nerve root involvement.

It may not be possible to differentiate degenerative lumbosacral disease, discospondylitis, and neoplasia on physical examination.

Radiography

Survey radiography

Interpretation of survey radiographs is difficult because many clinically normal dogs have radiographic abnormalities of the lumbosacral junction. Conversely, occasional dogs with lumbosacral disease will have normal survey radiographs. It is essential that the patient be anaesthetized when radiographing the lumbosacral joint (see **77, 78**). Rotation of the spine and pelvis must be avoided. Flexed and extended positional survey radiographs are difficult to interpret and the findings are of uncertain significance, thus we do not recommend that they be performed. Some specific diseases may be visible on survey radiographs, for example, discospondylitis (**281, 282**).

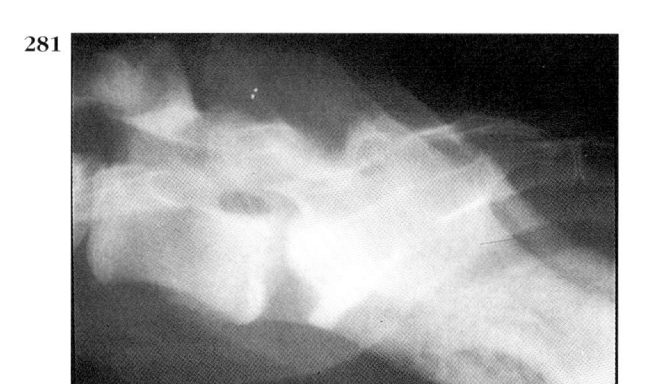

281 Lumbosacral discospondylitis. Early changes, with widening of the ventral intervertebral space.

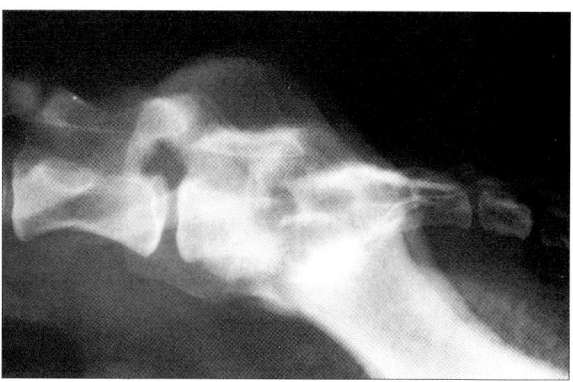

282 Lumbosacral discospondylitis. More severe changes, with collapse of the intervertebral space and marked destruction of the end plates.

Myelography

Myelography (**283–285**) is useful in assessing the low lumbar spine. Cervical injection is preferred, as it avoids the potential for epidural leakage of contrast in the area of interest. In the vast majority of dogs, the subarachnoid space extends beyond the lumbosacral junction. Dorsal elevation or attenuation of the column may be seen. Flexion-extension studies may be useful to demonstrate lesions (Lang, 1988), but false positive results may be found.

Epidurography

Epidurography may demonstrate some lesions, usually by obstruction or dorsal deviation of the column, indicating a space-occupying lesion on the floor of the vertebral canal (**286**). For some radiologists, epidurography is the preferred diagnostic method (Selcer *et al.*, 1988).

If both myelography and epidurography are planned, the myelogram should be performed first, as the presence of epidural contrast makes interpretation of the myelogram difficult.

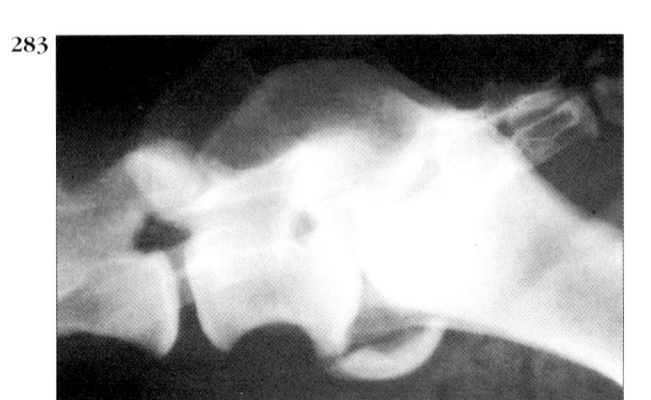

283 Lumbosacral spondylosis deformans and narrowing of the intervertebral space. This type of change is seen frequently in older, large breed dogs, but in itself is not diagnostic of clinical disease.

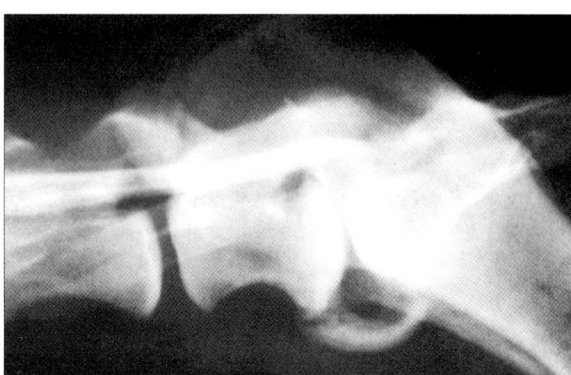

284 Myelogram of the dog in 283. Note dorsal elevation of the myelogram column over the lumbosacral disc protrusion. Compare with the normal myelogram shown in **82**.

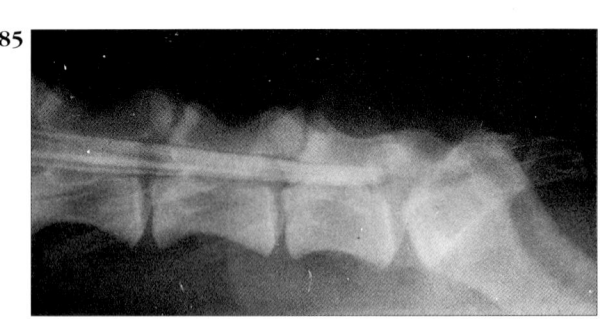

285 In this myelogram, there is abrupt termination of the myelogram column, with some dorsal elevation. Surgical exploration revealed a large Type II disc protrusion.

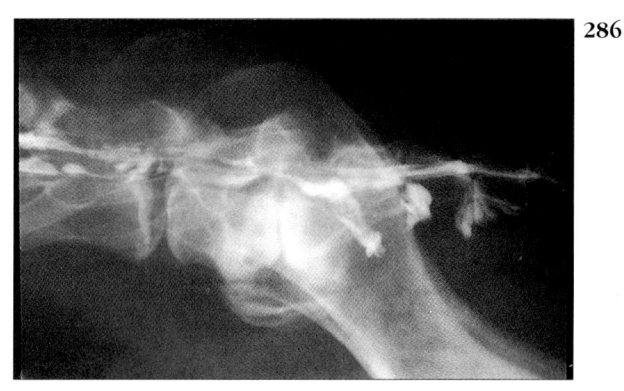

286 Epidurogram demonstrating a large disc protrusion.

10 LUMBOSACRAL DISEASE

Other techniques
Discography can be useful in demonstrating intervertebral disc lesions at this site (Sisson *et al.*, 1992). Linear tomography is helpful in discospondylitis and osteochondrosis. Other imaging modalities, such as CT and MRI, may also be useful (DeHaan *et al.*, 1993) (see **100**).

Clinical electrophysiological studies may provide important data (see Chapter 4) (Sisson *et al.*, 1992). Electromyography of the limbs, tail, and perineum may reveal denervation. Identification of spontaneous activity is a valuable positive finding, as it indicates LMN involvement. However, a normal electromyogram does not eliminate the possibility of lumbosacral disease. Nerve conduction studies and f-wave latencies may also be useful. Abnormal findings confirm the presence of neurological disease, but not the aetiology.

The choice of diagnostic test to be used is largely dependent on the preference of the clinician. The authors prefer survey radiography, CSF sampling, myelography (by cervical injection), and clinical electrophysiology. If additional information is required, epidurography or discography, or both are performed.

TREATMENT

Nonsurgical treatment
Most dogs are initially treated nonsurgically with rest and anti-inflammatory medication (see Chapter 15). If pain is the main clinical sign, this course may be successful. A lengthy period of inactivity can lead to improvement, but such a course may be unacceptable in working dogs.

In lumbosacral discospondylitis, medical management is the first course of action (page 194). Should this fail, ventral curettage of the intervertebral space via a ventral midline transabdominal approach is feasible.

Fractures of the caudal lumbar area are discussed in Chapter 13, and spinal tumours are discussed in Chapter 12.

Surgical treatment
Surgical treatment is indicated in dogs with motor deficits, or where nonsurgical treatment has failed. Decompression of the cauda equina and spinal nerves is achieved by dorsal laminectomy and foramenotomy. The anulus fibrosus of a protruded disc may be excised once the cauda equina is retracted laterally, and redundant joint capsule can also be removed. Decompression provides rapid relief of pain, with improvement of mild gait abnormalities and minor neurological deficits. It does not address the problem of instability where this is a contributing factor.

SURGERY

Dorsal laminectomy and foramenotomy (287–310)

287 Positioning of dog for lumbosacral dorsal laminectomy. Note that the pelvic limbs are drawn forward. The spine is extended over a sandbag, opening the dorsal space between the vertebral laminae. The dog's head is to the left in all illustrations.

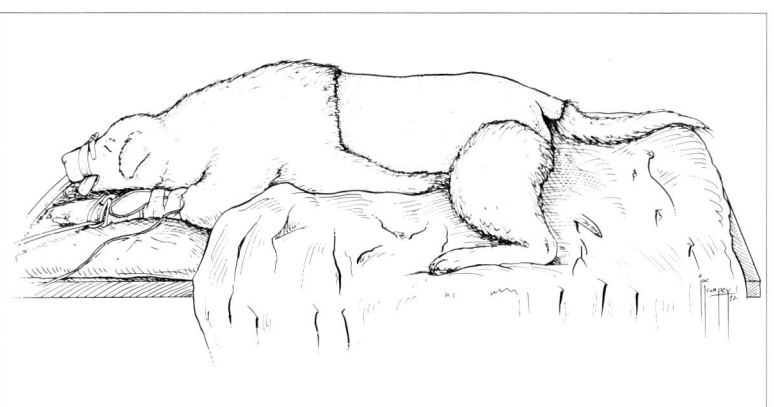

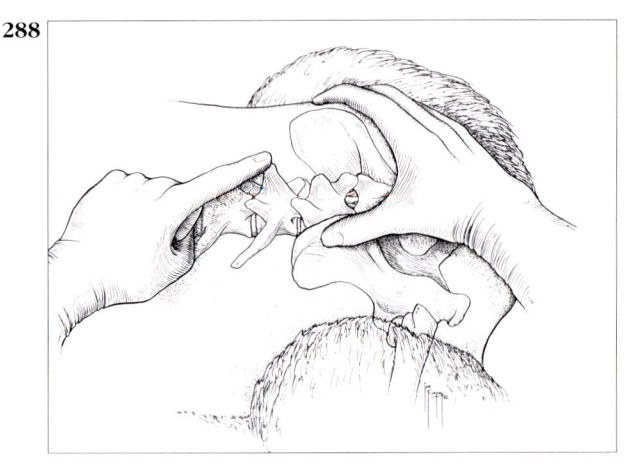

DIAGNOSIS AND SURGERY OF SMALL ANIMAL SPINAL DISORDERS

288 The important landmarks are being palpated. The surgeon's right hand is on the cranial dorsal iliac spines. The left index finger is on the spinous process of L_6. The spinous process of L_7 is shorter and often cannot be palpated (see **13**).

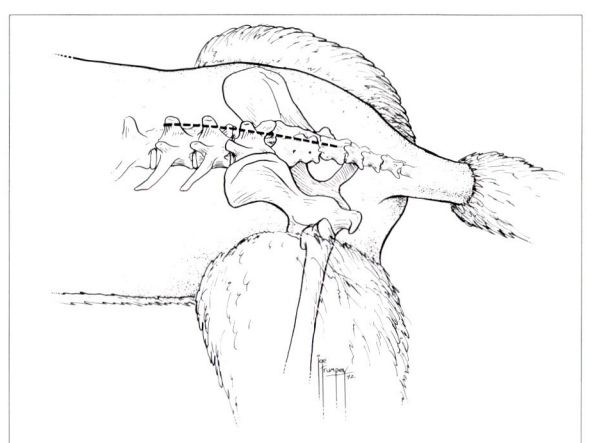

289 The incision is made just off the midline, from L_5 to the caudal sacrum.

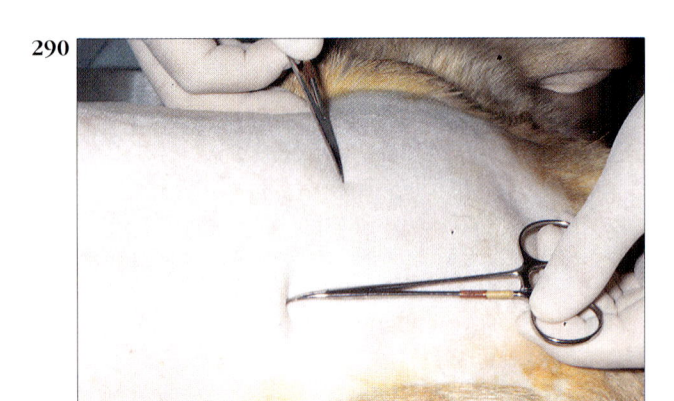

290 Here the upper instrument is on the lumbosacral space, and the lower instrument on the wing of the left ilium.

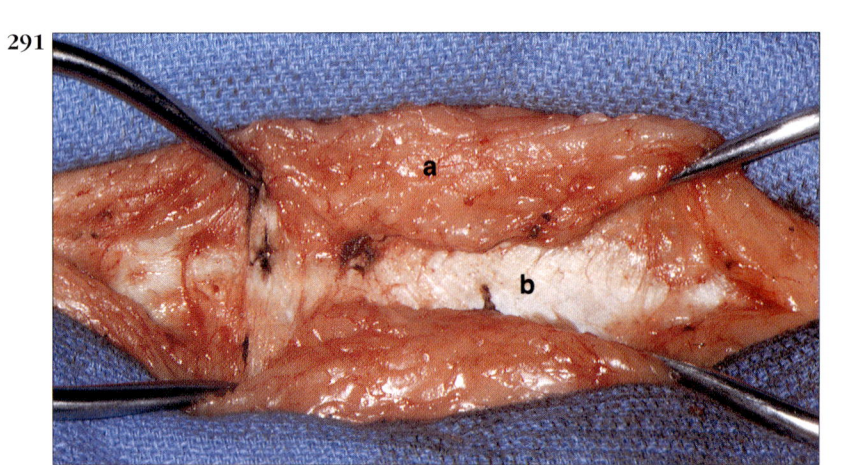

291 The skin incision is made just lateral to the midline. It extends from the spinous process of L_5 to the caudal end of the fused spinous processes of the sacrum. Here the skin and superficial fascia (**a**) have been incised revealing the deep lumbodorsal fascia (**b**). The superficial fascia, which may be quite thick, is undermined and retracted laterally with self-retaining retractors.

10 LUMBOSACRAL DISEASE

292 The lumbodorsal fascia is incised around and between the spinous processes (a). This reveals the epaxial musculature. Here the fascia has been incised and retracted on the lower side of the illustration, but is still intact on the upper side (**b**). The lumbodorsal fascia merges with the interspinous ligament that lies between the spinous processes. (**c**) Transverse process L$_6$. (**d**) Transverse process L$_7$. (**e**) Wing of ilium.

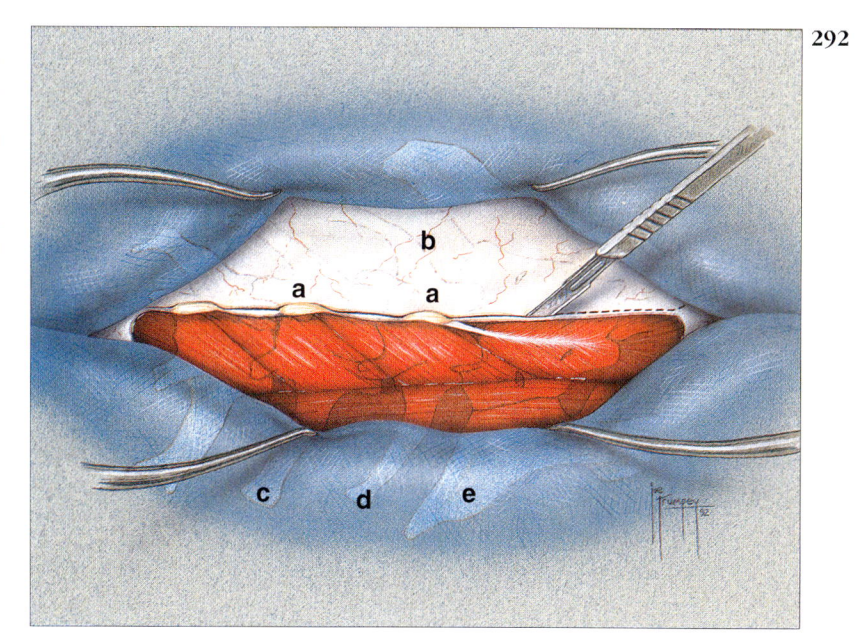

293 Here the fascia has been retracted on both sides, revealing the epaxial muscles. The spinous processes are seen in the midline (**a**). The interspinous fascia between the spinous processes is thick.

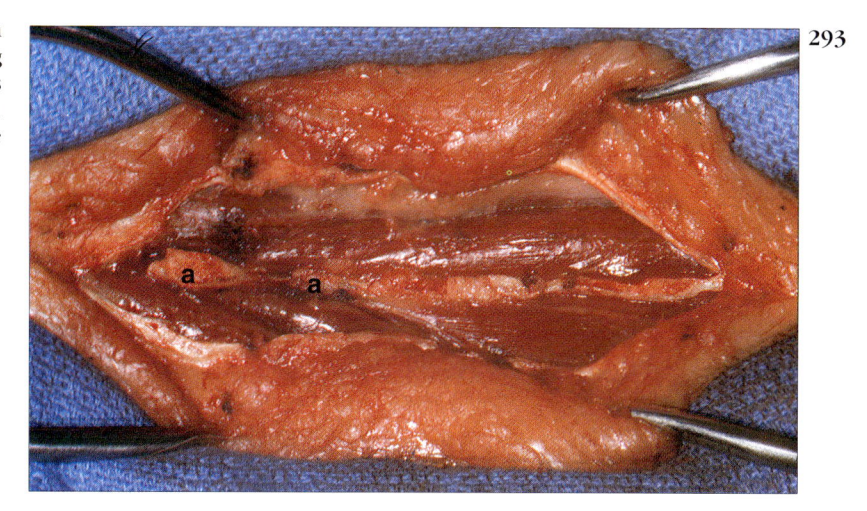

294 The muscles are elevated from the spinous processes and retracted. The L$_6$ (**a**), L$_7$ (**b**), and sacral (**c**) spinous processes are visible. Note that the spinous process of L$_6$ is taller than L$_7$.

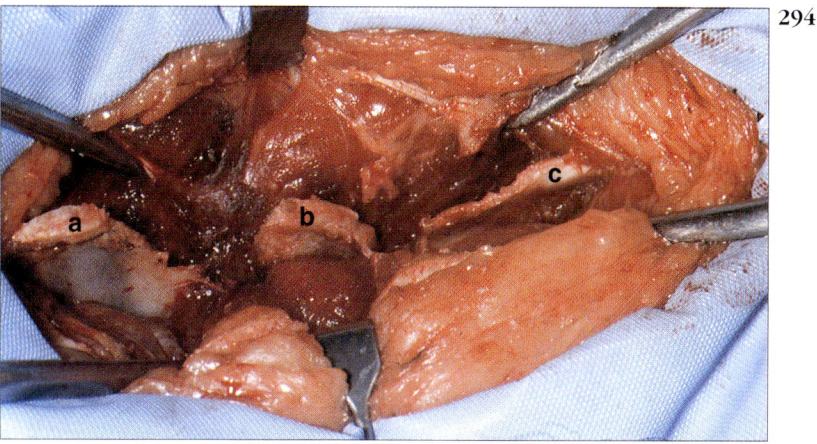

129

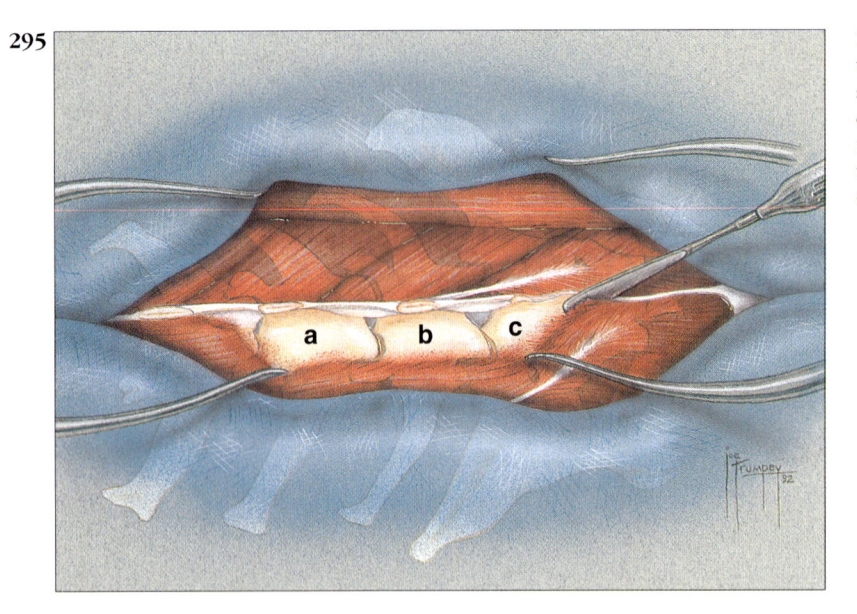

DIAGNOSIS AND SURGERY OF SMALL ANIMAL SPINAL DISORDERS

295 A periosteal elevator is used to remove the muscles from the spinous processes on both sides of the vertebral column. It is useful to insert self-retaining retractors to maintain the exposure (see **296** for key.)

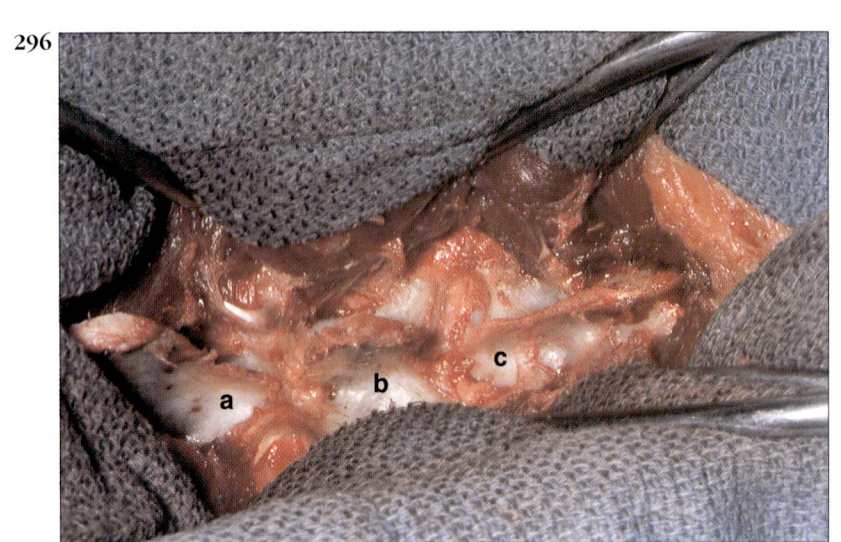

296 The muscles have been retracted from the dorsal arches of the vertebrae. In the illustration, L_6 (**a**), L_7 (**b**), and the sacrum (**c**) have been exposed.

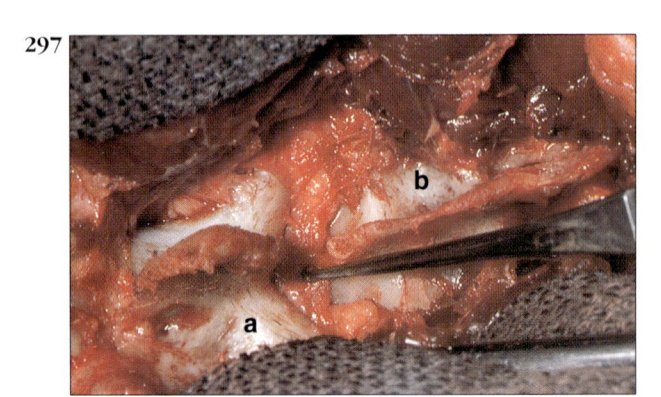

297 Closer view of 296. The curette is on the ligamentum flavum. (**a**) L_7 vertebra. (**b**) Sacrum.

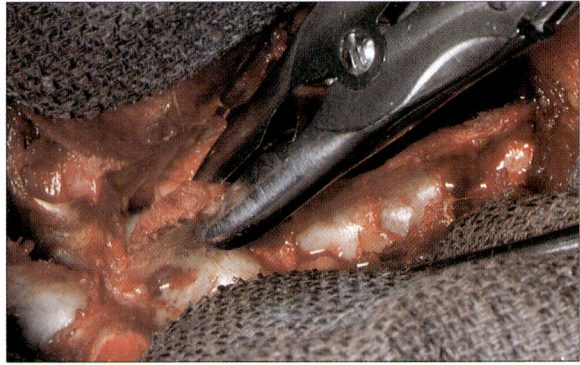

298 The spinous processes of L_7 (shown here) and S_1 are removed with rongeurs or bone cutters.

10 LUMBOSACRAL DISEASE

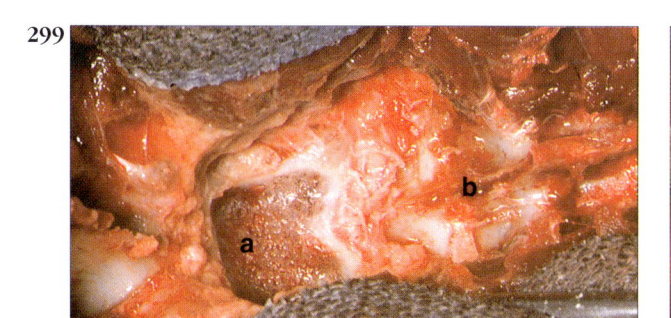

299 The laminectomy is made with a power bur. In this illustration, the laminectomy has been commenced in L_7; note the dark red cancellous bone (**a**). The site of removal of the spinous process of the sacrum is seen (**b**). The laminectomy should be restricted to the lamina at this stage, preserving the articular processes.

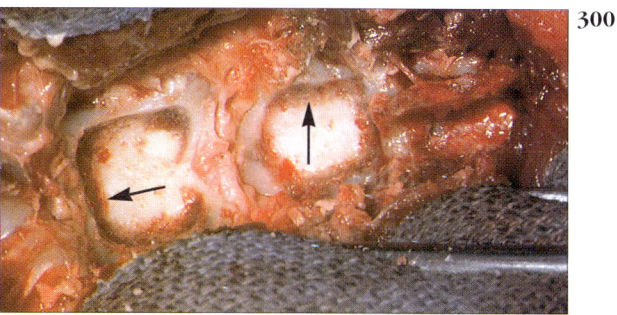

300 The laminectomy has been continued in both L_7 and the sacrum to the inner cortical bone. The margin between dark cancellous bone and white inner cortical bone is clearly seen (arrow).

301 In this illustration, taken at a slightly different angle, the ligamentum flavum is removed by sharp dissection. Great care must be taken not to penetrate too deeply, risking damage to the cauda equina, as there is no bony protection overlying the neural structures at this level. In some dogs with lumbosacral disease, the sacrum tips cranioventrally, and the dorsal lamina of the sacrum comes to lie adjacent to, or even under, the lamina of L_7. In these circumstances, the interarcuate space is not apparent.

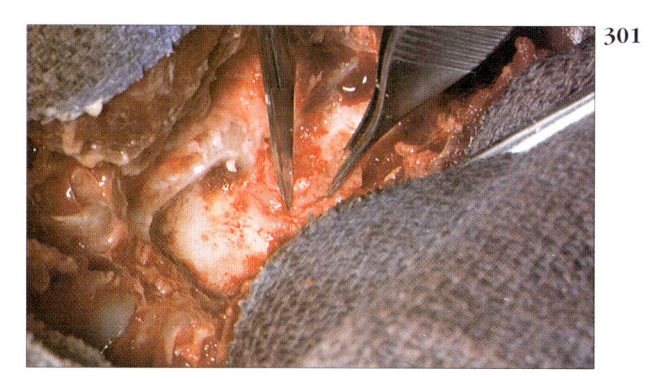

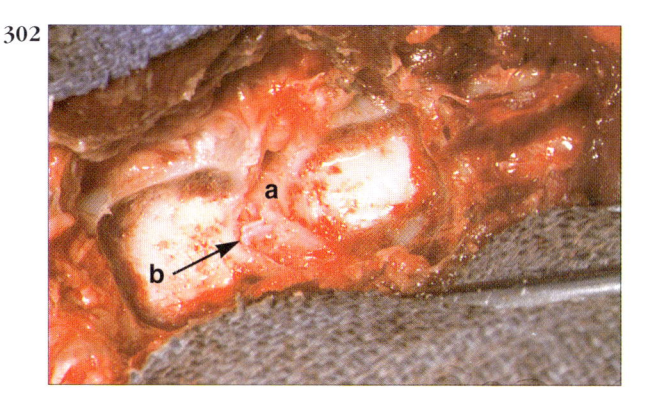

302 Removal of the ligamentum flavum exposes the epidural fat (a) and the cauda equina (b). Epidural fat should be removed only if necessary.

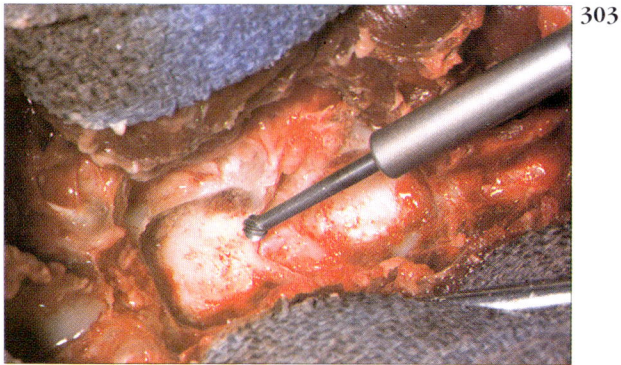

303 The final shelf of bone is thinned with the bur.

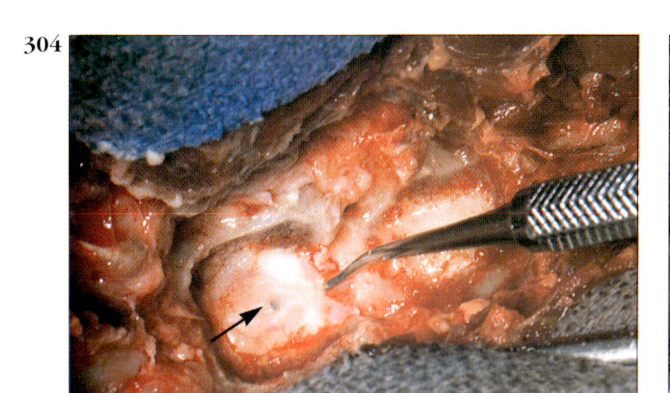

DIAGNOSIS AND SURGERY OF SMALL ANIMAL SPINAL DISORDERS

304 It is best to bur the bone to eggshell thickness to allow easy removal. As can be seen here, the tip of the probe is visible through the thinned bone (arrow).

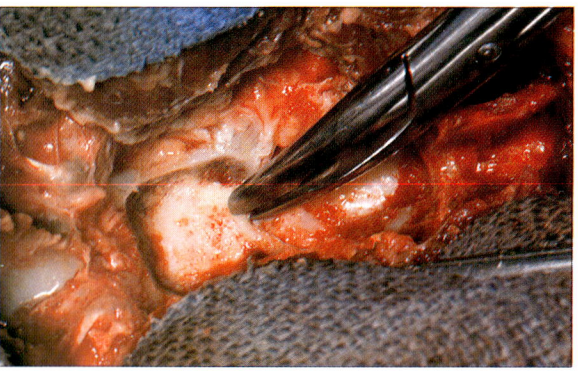

305 The inner shelf of bone is removed carefully with rongeurs.

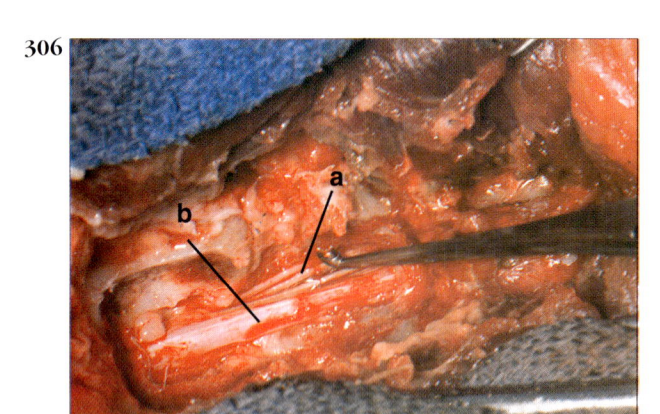

306 The laminectomy is completed with rongeurs or a curette. The cauda equina is then inspected. The S_1 spinal nerve root (**a**) is usually seen adjacent to the dural tube of the cauda equina (**b**). The L_7 nerve root lies further laterally, in a recess under the articular process (see also **13**).

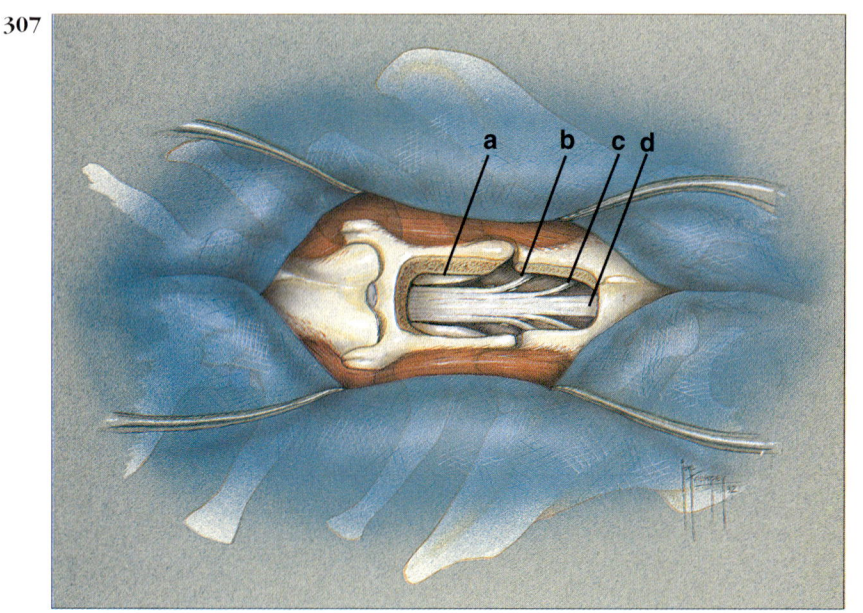

307 Laminectomy has been completed. The L_7 nerve root (**a**) is seen in the lateral recess, before traversing the intervertebral foramen.
(**b**) S_1 spinal nerve.
(**c**) S_2 spinal nerve.
(**d**) Remainder of cauda equina.
If power instruments are not available, the laminectomy can be performed with rongeurs and bone cutters. The ligamentum flavum is removed, as described in **302**.

10 LUMBOSACRAL DISEASE

308 If a foramenotomy is to be performed, the laminectomy is extended laterally. The articular processes should be preserved if possible. The intervertebral foramen can be explored with a probe and enlarged with a small curette. Note the relationship between the lumbosacral disc space and the foramen in **13**; the foramen lies cranial to the disc.

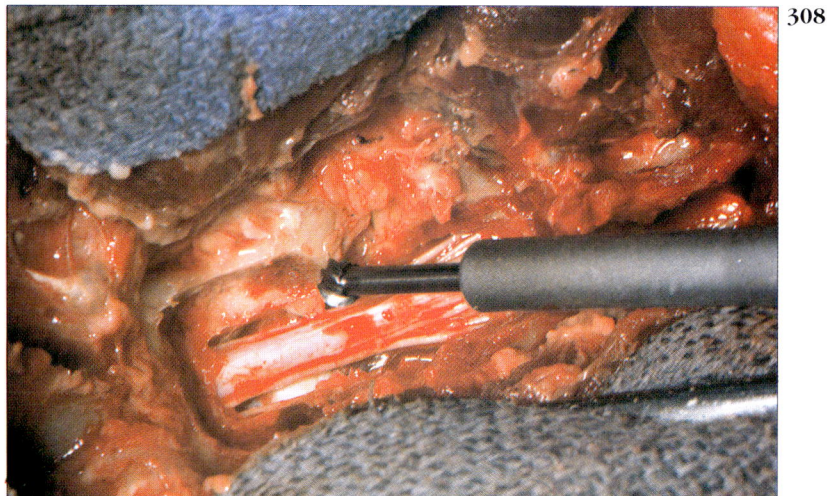

309 The cauda equina is quite resistant to blunt pressure, so some manipulation is possible. The laminectomy is continued cranially and caudally until normal non-compressed neural structures are seen. Here the cauda equina has been moved laterally to reveal the L_7/S_1 intervertebral disc. A protruded disc can be seen, or palpated by running a probe along the floor of the vertebral canal. The anulus fibrosus can be incised with a #11 blade and removed. The nucleus pulposus is then removed with a suitable instrument. Here the disc is seen between the dural covering of the remainder of the cauda equina and S_1 spinal nerve (arrow).

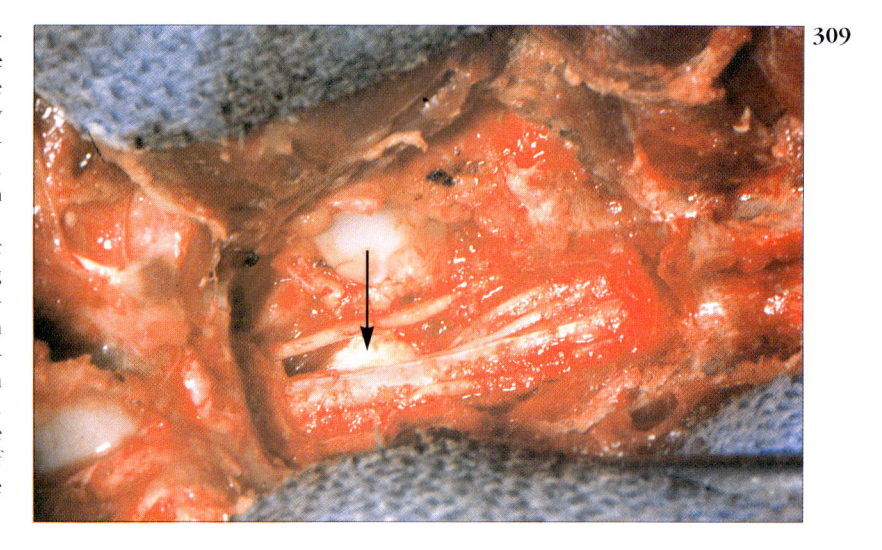

310 In this patient, the cauda equina is compressed by large, soft tissue proliferations of the joint capsule (arrow).

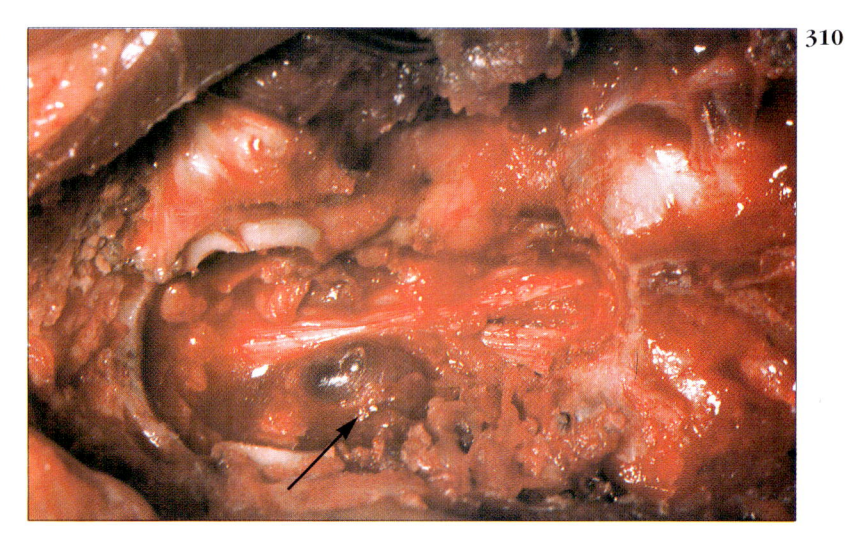

Wound closure is routine. A free fat graft, pedicle of subcutaneous fat, or a piece of surgical cellulose may be placed in the laminectomy site. The deep muscles are apposed with interrupted sutures. The lumbodorsal fascia is closed similarly. A simple continuous suture closes the subcutaneous tissue. In closing the skin it is useful to insert several tension sutures.

Other procedures

Dorsal fusion-fixation (Slocum and Devine, 1986)

Distraction of the dorsal aspect of L_7 and S_1 is achieved using pins placed through the spinous processes, the articular processes of L_7/S_1 and into the wings of the ilium. Fusion is promoted with cancellous bone placed over the dorsal lamina. The principle is to open the intervertebral foramen, relieving nerve root pressure, and to stabilize the lumbosacral articulation.

COMPLICATIONS

No particular complications should result from the surgical approach. Haemostasis during the approach must be meticulous to avoid seroma formation. Manipulation of the cauda equina when entering the vertebral canal must be undertaken with care. If disc fenestration is performed, the cauda equina must be adequately retracted.

Animals that are permitted to exercise excessively following surgery frequently experience a poor recovery.

Initial improvement may be followed by subsequent recurrence of clinical signs in some patients. This is usually a result of regrowth of soft tissue or bone (laminectomy membrane), compressing the cauda equina. Placement of a fat graft may reduce the likelihood of this complication (see Chapter 6).

POSTOPERATIVE CARE (see Chapter 15)

Strict rest is enforced for a month following surgery, followed by a gradual return to fitness over a further two months. In severely disabled patients, the general nursing considerations described in Chapter 15 are applicable.

PROGNOSIS

Laminectomy and foramenotomy provide rapid relief from pain in most dogs. Similarly, lameness and mild neurological deficits usually recover rapidly. More severe LMN deficits carry a less favourable prognosis (Denny et al., 1982; Chambers et al., 1988; Chambers, 1989).

REFERENCES AND FURTHER READING

Chambers, J.N. (1989) Degenerative lumbosacral stenosis in dogs. *Veterinary Medicine Report* **2**, 166–180.

Chambers, J.N., Selcer, B.A. and Oliver, J.E. (1988) Results of treatment of degenerative lumbosacral stenosis in dogs by exploration and excision. *Veterinary Comparative Orthopaedics and Traumatology* **3**, 130–133.

DeHaan, J.J., Shelton, S.B. and Ackerman, N. (1993) Magnetic resonance imaging in the diagnosis of degenerative lumbosacral stenosis in four dogs. *Veterinary Surgery* **22**, 14.

Denny, H.R., Gibbs, C. and Holt, P.E. (1982) The diagnosis and treatment of cauda equina lesions in the dog. *Journal of Small Animal Practice* **23**, 425–443.

Hurov, L. (1985) Laminectomy for treatment of cauda equina syndrome in a cat. *Journal of the American Veterinary Medical Association* **186**, 504–505.

Lang, J. (1988) Flexion extension myelography of the canine cauda equina. *Veterinary Radiology* **210**, 242–257.

Lang, J., Hani, H. and Schawalder, P. (1992) A sacral lesion resembling osteochondrosis in the German shepherd dog. *Veterinary Radiology and Ultrasound* **33**, 69–76.

Oliver, J.E., Selcer, R.R. and Simpson, S. (1978) Cauda equina compression from lumbosacral malarticulation and malformation in the dog. *Journal of the American Veterinary Medical Association* **173**, 207–214.

Selcer, B.A., Chambers, J.N., Schwensen, K. and Mahaffey, M.B. (1988) Epidurography as a diagnostic aid in canine lumbosacral compressive disease: 47 cases (1981–1986). *Veterinary and Comparative Orthopaedics and Traumatology* **2**, 97–103.

Sisson, A.F., LeCouteur, R.A., Ingram, J.T., Park, R.D. and Child, G. (1992) Diagnosis of cauda equina abnormalities by using electromyography, discography, and epidurography in dogs. *Journal of Veterinary Internal Medicine* **6**, 253–263.

Slocum, B. and Devine, T. (1986) L_7/S_1 fixation fusion for the treatment of cauda equina compression in the dog. *Journal of the American Veterinary Medical Association* **188**, 31–35.

Wheeler, S.J. (1990) Lumbosacral disorders in dogs. *Veterinary Annual* **30**, 262–268.

Wheeler, S.J. (1992) Lumbosacral disease. *Veterinary Clinics of North America, Small Animal Practice* **22(4)**, 937–950.

11. CAUDAL CERVICAL SPONDYLOMYELOPATHY

Caudal cervical spondylomyelopathy (CCSM, Wobbler syndrome) is a syndrome of large and giant breed dogs, particularly Dobermanns and Great Danes (**311**). Signs of ataxia, paresis, and cervical pain are caused by spinal lesions that mainly affect the caudal cervical spine.

The cause of CCSM is multifactorial, but some of the important contributing factors are as follows.
- Stenosis of the vertebral canal.
- Vertebral instability.
- Disc herniation.
- Ligamentous hypertrophy.
- Joint capsule proliferation.
- Osteophyte production.

The exact role of each of these factors remains largely speculative in the pathogenesis of CCSM (Seim and Withrow, 1982).

Stenosis is seen at the cranial aspect of the cervical vertebra, and occurs most commonly from C_4–C_6 vertebrae in the Great Dane and C_5–C_7 in the Dobermann (Lewis, 1989). Clinical signs may be seen in young dogs, particularly Great Danes with severe vertebral canal stenosis (**312**). Most other breeds show signs from middle age onwards. Older dogs have less severe vertebral canal stenosis, and the later onset of clinical signs depends on secondary factors that are probably a consequence of low-grade instability.

Consideration of the pathogenesis of this complex condition is important when considering surgical treatment. It is sensible to choose a technique appropriate for the specific type of spinal cord compression affecting that individual dog, for example, ventral slot to decompress a disc herniation or dorsal laminectomy to remove proliferation of the dorsal articular processes (see 'Treatment,' below).

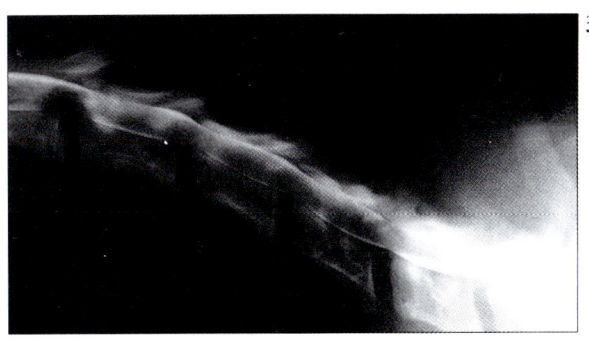

312 Cervical myelogram of an 11-month-old Great Dane. This shows extradural spinal cord compression at multiple levels of the vertebral canal, associated with stenosis.

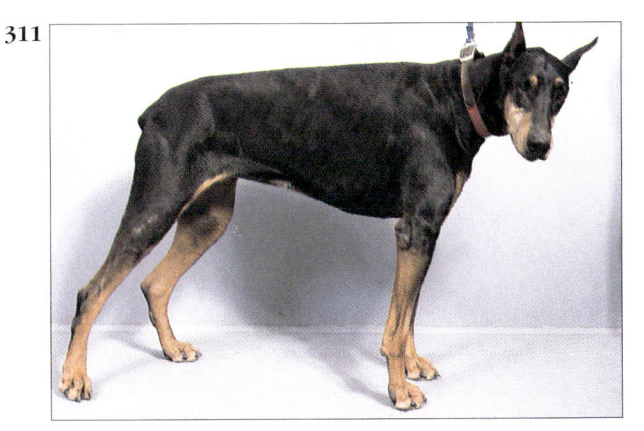

311 Dobermann with CCSM. Note the broad-based pelvic limb stance and low head position. This dog was also hypothyroid.

CLINICAL SIGNS

The clinical signs reflect either damage to the spinal cord (myelopathy) or the spinal nerve roots (radiculopathy), or both. Radiculopathy is probably an important contributory factor to the pain, lameness and shoulder muscle atrophy.

The most common presentation is a gait disturbance that is most severe in the pelvic limbs. This ranges in severity from mild ataxia and paresis, to marked pelvic limb hypermetria and an associated short-stepping thoracic limb gait. Eventually, the dog may become sufficiently tetraparetic to have difficulty rising or be unable to walk. Cervical hyperaesthesia, guarding of the neck, or a low carriage of the head may be seen. Lameness and muscle atrophy in one thoracic limb, or pain when traction is applied to the limb (root signature), suggest that nerve root compression is present.

The neurological examination shows normal or exaggerated pelvic limb reflexes, and usually increased tone in the thoracic limbs. Conscious proprioceptive deficits are more pronounced in the pelvic limbs. Evidence of LMN disease in the thoracic limbs is usually restricted to muscle atrophy of the spinatus muscles.

DIAGNOSIS

Although the gait abnormalities are suggestive of CCSM, a careful history and thorough physical and neurological examinations are important to help rule out the differential diagnoses listed in **Table 22**. The clinician should always consider the possibility of a thoracolumbar lesion being present in a dog with signs restricted to the pelvic limbs.

Table 22 Differential diagnosis for CSSM

Degenerative spinal cord disease
Ischaemic myelopathy
Congenital anomaly
Discospondylitis
Inflammatory CNS disease
Spinal neoplasia
Brachial plexus tumour
Arachnoid cyst
Trauma
Thoracolumbar lesion (if signs are restricted to pelvic limbs)

Radiography

Survey radiography

Survey radiographs are useful for excluding other conditions, but do not accurately locate the site of cord compression (Seim and Withrow, 1982; Lewis, 1992). They must always be taken under general anaesthesia. We do not feel that flexed and extended positional views are useful in the survey series.

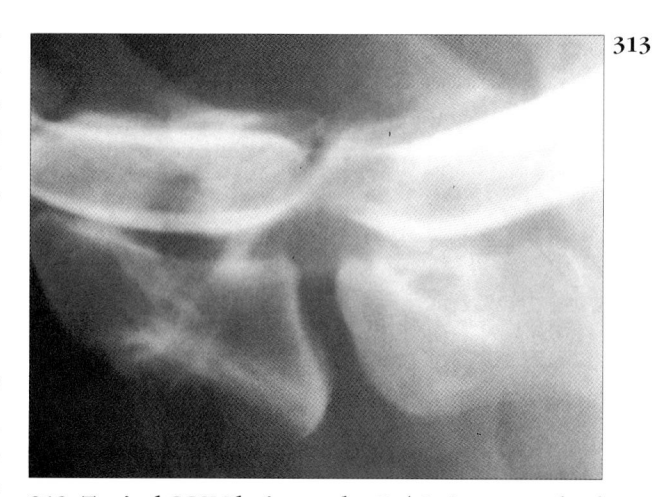

313 Typical CCSM lesion at the C_6/C_7 intervertebral disc in a Dobermann with sudden onset of severe tetraparesis. Traction applied to the vertebral column did not change the degree of spinal cord compression, indicating a static lesion. A large amount of herniated disc material was removed from the vertebral canal during ventral decompression.

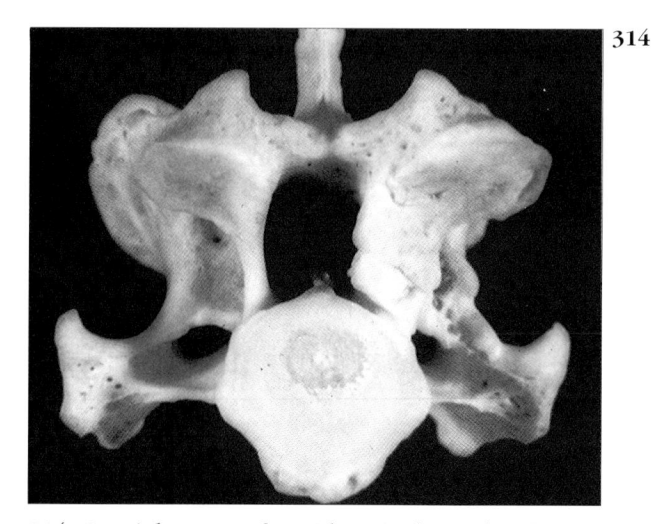

314 Cranial aspect of a midcervical vertebra from a one-year-old Great Dane. This dog has severe stenosis of the vertebral canal, caused by marked proliferation of bone around the articular process.

11. CAUDAL CERVICAL SPONDYLOMYELOPATHY

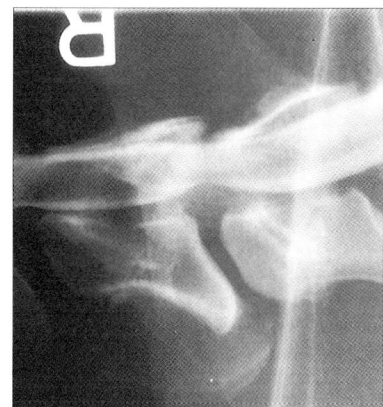

315 Ventral spinal cord compression over C_6/C_7 intervertebral space due to disc herniation in a Dobermann.

316 Same dog as in 315, with traction applied to the vertebral column. This has resulted in marked relief of spinal cord compression (dynamic lesion).

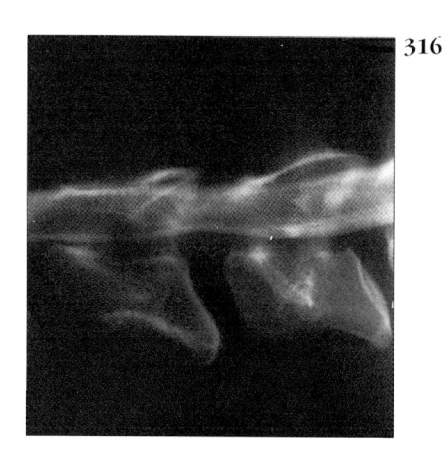

Myelography

The most important diagnostic aid is myelography, and both lateral and ventrodorsal projections should be taken. Also the traction view should be included (see Chapter 4). Traction usually results in a marked reduction of spinal cord compression caused by redundant anulus fibrosus or ligamentous tissue. A lesion that improves in this manner is termed 'dynamic'. In contrast, herniation of nucleus pulposus is not significantly improved by traction (see **313**) and is termed 'static'. Differentiation between static and dynamic compression has an important bearing on the choice of surgical procedure.

The extension view is less useful, but may help the surgeon to decide which is the most significant lesion when compression exists at more than one site. Also, extension may identify other lesions, which could become clinically significant in the future. Cervical extension exacerbates spinal cord compression and should be undertaken with great care, preferably under fluoroscopy. Otherwise, the dog should be positioned in moderate (not extreme) extension for as short a period as possible.

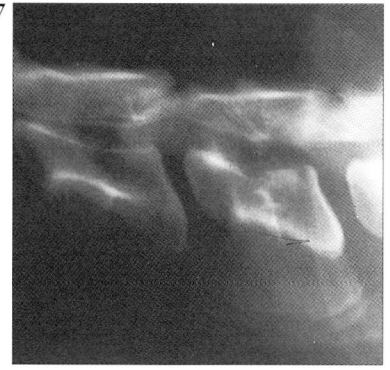

317 Cervical myelogram of a Dobermann with the vertebral column in a neutral position; a single lesion at C_5/C_6 intervertebral space is seen. There is ventral compression associated with a disc lesion and dorsal compression related to ligamentum flavum.

318 Extension applied to the vertebral column; an additional compressive lesion is seen at the C_6/C_7 intervertebral space.

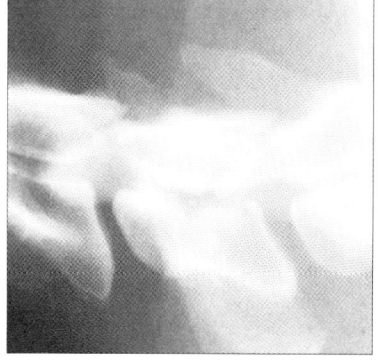

CT myelography

Where available, CT myelography is a useful addition to the conventional study (Sharp *et al.*, 1992). The main advantage is the graphic transverse image that it provides of any spinal cord distortion. This information can help the clinician choose the most appropriate surgical procedure for that individual dog. It may also provide prognostic information by detecting spinal cord atrophy.

It is wise to perform radiographic evaluations at least 48 hours before surgery. A temporary worsening of the neurological deficit may occur in dogs with CCSM following myelography, and a delay allows the patient to recover. Also, this time gives ample opportunity to decide on the best treatment based on all the information gained, and to discuss this with the owner. It also permits a thorough presurgical evaluation.

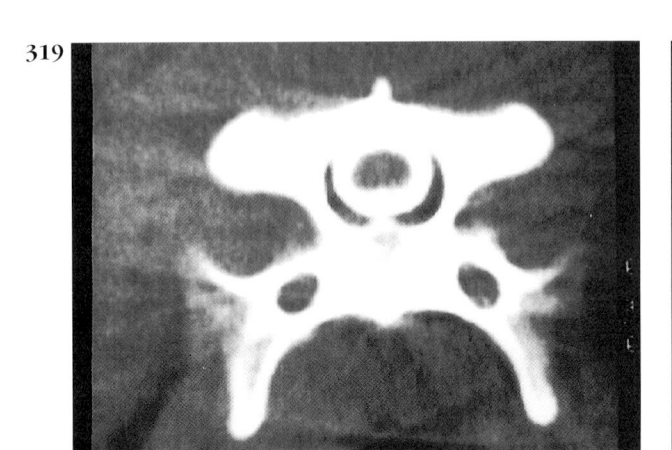

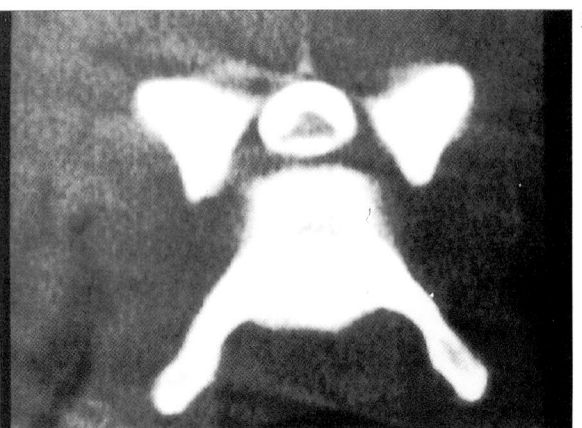

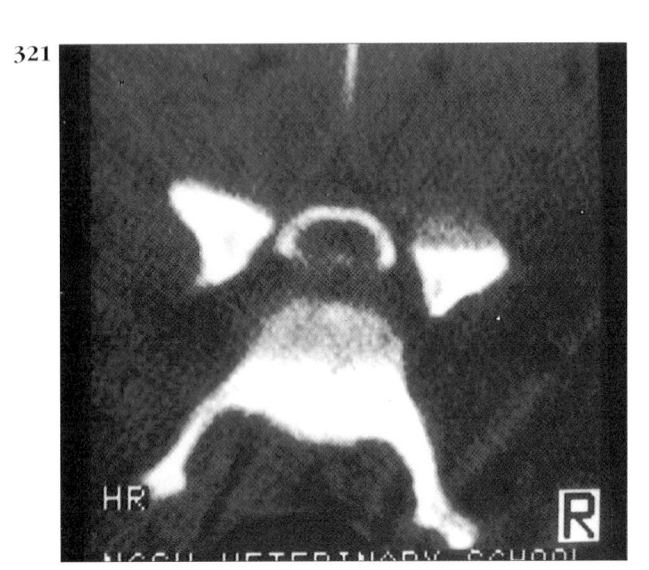

319 Transverse CT myelogram from the same dog shown in 315 and 316. This image is made at the midpoint of the sixth cervical vertebra where the spinal cord and subarachnoid space are of normal appearance.

320 Transverse CT myelogram. This image is made at the C_6/C_7 intervertebral disc of the dog in **319**, 10mm caudal to the image shown in **319**. Note that the spinal cord does not appear to be compressed, although the dural tube is lifted slightly above the floor of the vertebral canal. The spinal cord is thin and has an abnormal shape, which is consistent with spinal cord atrophy. Contrast this atrophic spinal cord with the obviously compressed spinal cord shown in **321**.

321 CT myelogram from a different dog taken at C_6/C_7. The spinal cord has been compressed by a ventral extradural mass of bulging anulus fibrosus (subsequently confirmed at surgery).

11. CAUDAL CERVICAL SPONDYLOMYELOPATHY

PRESURGICAL EVALUATION

During the recovery period after myelography, medical problems that may complicate the situation should be assessed **(Table 23)**.

Table 23 Important diseases that may coexist with CSSM

Hypothyroidism
Von Willebrand's disease (Dobermanns)
Cardiomyopathy
Chronic active hepatitis

Hypothyroidism
Dobermanns are predisposed to hypothyroidism, which is easily overlooked as the signs are nonspecific. Lethargy, muscle weakness, and peripheral neuropathy may occur, all of which are undesirable in a surgical candidate. There also seems to be a negative effect of hypothyroidism on VW factor, such that dogs with even subclinical VW disease can become predisposed to overt bleeding (Dodds, 1984). We screen all surgical candidates by the thyroid stimulating hormone test. Hypothyroid dogs are given hormone supplement for at least 48 hours before surgery if possible, and this should be continued indefinitely after surgery.

Bleeding disorders
It has been estimated that 16% of Dobermanns in the USA have a bleeding tendency related to VW disease (Dodds, 1989). Bleeding from the internal vertebral venous plexus is a potential problem during ventral decompression, and can be almost impossible to arrest unless the dog has normal haemostatic abilities. In all techniques using a ventral approach to the neck, inability to close dead space can cause haematoma formation several days after surgery (**322, 323**). The easiest way to test an animal's VW status is to perform a standardized bleeding time test (**324, 325**).

Dobermanns with prolonged bleeding times, or those with known VW disease, can be given desmopressin (DDAVP, Rhone Poulenc Rorer, 1.0 microgram/kg SQ) immediately before surgery. Cryoprecipitate is the optimal therapy, although

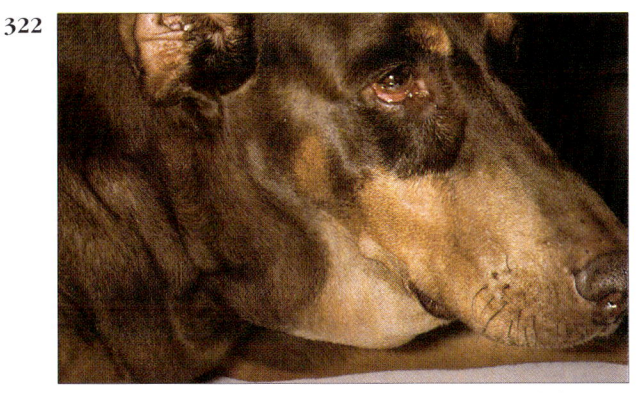

322 Dobermann that had undergone ventral decompression for CCSM 10 days previously. It presented with intermandibular oedema and a firm swelling in the ventral cervical region. Horner's syndrome (note prolapse of the third eyelid), laryngeal paralysis, megaoesophagus, and mild aspiration pneumonia were also present.

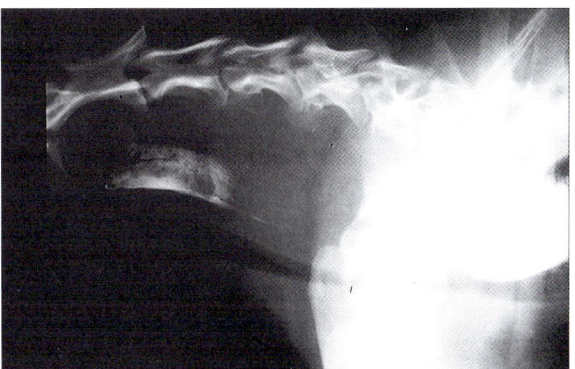

323 The cervical swelling, dramatically illustrated by this barium oesophagram, was felt to be the cause of all complications, including the megaoesophagus. A large volume of sanguinopurulent fluid was drained from the swelling at surgery, which had probably accumulated because of bleeding and then become infected.

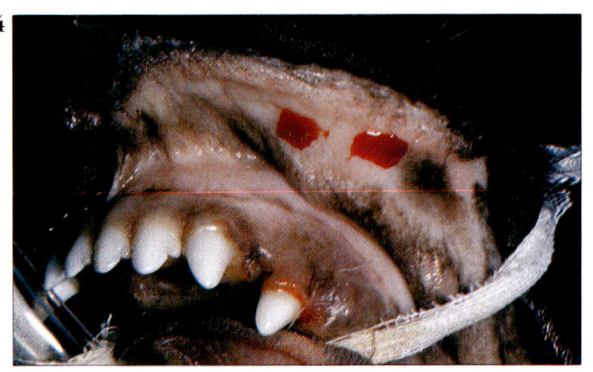

324 Illustration of a buccal mucosal bleeding time being performed in a dog. This can be performed in the conscious or the anaesthetized patient. The gauze strip has been used to keep the lip turned over and to cause slight venous engorgement. A two-blade, spring-loaded device (Simplate II Organon Teknika, General Diagnostics, Cambridge, UK; Jessup, MD, USA) has been used to make two 6 mm long by 1 mm deep incisions in the upper lip mucosa. Any obvious blood vessels should be avoided. A stopwatch is started just as the incisions are made. Blood is blotted at five second intervals using filter paper, taking care not to touch the incision itself. The mean buccal mucosa bleeding time for normal dogs is 2.62 minutes, with a range of 1.7–4.2 minutes (Jergens *et al.*, 1987).

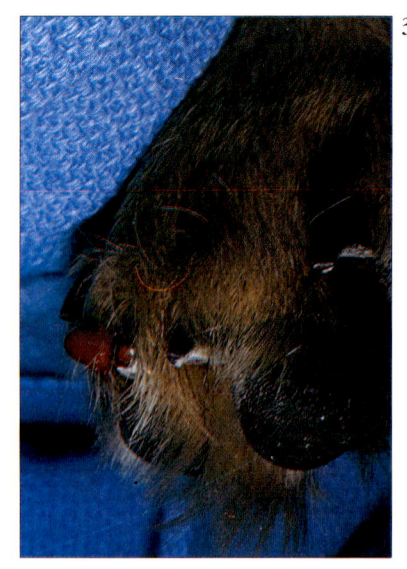

325 Illustration of a cuticle bleeding time being performed in a dog. A cut is made using a guillotine nail clipper at the apex of the cuticle. In normal dogs, bleeding stops within eight minutes, but occasionally continues for up to 12 minutes (Giles *et al.*, 1982). This test is harder to standardize than the buccal mucosa bleeding time, but should identify severe bleeding disorders.

fresh or frozen plasma (10 ml/kg of plasma, taken 30–60 minutes after the donor has been given desmopressin) may also be useful (Littlewood, 1991; Meyers *et al.*, 1992). As a precaution, dogs at known risk can be crossmatched if they are to undergo ventral decompression. Dogs with prolonged bleeding times should receive thyroid hormone supplementation for 48 hours before surgery, which improves the function of VW factor in hypothyroid dogs and may even benefit euthyroid dogs (Dodds, 1984; Peterson and Ferguson, 1989).

Other disorders

Chronic active hepatitis of Dobermanns may be identified by standard biochemical evaluation (Franklin and Saunders, 1988).

Cardiomyopathy is seen in many large and giant breed dogs, and is invariably fatal within six months of diagnosis (Fox, 1989). Even a subtle arrhythmia should not be discounted, and an ECG and echocardiogram should be performed as indicated.

TREATMENT

The decision regarding the best way to treat each patient is based on the presenting history, neurological status, radiological findings, and the owner's expectations and their ability to undertake any necessary aftercare. Most dogs that show neurological deficits are surgical candidates, but consideration will be given here to nonsurgical treatment.

Nonsurgical treatment

Dogs that develop mild neurological deficits following minor trauma may respond favourably to nonsurgical treatment. However, surgery should be considered for most other dogs as they will undergo a slow but steady deterioration (Denny *et al.*, 1977). As surgery is elective for the majority of dogs with CCSM, a 2–4 week course of severe exercise reduction and use of a chest harness can usually be justified (see **482**).

11. CAUDAL CERVICAL SPONDYLOMYELOPATHY

SURGERY

A large number of different surgical techniques have been proposed for CCSM, with many of the authors claiming a 70–80% success rate (**Table 24**).

We feel that the way to obtain the best overall results is to consider three basic types of surgery and to perform these for certain, relatively well-defined indications. The three types of surgery are:
- Ventral decompression.
- Vertebral distraction/fusion.
- Dorsal decompression.

The basic indications for each surgical procedure are summarized in **Table 25**.

The main factor governing the choice of surgical procedure is the appearance of the spinal cord on myelography, particularly the traction view. Many lesions, when evaluated by traction, show a combination of both static and dynamic compression. A judgement must then be made as to which is the major component.

An algorithm for surgical decision making, based on the myelogram, is provided in **326**. All the surgical techniques described below are technically challenging.

Table 24 Reported results for surgical treatment of CSSM

	Ventral slot		Metal and cement	Screw and washer	Dorsal laminectomy*
Number	18[1]	27[2]	41[3]	20[4]	18[5]
Successes	14	18	37	17	14
(as %)	(78)	(67)	(90)	(85)	(78)
Follow up in months	10–60	6–48	3–50	3–30	1.5–53
(mean)	(29)	(N/A)	(20)	(21)	(17)**
Dogs with repeat episode	4/14***	N/A	8/37[+]	1[++]	2
(as %)	(28)		(22)		
Months to repeat episode	12–60		5–42		1[+++]
(mean)	(32)		N/A		

* Eight additional dogs have been reported to have undergone continuous dorsal laminectomy from C_4–C_7. Follow-up over a mean period of 3.5 years revealed good recoveries in all dogs, with one dog suffering a repeat period of tetraparesis. The total number of dogs undergoing this procedure and the selection criteria were not noted (Lyman and Seim, 1991).
**Recorded in only 9 of the 14 dogs.
***One confirmed to have a domino lesion.
[+]Three confirmed to have a domino lesion.
[++]Not due to domino; screw needed shortening.
[+++]Confirmed to be due to a constrictive fibrosis at surgery site in one dog.
[1] Bruecker et al., 1989b; [2] Chambers et al., 1986; [3] Bruecker et al., 1989a; [4] McKee et al., 1990; [5] Trotter et al., 1976.

Table 25 General indications for surgical procedures in CSSM

Procedure	Indication	Lesion
Ventral decompression	1. STATIC lesion (ventral)	Disc herniation
Distraction/fusion		
Metal and bone cement (or screw and washer)	1. SINGLE DYNAMIC lesion	Bulging anulus fibrosus or ligamentum flavum
Screw and washer	2. MULTIPLE DYNAMIC lesions	Bulging anulus fibrosus or ligamentum flavum
Dorsal decompression	1. STATIC lesion (dorsal)	Osseous vertebral canal stenosis, articular process osteophytosis
	2. MULTIPLE sites of compression	All types of lesion

141

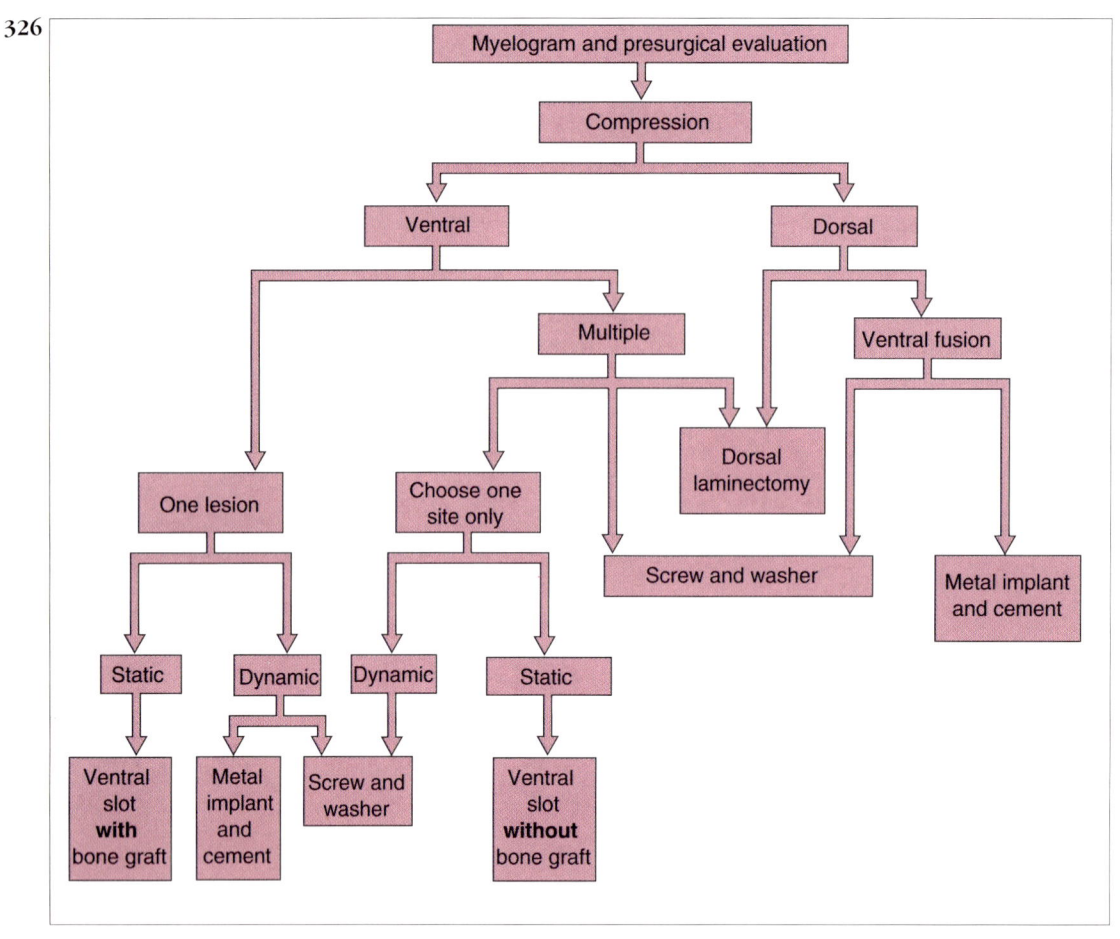

DIAGNOSIS AND SURGERY OF SMALL ANIMAL SPINAL DISORDERS

326 Surgical decision making for an adult dog with CSSM.

Operative considerations

As some dogs with CCSM deteriorate postoperatively for obscure reasons, methylprednisolone given before dorsal or ventral decompression may be useful. It should also be remembered that prolonged excessive extension of the neck during surgery is undesirable. In addition, overzealous retraction of soft tissues during a ventral approach to the neck can damage any of the nerves in the cervical region. This can induce arrhythmia, Horner's syndrome (see **322, 323**), or laryngeal paralysis, and retraction may also exacerbate bleeding from the internal vertebral venous plexus (vertebral sinuses) by compressing the jugular veins.

Ventral decompression (see Chapter 7)

Ventral decompression (ventral slot) is indicated primarily for the relief of static ventral lesions such as herniated disc material, although some surgeons also use it for dynamic lesions. The surgical approach is described in Chapter 7. In CCSM it may be complicated by ventral osteophytosis or a misshapen C_7 vertebra. Access to the C_6/C_7 site may be restricted, but this problem is minimized by taking particular care with patient positioning (**327**).

In general, ventral decompression can only be considered to have been completed satisfactorily when the dura is clearly visible in the depths of the slot. In CCSM, it is uncommon to identify an obvious

11. CAUDAL CERVICAL SPONDYLOMYELOPATHY

327 Patient positioning for a ventral decompression or distraction by screw and washer. If distraction/fusion by metal implant and bone cement is to be performed, the patient is positioned with the neck flat on the operating table to enable traction to be applied. The relationship of the proximal humerus to the operative field is shown, with the prepared area of the ventral neck extended to include the proximal humerus.

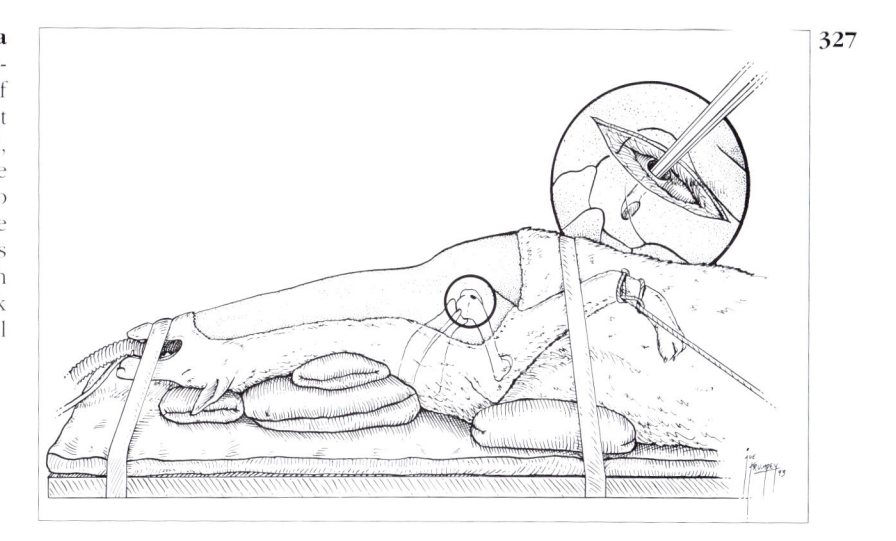

328 Harvesting of cancellous bone from the proximal humerus.

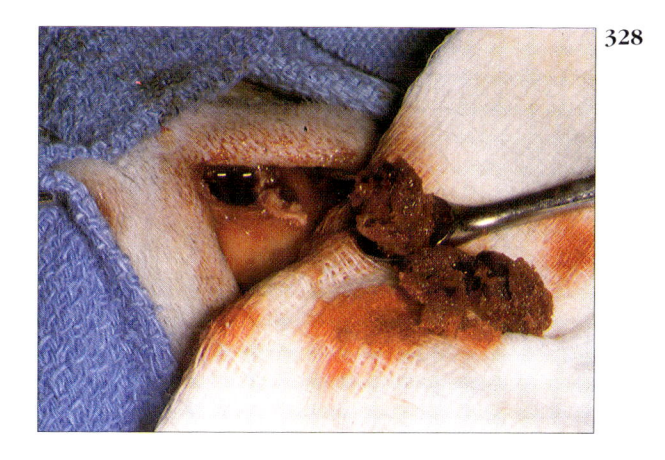

mass of herniated disc material as seen with a classic Type I disc extrusion in a chondrodystrophoid dog. Rather, the compression often appears to be caused by fibres of the anulus fibrosus infiltrated by degenerate nuclear material.

To promote vertebral fusion at the surgical site, cancellous bone may be packed around the slot (**328**). Cancellous bone enhances fusion, which usually occurs within eight weeks. Without grafting, osseous fusion is delayed and occurs in only about 50% of dogs, with the others presumably undergoing fibrous union. Thus some range of motion may be preserved by not using a graft. This could be advantageous in a dog where only one of two adjacent lesions is operated on with this technique, to try and lessen the potential for the domino effect (Chambers *et al.*, 1982; Van Gundy, 1988, 1989).

Vertebral distraction and fusion

The primary indication for distraction and fusion is the presence of a dynamic component to the spinal cord compression (see **Table 25**). This can cause dorsal, ventral, or annular compression of the vertebral canal. Distraction has been attempted in the past using a number of different techniques, but the two methods described here are the use of metal implants and bone cement, and a screw and washer technique. An advantage of both of these distraction methods is that they often provide rapid relief of cervical hyperaesthesia, probably because of decompression of nerve roots at the distracted interspace. Both techniques have the potential for implant failure, which can be catastrophic (Ellison *et al.*, 1988; Bruecker *et al.*, 1989a; McKee *et al.*, 1990). Other methods have been described, for example the use of Harrington rods (Walker, 1989).

Metal implant and bone cement method (329–335)

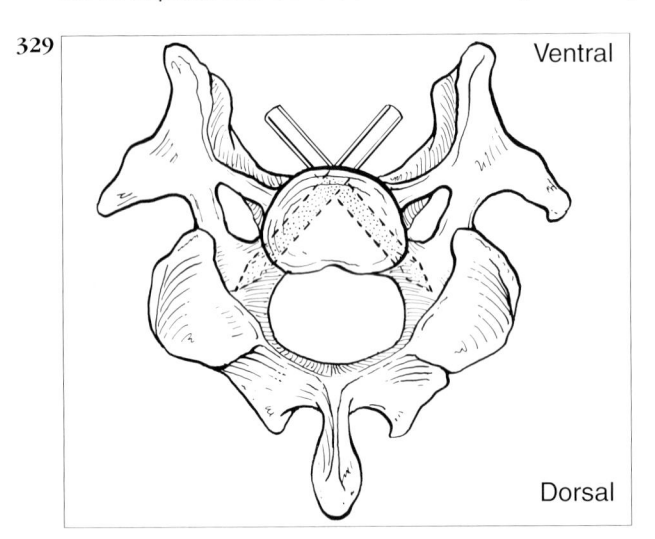

329 Placement of pins or screws in cervical vertebra for distraction/fusion. The ventral approach to the neck is illustrated in Chapter 7. The implants are placed close to the midline and then driven across the midline towards the contralateral transverse process, away from the vertebral canal. It is important that the distal cortex is penetrated. Two implants are placed in the vertebrae each side of the spinal cord compression (see **332**). The vertebrae are then distracted (see **330, 331**). The position is maintained by methylmethacrylate bone cement placed around the pins or screws (see **333**).

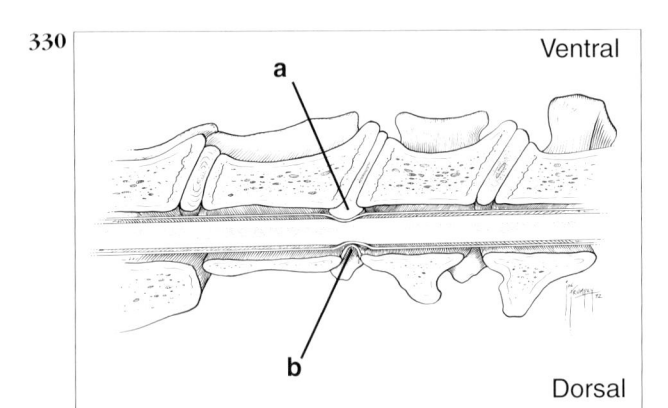

330 Principle behind the vertebral distraction/fusion technique. Sagittal section through the cervical spine to show compression ventrally from disc (**a**) and dorsally from ligamentum flavum (**b**).

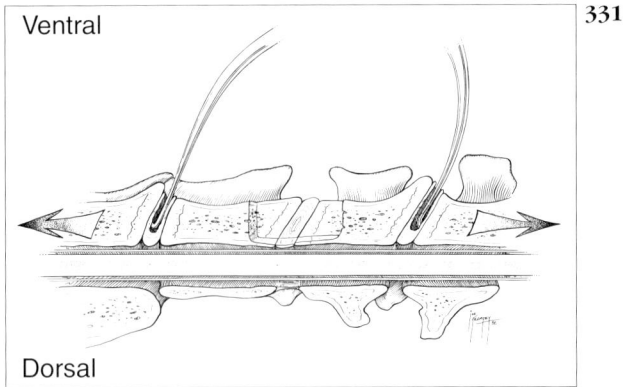

331 Principle behind the vertebral distraction/fusion technique. A partial ventral slot has been created at the site of spinal cord compression. Traction is applied to the intervertebral space by a combination of modified Gelpi retractor placed in the adjacent intervertebral spaces, and traction applied to the maxilla. This relieves the compression shown in **330**.

11. CAUDAL CERVICAL SPONDYLOMYELOPATHY

332 Placement of screws; the dog's head is to the left in all surgical illustrations. The screws diverge from the midline towards the transverse processes. A partial ventral slot has been created at the C_6/C_7 intervertebral space.

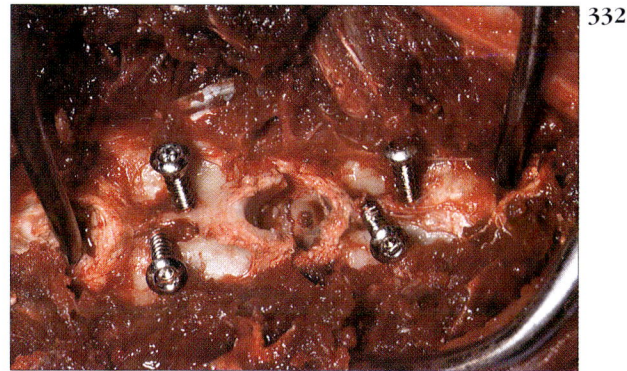

333 Bone cement in place to incorporate the screws.

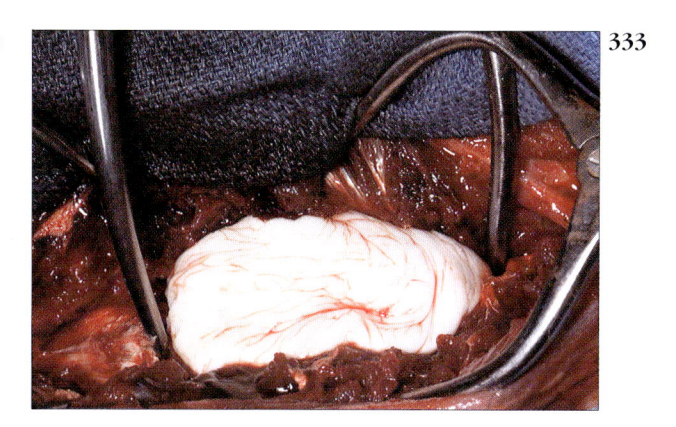

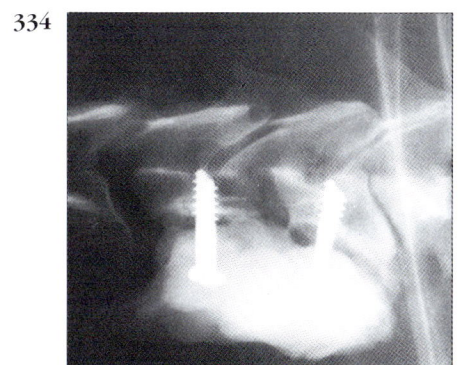

334 Postoperative radiograph of a dog with screws and bone cement in place. This is the same dog as shown in **365**. Fully threaded screws are preferred to the partially threaded screws shown here.

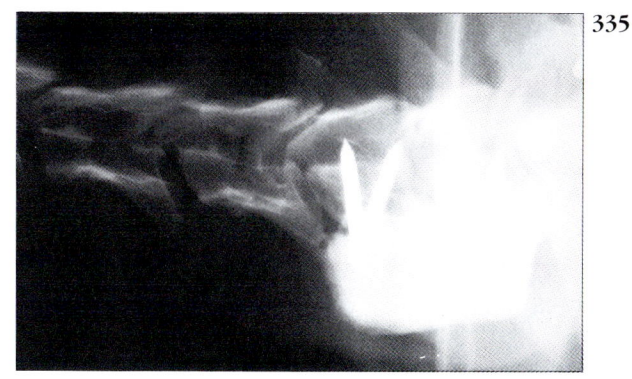

335 Postoperative radiograph of a dog with pins and bone cement in place.

In the metal implant and bone cement technique, the cement renders revision of a surgical failure difficult, and also raises the risk of implant infection. The dog should receive intravenous intraoperative antibiotic against staphylococci (such as cephazolin 20 mg/kg, every 1–2 hours during surgery). Despite potential disadvantages, metal implant and bone cement distraction is well tested with good long term results (see **Table 24**). The implants can be Steinmann pins (**329**) or bone screws (**332–334**), but neither are suitable for distraction at more than one interspace (Ellison *et al.*, 1988; Van Gundy, 1988).

DIAGNOSIS AND SURGERY OF SMALL ANIMAL SPINAL DISORDERS

Screw and washer (336–344)

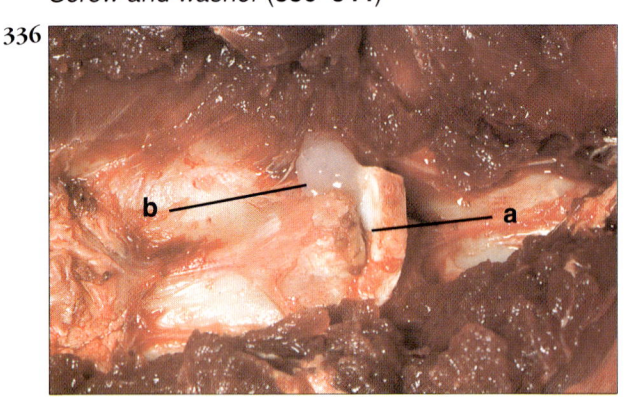

336 The ventral approach to the neck is illustrated in Chapter 7. A wide fenestration has been performed at the C_6/C_7 disc. The window in the anulus fibrosus (**a**) and nucleus pulposus (**b**) are visible.

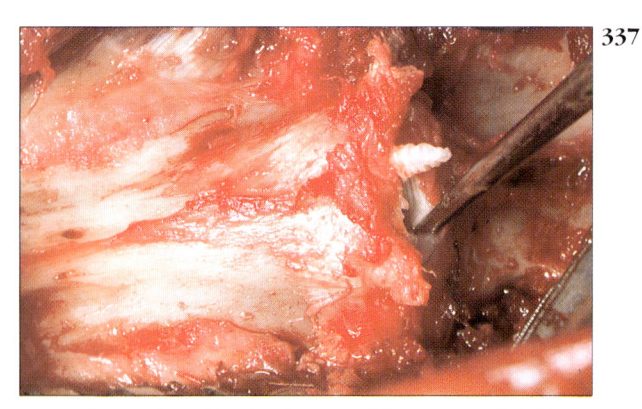

337 The C_6/C_7 disc is thoroughly curetted following fenestration.

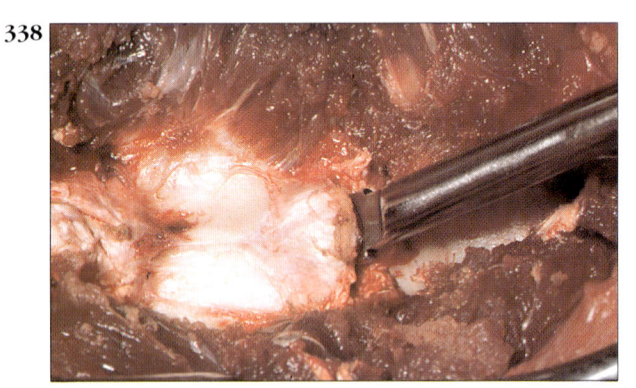

338 The distraction device has been introduced into the intervertebral space.

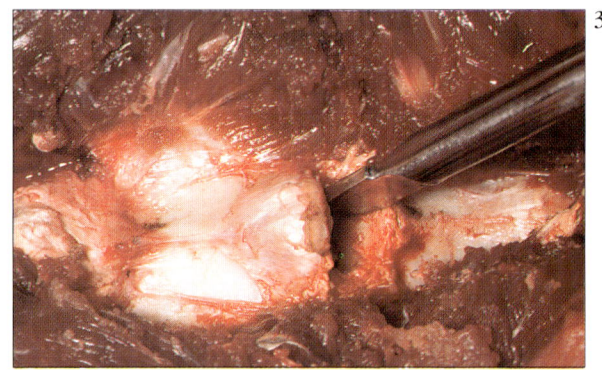

339 The device has been turned through 90° to distract the two vertebrae. Note the widening of the intervertebral space.

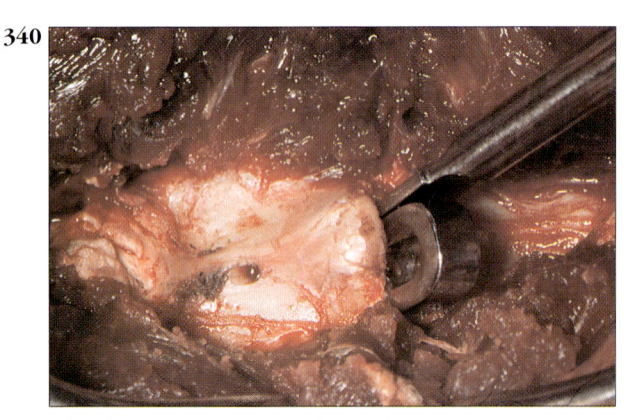

340 The washer is inserted into the distracted intervertebral space to ensure a correct fit, then removed. A 1.5 mm pilot hole has been drilled through C_6 to ensure that the screw will pass through the centre of the C_6 endplate, and therefore through the hole in the washer. A 2.5 mm drill bit is then used to enlarge the hole in C_6. The washer is repositioned and a tapped hole created through the washer into C_7 using a 2.5 mm drill followed by a 3.5 mm tap.

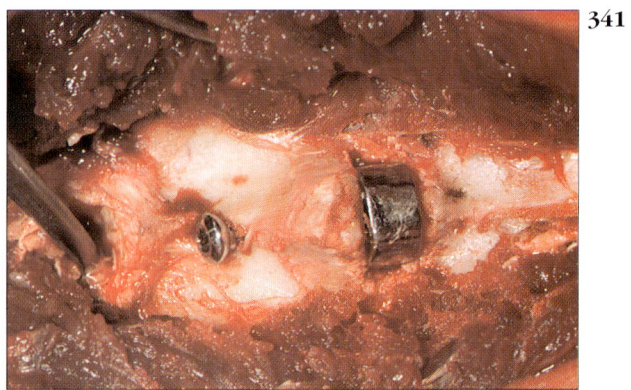

341 A 26–30 mm long, 3.5 mm diameter, cortical bone screw is engaged as a positional screw through the washer and across the intervertebral space. A cancellous bone graft obtained from the proximal humerus is then packed over the exposed vertebrae and implants. (A 7.5 mm thick washer is used for Great Danes, and a 6 mm thick washer is used for other dogs).

11. CAUDAL CERVICAL SPONDYLOMYELOPATHY

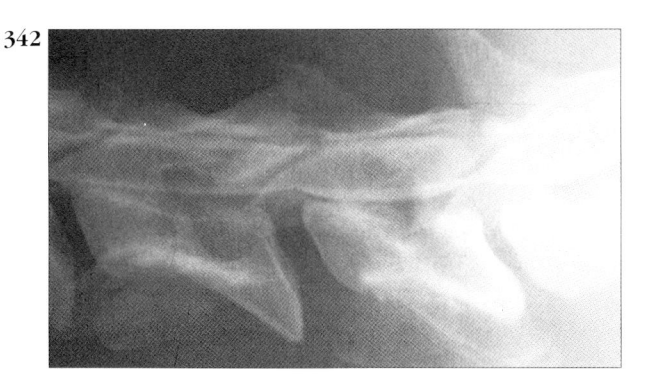

342 Preoperative appearance of a Dobermann with a lesion at both C$_5$/C$_6$ and C$_6$/C$_7$.

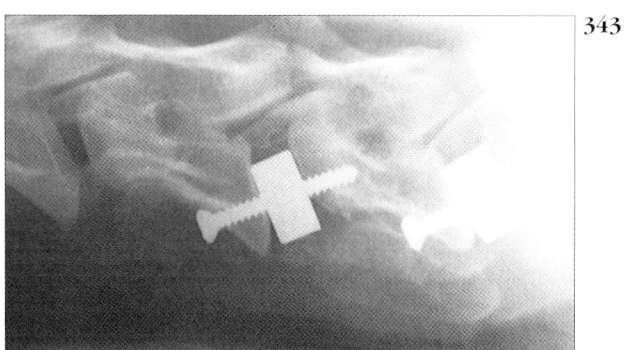

343 Postoperative radiograph showing a 6 mm washer at C$_5$/C$_6$ and a 7.5 mm washer at C$_6$/C$_7$.

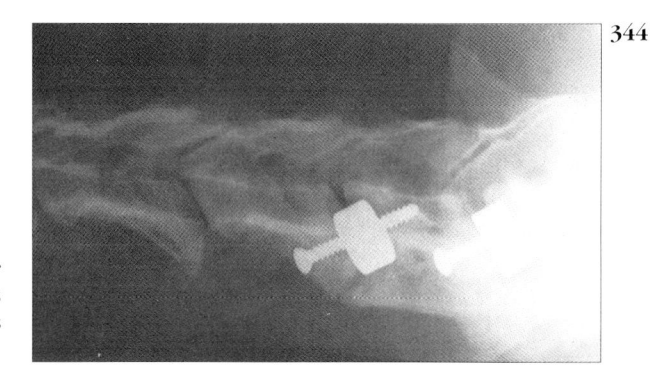

344 Same dog as in 342 and 343 three months after surgery. Despite the collapse of the vertebral endplates and loss of distraction, the dog's clinical status was markedly improved.

The screw and washer technique will probably benefit from further modification to overcome its main problem of vertebral endplate resorption, with subsequent collapse of the distracted interspace. The collapse appears to be caused by suboptimal washer design, so that all of the force resulting from distraction is concentrated on relatively small areas of contact between the endplate and washer. However, the temporary stability provided by the implants seems to allow fusion to occur. This provides long-term relief of spinal cord compression, despite the subsequent collapse of the distracted site (**342–344**). The reported results are very good (see **Table 24**). A major advantage is that, unlike metal implant and cement distraction, the screw and washer technique can be applied to more than one site. The surgeon can therefore be more aggressive in dealing with a dog that has two adjacent lesions, one of which could go on to cause a domino problem in the future if not treated (see **364**). The disadvantage is that 10 percent of dogs show a marked, early deterioration in neurological status, presumably because of endplate collapse or implant failure (McKee *et al.*, 1990).

147

DIAGNOSIS AND SURGERY OF SMALL ANIMAL SPINAL DISORDERS

Lag Screw Fixation (345–347)

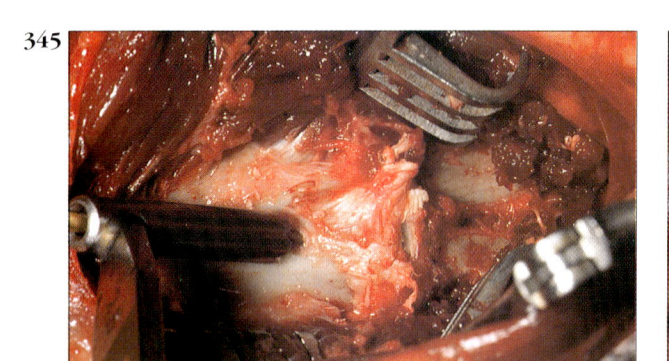

345 Surgical procedure for transvertebral lag screw fixation at C_6/C_7. Following fenestration and curettage of the space as shown in **336** and **337**, a 2.5 mm pilot hole is drilled through C_6 and C_7. A 3.5 mm tap is used to create the thread and the hole in C_6 is over drilled with a 3.5 mm diameter drill bit.

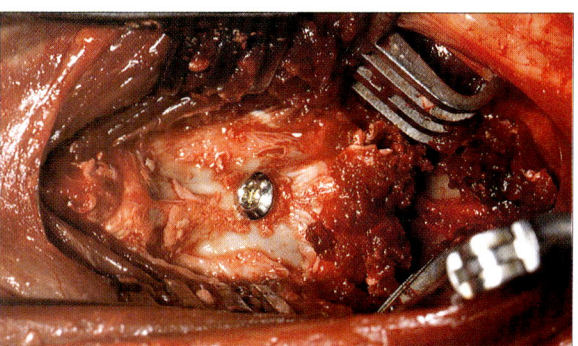

346 A 3.5 mm cortical bone screw is placed as a lag screw to compress the two vertebrae. Cancellous bone graft from the proximal humerus is packed over the intervertebral space (shown partially completed). Sufficient graft is used to cover the space and screw head.

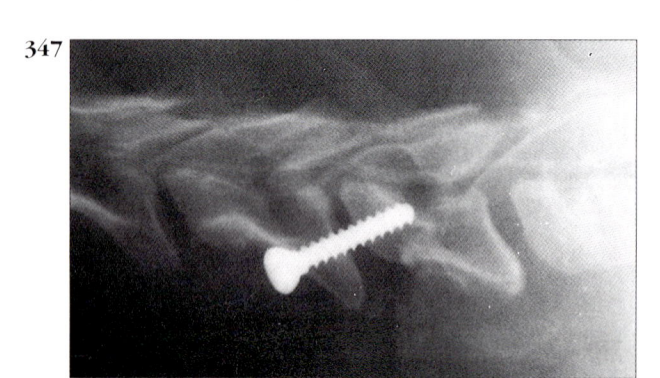

347 Radiograph of a dog that has undergone lag screw fixation at C_5/C_6. Residual contrast medium following the myelogram shows that there is still spinal cord compression at the site. However, the dog improved following surgery, and this improvement was maintained.

Use of bone screws without washers (**345–347**) may also reduce instability and so relieve dynamic spinal cord compression (Denny et al., 1977). It often results in fusion and can be used at multiple sites.

The screw and washer technique is preferable to lag screw fixation because the washer shares the load of distraction, which should lower the risk of implant failure and enhance fusion. In addition, the washer causes distractive fixation (versus compressive fixation), which is more appropriate for a dynamic lesion.

Ventral fusion performed in horses with Wobbler syndrome, an equivalent condition to CCSM in dogs, can cause new bone around the articular processes to regress (Grant et al., 1985). Similarly, ventral fusion in dogs might also relieve compression caused by dorsally located osteophytes (see **314, 348**), especially as ligamentum flavum has been shown to atrophy in dogs following fusion (Bruecker et al., 1989a; McKee et al., 1990). Using a ventral approach in these patients may avoid the morbidity problems sometimes associated with dorsal laminectomy in dogs.

11. CAUDAL CERVICAL SPONDYLOMYELOPATHY

Dorsal decompression (349–362)

This technique would seem to be the logical treatment for dogs with multiple sites of vertebral canal stenosis (see **312**), and for those with osteophytes in the region of the dorsal articular processes (see **314** and **348**). It is also an option for dogs with ventral lesions at two or more intervertebral spaces.

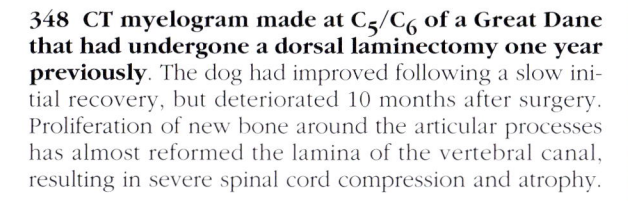

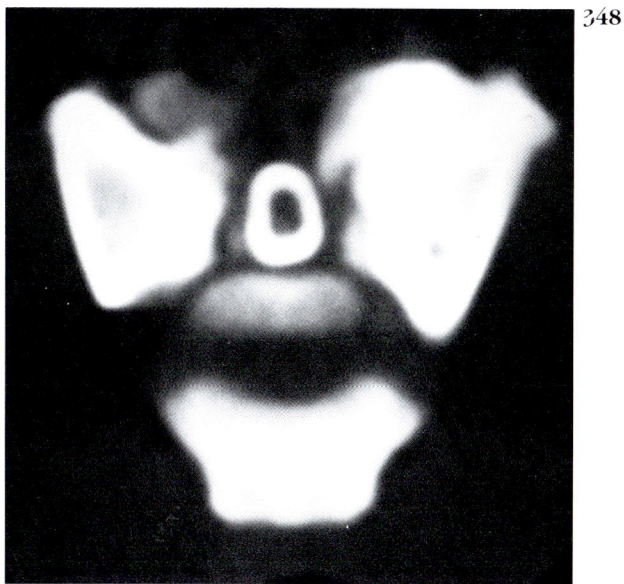

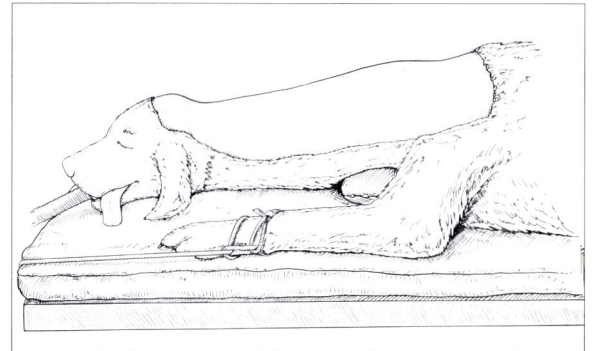

348 CT myelogram made at C_5/C_6 of a Great Dane that had undergone a dorsal laminectomy one year previously. The dog had improved following a slow initial recovery, but deteriorated 10 months after surgery. Proliferation of new bone around the articular processes has almost reformed the lamina of the vertebral canal, resulting in severe spinal cord compression and atrophy.

349 Positioning of dog: dorsal cervical laminectomy.

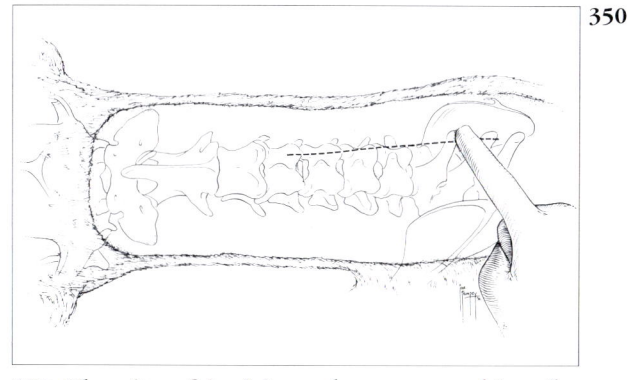

350 The site of incision when approaching the caudal cervical vertebrae is from C_4 to T_2 or T_3.

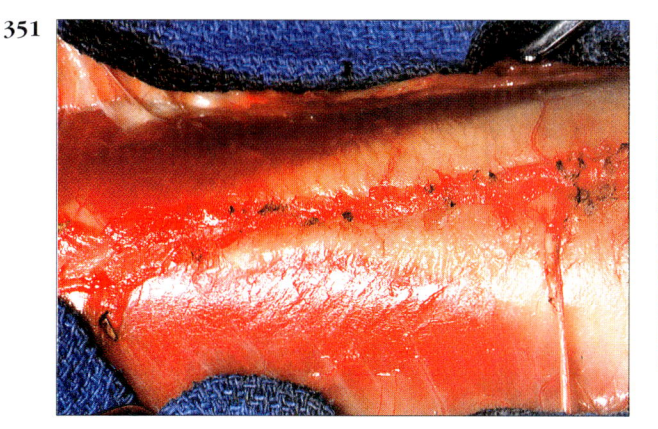

351 Skin and superficial fascia incised and retracted to reveal the aponeuroses of the rhomboideus and trapezius muscles.

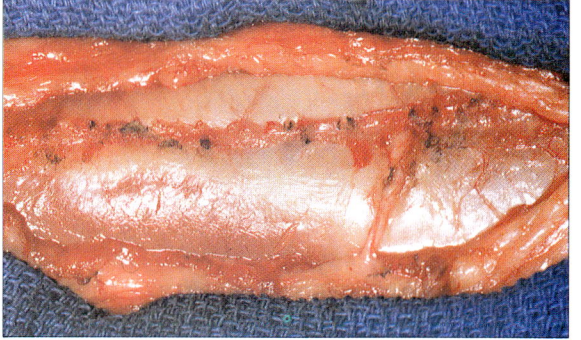

352 The muscles are divided in the midline. There are numerous blood vessels in the fascia and these must be controlled. Most anatomical descriptions indicate that the muscles are arranged symmetrically, but often some layers are somewhat oblique, which can be confusing. Several smaller muscles overlie the nuchal ligament, which can be palpated at this stage.

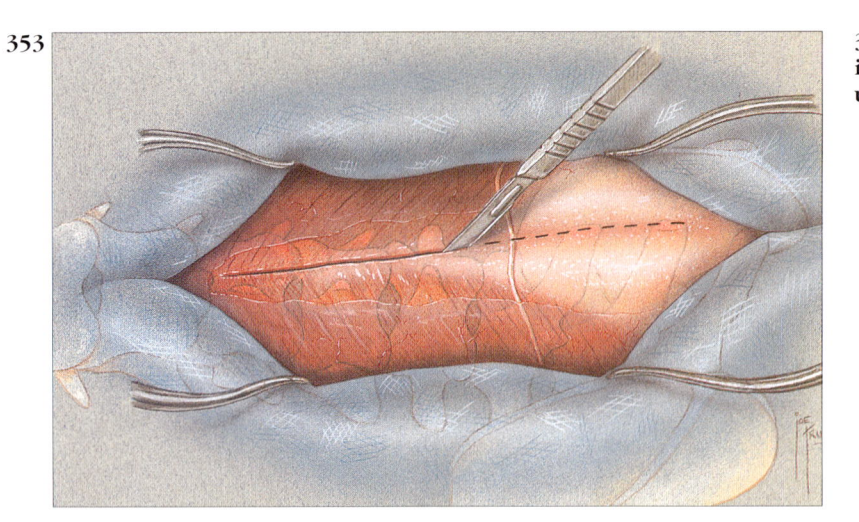

353 Diagram to show the position of muscles relative to underlying skeletal structures.

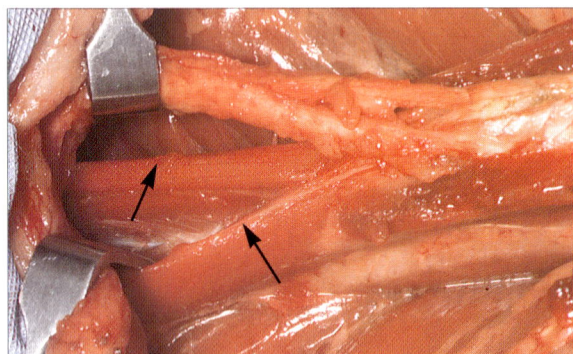

354 The fascia overlying the nuchal ligament is divided and cleared. The ligament is freed back to the prominent spinous process of T₁. Here the nuchal ligament is mobilized, revealing the paired spinalis muscles (arrows).

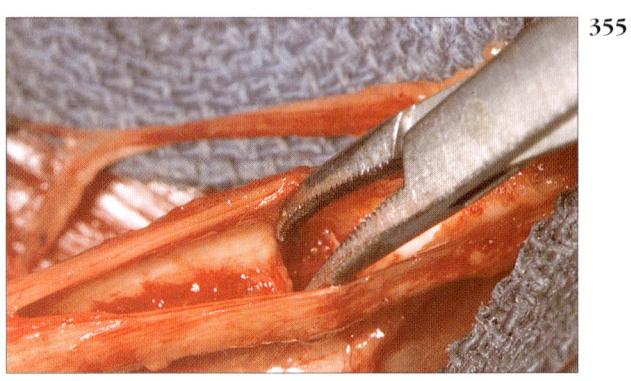

355 The nuchal ligament attaches to the prominent spinous process of T₁ and continues caudally with the interspinous ligament. Here it is being divided in the midline. It is possible to make the approach alongside the nuchal ligament rather than in the midline. The ligament may even be sectioned if additional exposure is required; it may be repaired later.

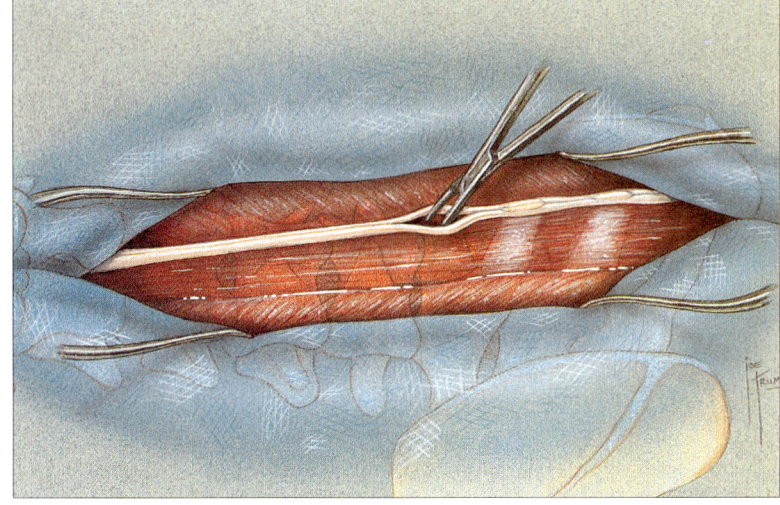

356 The nuchal ligament and the spinalis muscles are divided and retracted with Gelpi retractors. The spinous process of C₇ can be palpated.

11. CAUDAL CERVICAL SPONDYLOMYELOPATHY

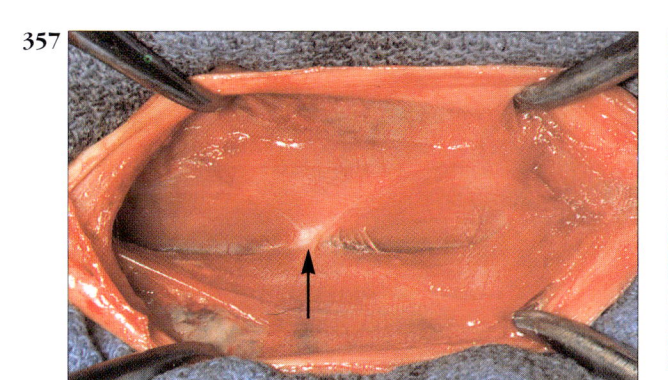

357 Closer view showing spinalis muscles attached to spinous process of C_7 (arrow).

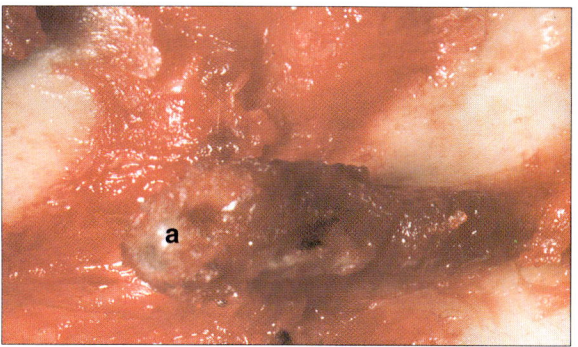

358 The muscles are elevated from the spinous process (a) and lamina of the vertebra. Exposure is maintained with two pairs of Adson–Baby retractors.

359 The spinous process is removed with bone cutters. There is a layer of fascia associated with the ligamentum flavum. This is removed by sharp dissection, using a #11 blade and must be performed with care as the spinal cord is unprotected by bone between the vertebral arches. The spinal cord is visible (**a**). Large blood vessels may be present associated with this layer of soft tissue; haemorrhage is controlled with bipolar cautery.

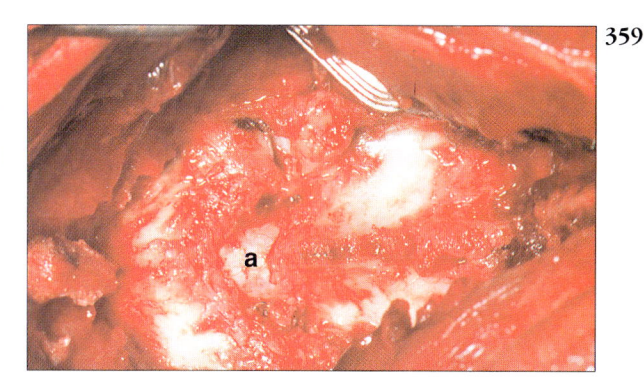

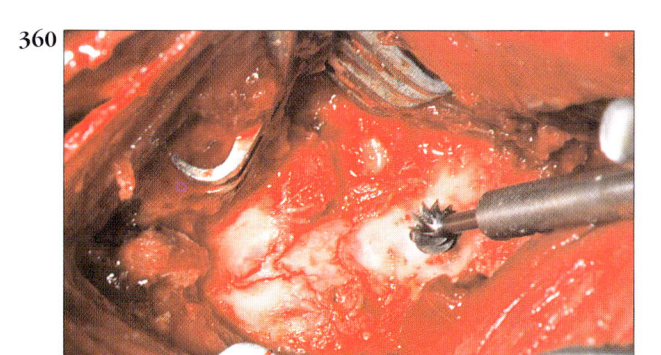

360 The laminectomy is performed with a bur. Close attention is paid to the layers of bone as they are removed (see Chapter 10).

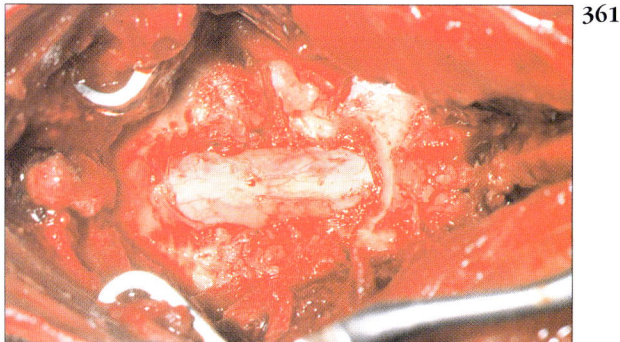

361 Spinal cord exposed. The laminectomy may be continued laterally to remove proliferated articular processes or to gain access to the nerve roots. Again, significant haemorrhage may result from the soft tissues.

151

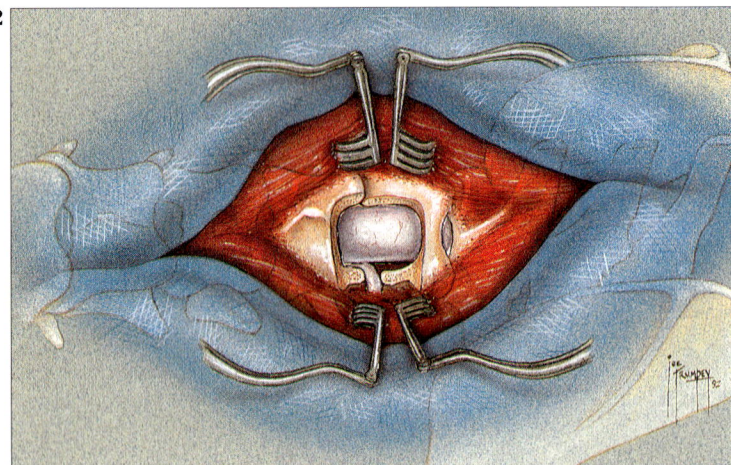

362 Diagram to show laminectomy continued to one side to reveal the nerve root.

Long-term results of dorsal laminectomy have been reported to be favourable (Lyman and Seim, 1991), but several authors have reported significant postoperative morbidity and deterioration in neurological status (Trotter *et al.*, 1976; De Lahunta, 1983; Trotter, 1985; Walker *et al.*, 1985). In general, for these reasons, we are reluctant to perform dorsal decompression when other techniques can be used.

In a survey of perioperative mortality associated with cervical decompressive surgery, dorsal laminectomy was associated with three times the mortality rate of ventral decompression (Clark, 1986). Another potential complication is constrictive fibrosis at the surgical site by so called 'laminectomy membranes' (see Chapter 6). Dorsal decompression should not cause the domino effect, as the vertebrae do not usually fuse together. Fusion can be encouraged, if necessary, by screwing and then bone grafting the dorsal articular processes.

Ventral fenestration
Fenestration is not a suitable treatment for adult dogs with CCSM. It has been proposed as an effective treatment for young Dobermanns with this condition, although others have reported mixed results (Mason, 1979; Lincoln and Pettit, 1985; Lewis, 1992).

Dogs with multiple lesions
Between 15 and 50% of Dobermanns present with compression at both C_5/C_6 and C_6/C_7 intervertebral spaces (Bruecker *et al.*, 1989b; McKee *et al.*, 1989).

Dogs with more than one lesion may be treated in one of several ways.

- **Perform surgery at both sites**. This increases the overall complication rate, and is contraindicated for the metal implant and bone cement technique of distraction because of the high risk of implant failure. Screw and washer distraction can be used on two adjacent lesions without increasing the complication rate.
- **Try to determine which lesion is more significant, perhaps with the help of an extension view during myelography, and then correct this lesion in isolation**. Correcting the worst lesion might be successful with ventral decompression, but distraction at only one site may well exacerbate the adjacent lesion (domino effect), and should be undertaken with great circumspection. If only one of two lesions is corrected, dogs that deteriorate or do not respond after surgery should undergo repeat myelography within seven days.
- **Perform a continuous dorsal decompression over both sites**. This avoids the risk of a domino lesion, but can cause significant morbidity.

COMPLICATIONS

Seizures following myelography (**Table 26**) may be more common in Dobermanns with CCSM than in other breeds or other diseases (Lewis and Hosgood, 1992). This highlights the need for constant monitoring during recovery, with diazepam on hand to control any seizures, which could have an adverse effect on the spinal lesion.

Table 26 Postoperative complications associated with CSSM

Seizures following myelography
Horner's syndrome/laryngeal paralysis
Haematoma
Pneumonia
Bone cement infection
Deterioration of neurological status
Implant failure
Discospondylitis
Domino lesion
Gastric dilation and volvulus
Decubital ulcers

Bleeding from the venous plexus is the major complication of ventral decompression. Usually, the haemorrhage can be arrested by employing a small piece of muscle tissue to promote coagulation of the leaking vessel (see **208**). Haematoma formation is most likely in Dobermanns with defective clotting, and if present should be managed with a drain (see **129** and **130**).

Dogs that remain recumbent after surgery require a very high level of nursing care (see Chapter 15). A particular risk for these dogs is pneumonia, which caused the majority of deaths related to surgery in one series (Bruecker *et al.*, 1989b).

Postoperative deterioration

Postoperative deterioration occurs with sufficient frequency in CCSM to warrant further discussion. A repeat myelogram should be performed in any dog that deteriorates after surgery. Potential reasons for deterioration include the following.

- **Inadequate removal of disc material** during ventral decompression can increase spinal cord compression as the intervertebral space collapses. This was seen in over 20% of dogs in one study that did not respond to ventral decompression (Chambers *et al.*, 1986). Collapse can also compress the nerve roots in the intervertebral foramen, thereby increasing cervical hyperaesthesia.
- **Decompression** via either a dorsal or ventral approach may exacerbate any instability.
- **Ischaemic or reperfusion injury** of the spinal cord could occur either during surgery or the immediate postoperative period.
- **Self-induced trauma** seems to occur as some dogs recover from anaesthesia (**365**), or when they make efforts to stand up as their neurological status improves (Bruecker *et al.*, 1989b). As a minimum precaution, neck collar restraint and vigorous exercise should be avoided for four months. The first 6–8 weeks are the most crucial, until significant bony or fibrous union has occurred. In the immediate postoperative period activity must be severely restricted, and some surgeons even confine the patient to a small kennel for one to two weeks. Activity is then gradually increased. Protective neck braces can be used but are often poorly tolerated.

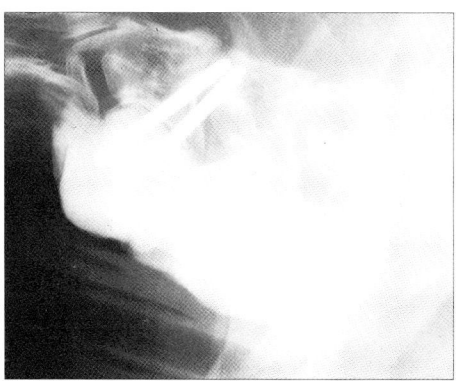

363 An excess of bone cement (or postoperative swelling as shown in 322 and 323) can cause compression of the structures in the thoracic inlet. Note that in this dog, the pins and bone cement have been used to bridge two intervertebral spaces, which is not recommended as the cement may fracture (Ellison *et al.*, 1988). In this patient, the pins are incorrectly positioned, pointing caudally in C_5.

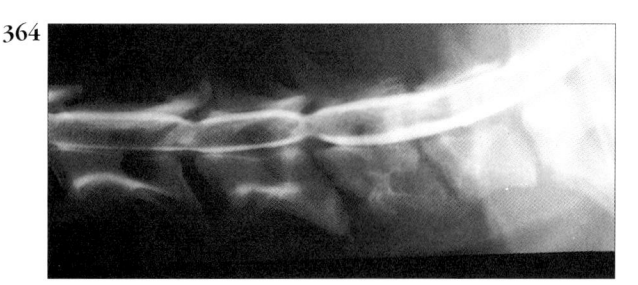

364 This dog had undergone a ventral decompression at C_6/C_7 one year previously. It suffered a second episode of tetraparesis, which was caused by a new lesion at C_5/C_6. This is an example of the domino effect.

- **Implant failure** can cause spinal cord trauma or postoperative pain. Excessive bone cement can also cause postoperative problems (**363**).
- **Any technique** can change the stresses placed on adjacent intervertebral spaces, causing spinal cord compression at a second site ('domino effect').

The domino effect

The domino effect (**364**) results from abnormal stresses imposed on an intervertebral space by fusion of the interspace immediately cranial or caudal to it. These stresses can exacerbate a subclinical instability and so result in disc protrusion or hypertrophy of ligamentous structures.

Domino lesions occur in about 20% of dogs after either ventral decompression or metal implant and bone cement fixation (see **Table 24**, page 141). They manifest as a second episode of paraparesis or tetraparesis occurring 6 months–4 years after the surgery, with a mean of 1.75–2.5 years (Seim, 1986; Bruecker *et al.*, 1989a ; Bruecker *et al.*, 1989b). Domino lesions do not seem to be a major complication of the screw and washer technique.

PROGNOSIS

The seriousness of this condition is illustrated by the fact that a quarter of dogs with CCSM in one series were euthanatized within six weeks of surgery for neurological problems (Seim, 1986). Dogs with more than one lesion generally have a worse prognosis than dogs with single lesions, and dogs with chronic tetraparesis have a very guarded prognosis. In contrast, dogs with a sudden onset of tetraparesis often respond well to surgery if treated promptly. Most severely tetraparetic dogs that will

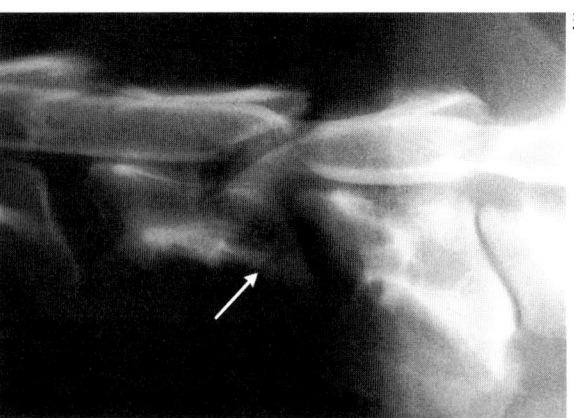

365 Radiograph of a dog with CCSM that made a good recovery following ventral decompression at C_5/C_6, but which then became severely tetraparetic while still in the hospital 36 hours after surgery. A small fracture is visible at the ventral aspect of C_5, presumably the result of a fall. The spinal cord compression that is apparent on the myelogram was confirmed at surgery to be due largely to rotational instability at the previously decompressed interspace. Distraction and stabilization was performed with screws and bone cement (see **332–334**), and the dog made a slow, but complete, recovery over the next four months (see also **482**).

recover do so within six weeks (Trotter, 1985).

A useful general estimate of the likely outcome in this condition has been provided by Seim (1986). For dogs with single lesions, about 80% of those that are walking before surgery will have a favourable outcome. However, only about 40% of those that cannot walk will recover. These success rates are some 20% lower for dogs with two lesions. It is hoped that careful tailoring of the surgical procedure to the exact type of lesion may be able to improve on these figures.

REFERENCES

Bruecker, K.A., Seim, H.B. and Blass, C.E. (1989a) Caudal cervical spondylomyelopathy: Decompression by linear traction and stabilization with Steinmann pins and polymethylmethacrylate. *Journal of the American Animal Hospital Association* **25**, 677–683.

Bruecker, K.A., Seim, H.B. and Withrow S.J. (1989b) Clinical evaluation of three surgical methods for treatment of caudal cervical spondylomyelopathy of dogs. *Veterinary Surgery* **18**, 197–203.

Chambers, J.N., Oliver, J.E., Kornegay, J.N. and Malnati, G.A. (1982) Ventral decompression for caudal cervical disk herniation in large and giant breed dogs. *Journal of the American Veterinary Medical Association* **180**, 410–414.

Chambers, J.N., Oliver, J.E. and Bjorling, D.E. (1986) Update on ventral decompression for caudal cervical disk herniation in Dobermann pinschers. *Journal of the American Animal Hospital Association* **22**, 775-778.

Clark, D.M. (1986) An analysis of intraoperative and early postoperative mortality associated with cervical spinal decompressive surgery in the dog. *Journal of the American Animal Hospital Association* **22**, 739–744.

DeLahunta, A. (1983) *Veterinary Neuroanatomy and Clinical Neurology*, 2nd edn, p. 204. W.B. Saunders Co., Philadelphia.

Denny, H.R., Gibbs, C. and Gaskell, C.J. (1977) Cervical spondylopathy in the dog – a review of thirty-five cases. *Journal of Small Animal Practice* **18**, 117–132.

Dodds, W.J. (1984) Von Willebrand's disease in dogs. *Modern Veterinary Practice* **65**, 681–686.

Dodds, W.J. (1989) Acquired von Willebrand's disease. *Proceedings of the 56th Annual Meeting of the American Animal Hospital Association.* pp 614–619.

Ellison, G.W., Seim, H.B. and Clemmons, R.M. (1988) Distracted cervical spinal fusion for management of caudal cervical spondylomyelopathy in large-breed dogs. *Journal of the American Veterinary Medical Association* **193**, 447–453.

Fox, P.R. (1989) Myocardial diseases. In *Textbook of Veterinary Internal Medicine*, 3rd edn, p. 1104. (Ed. S. J. Ettinger.) W. B. Saunders Co., Philadelphia.

Franklin, J.E. and Saunders, G.K. (1988) Chronic active hepatitis in Dobermann pinschers. *Compendium on Continuing Education for the Practicing Veterinarian* **10**, 1247–1254.

Giles, R., Tinlin, S. and Greenwood, R. (1982) A canine model of haemophilic (Factor VIII:C deficiency) bleeding. *Blood* **60**, 727–730.

Grant, B.D., Hoskinson, J.J., Barbee, D.D., Gavin, P.R., Sande, R.D. and Bayly, W.M. (1985) Ventral stabilization for decompression of caudal cervical spinal cord compression in the horse. *Proceedings of the 31st Annual Convention of the American Association of Equine Practitioners.* pp 75–103.

Jergens, A.E., Turrentine, M.A., Kraus, K.H. and Johnson, G.S. (1987) Buccal mucosal bleeding times of healthy dogs and of dogs in various pathologic states, including thrombocytopenia, uraemia and von Willebrand's disease. *American Journal of Veterinary Research* **48**, 1337–1342.

Lewis, D.D. and Hosgood, G. (1992) Complications associated with the use of iohexol for myelography of the cervical vertebral column in dogs: 66 cases (1988–1990). *Journal of the American Veterinary Medical Association* **200**, 1381–1384.

Lewis, D.G. (1989) Cervical spondylomyelopathy (wobbler's syndrome) in the dog: A study based on 224 cases. *Journal of Small Animal Practice* **30**, 657–665.

Lewis, D.G. (1992) Cervical spondylomyelopathy (wobbler' syndrome) in the dog: *In Practice* **14**, 125–130.

Lincoln, J.D. and Pettit, G.D. (1985) Evaluation of fenestration for treatment of degenerative disc disease in the caudal cervical region of large dogs. *Veterinary Surgery* **14**, 240–246.

Littlewood, J.D. (1991) Von willebrand disease in the dog. *Veterinary Annual* **31**, 163–172.

Lyman, R. and Seim, H.B. (1991) Viewpoint: Wobbler syndrome. Progress in Veterinary Neurology, **2**, 143–150.

Mason, T.A. (1979) Cervical vertebral instability (wobbler syndrome) in the dog. *Veterinary Record* **104**, 142–145.

McKee, W.M., Lavelle, R.B. and Mason, T.A. (1989) Vertebral stabilisation for cervical spondylopathy using a screw and washer technique. *Journal of Small Animal Practice* **30**, 337–342.

McKee, W.M., Lavelle, R.B., Richardson, J.L. and Mason, T.A. (1990) Vertebral distraction-fusion for cervical spondylopathy using a screw and double washer technique. *Journal of Small Animal Practice* **31**, 22–27.

Meyers, K.M., Wardrop, K.J. and Meinkoth, J. (1992) Canine von Willebrand's disease: Pathobiology, diagnosis and short-term treatment. *Compendium on Continuing Education for the Practicing Veterinarian* **14**, 13–21.

Peterson, M.E. and Ferguson, D.C. (1989) Thyroid diseases. In *Textbook of Veterinary Internal Medicine*, 3rd edn, p. 1644. (Ed. S. J. Ettinger.) W. B. Saunders Co., Philadelphia.

Seim, H.B. (1986) Caudocervical spondylomyelopathy. *Proceedings of the 14th Annual Veterinary Surgical Forum.* pp 72–78.

Seim, H.B. and Withrow, S.J. (1982) Pathophysiology and diagnosis of caudal cervical spondylomyelopathy with emphasis on the Dobermann pinscher. *Journal of the American Animal Hospital Association* **18**, 241–251.

Sharp, N.J.H., Wheeler, S.J. and Cofone, M. (1992) Radiological evaluation of `wobbler' syndrome–caudal cervical spondylomyelopathy. *Journal of Small Animal Practice* **333**, 490–499.

Trotter, E.J., deLahunta, A., Geary, J.C. and Brasmer, T.H. (1976) Caudal cervical vertebral malformation-malarticulation in Great Danes and Dobermann pinschers. *Journal of the American Veterinary Medical Association* **168**, 917–930.

Trotter, E.J. (1985) Canine wobbler syndrome. In *Textbook of Small Animal Orthopaedics*, pp 765–790. (Eds. C. D. Newton and D. M. Nunamaker.) J.B. Lippincott Co., Philadelphia.

Van Gundy, T.E. (1988) Disc-associated wobbler syndrome in the Dobermann pinscher. *Veterinary Clinics of North America, Small Animal Practice* **18**, 667–696.

Van Gundy, T.E. (1989) Canine wobbler syndrome. Part II. Treatment. *Compendium on Continuing Education for the Practicing Veterinarian* **11**, 269–284.

Walker, T.L. (1989) Use of Harrington rods in caudal cervical spondylomyelopathy. In *Current Techniques in Small Animal Surgery*, pp 584–586. (Ed. M. J. Bojrab.) Lea and Febiger, Philadelphia.

Walker, T.L., Tomlinson, J.Jr., Sorjonen, D.C. and Kornegay, J.N. (1985) Diseases of the spinal column. In *Textbook of Small Animal Surgery*, pp 1385–1391. (Ed.D. H. Slatter). W.B. Saunders Co., Philadelphia.

12. NEOPLASIA

Although spinal tumours are uncommon causes of spinal disease, they are significant once the common problems such as disc disease (in dogs) and trauma have been eliminated. Older animals are usually affected, although certain tumour types do occur in young individuals, notably lymphoma in cats.

CLINICAL SIGNS

Clinical signs produced by tumours of the spine are the same as those seen for any spinal disorder. Animals with spinal tumours often have a fairly typical pattern of initial nonspecific discomfort, followed by development of progressive neurological deficits and more definitive evidence of spinal pain. Severe neurological disabilities eventually develop if the case is allowed to progress. Marked muscle atrophy is often seen caudal to the lesion (**366**).

There are exceptions to this pattern. Sometimes there is a precipitous worsening following initially mild or even imperceptible signs. This can occur with vertebral body tumours where a pathological fracture develops, or in soft tissue tumours where the animal tolerates a slowly progressing degree of spinal cord compression well, until it reaches a critical point and there is severe deterioration in the neurological status. Vascular interference by the tumour may be responsible for this acute deterioration.

Tumours involving the brachial or lumbosacral plexus may present first as progressive unilateral lameness, and later with LMN deficits and spinal cord dysfunction if the vertebral canal is invaded.

Involvement of other body systems in diffuse neoplasia or metastasis may cause clinical signs unrelated to the nervous system. This is most common in cats with lymphoma. Paraneoplastic effects may also occur, particularly lymphoma-related hypercalcaemia.

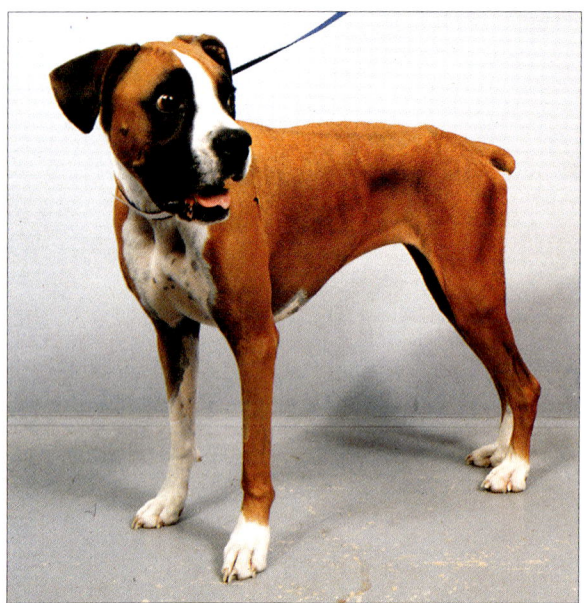

366 Six-year-old Boxer with osteosarcoma of the lumbar spine. Note the marked muscle atrophy in the pelvic limbs.

DIAGNOSIS

Spinal tumours can be diagnosed relatively easily using standard methods. Following a clinical and neurological examination, haematology, biochemistry and urinalysis are performed. Radiography is the technique with the highest diagnostic yield and will prove useful in the majority of cases. Survey radiographs of the spine are taken, although these may not be diagnostic of neoplasia. Part of the value of negative findings lies in the elimination of other conditions such as discospondylitis. Bony changes will be seen mainly in vertebral body tumours and occasionally in other tumours affecting bone (**367–369**).

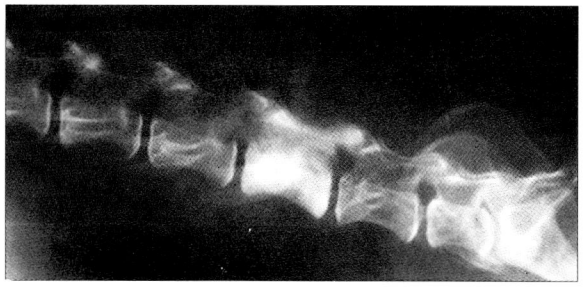

367 Survey radiograph of a six-year-old Spaniel with lumbar pain and paraparesis. Note the alteration in bone opacity in the vertebral body L$_5$. The histological diagnosis was osteosarcoma.

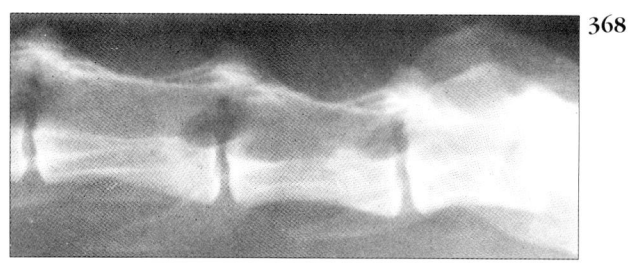

368 Survey radiograph of a nine-year-old cat with LMN signs in the pelvic limbs. Note widening of the vertebral canal in L$_6$ and enlargement of the L$_5$/L$_6$ intervertebral foramen. Histological diagnosis was neurofibrosarcoma of the L$_5$ spinal nerve. This type of tumour is generally slow growing and causes loss of bone by pressure atrophy rather than destruction.

369 Survey radiograph of the thoracic spine of a nine-year-old mixed breed dog with acute paraplegia preceded by a one-week history of spinal pain. There is collapse of the tumour-affected vertebral body. The histological diagnosis was osteosarcoma.

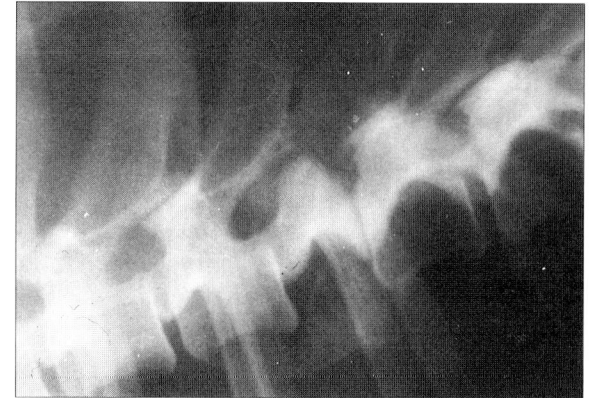

Most cases require myelography to reach a diagnosis (Wright *et al.*, 1979). Evaluation of the myelogram provides information about the location of the tumour, and also its position within the vertebral canal relative to the dura mater and spinal cord (see **84**). It is important to take two views (lateral and ventrodorsal) to allow correct evaluation of the myelogram. Other radiographic techniques may be useful to clarify the diagnosis or for surgical planning, such as CT (see **95–99**).

A CSF sample should be collected as occasionally neoplastic cells will be identified.

If a soft tissue extradural lesion is identified by myelography, collection of tissue from within the vertebral canal by needle aspiration may be attempted, thus potentially avoiding surgical intervention. This is facilitated by use of fluoroscopy (Irving and McMillan, 1990) (see **103–105**).

Spinal tumours do not often metastasize to the thorax but chest radiographs (three projections - both right and left laterals, and a ventrodorsal or dorsoventral) should always be taken with this possibility in mind.

Bone scanning may be useful to survey the entire skeleton in animals with tumours (see **101**).

The final stage of investigation may involve exploratory surgery and biopsy of the mass. In these circumstances, surgical debulking of the mass and adequate spinal cord decompression should be part of the procedure, but surgery should not be considered a definitive treatment for most spinal tumours.

PATHOLOGY

A large number of tumour types affect the spine. Many are only reported in small numbers, and these have been reviewed elsewhere (Bagley et al., 1993). The common types are given in **Table 27**. Spinal tumours are classified according to their location in the spine (see **84**) as extradural, intradural-extramedullary, or intramedullary.

Extradural tumours are the most prevalent type in dogs, accounting for approximately 50% of the cases. Intradural-extramedullary tumours make up one third and intramedullary tumours the remainder (Prata, 1977). Tumours of bone and nerve roots are most common in dogs; extradural lymphoma is most common in cats (Wheeler, 1989).

Table 27 Classification of major spinal tumour types according to location within the spine and histological type

Location	Type	Tumour
Extradural	Primary	Osteosarcoma Fibrosarcoma Chondrosarcoma Lymphoma Haemangiosarcoma Myeloma
	Secondary	Carcinoma Sarcoma Melanoma Lymphoma

Intradural–extramedullary	Primary	Meningioma
		Nerve sheath tumours
		  (schwannoma,
		  neurofibroma,
		  neurofibrosarcoma)
		Neuroepithelioma
		Sarcoma
		Lymphoma

	Secondary	Metastatic
Intramedullary	Primary	Glioma Lymphoma Haemangiosarcoma Reticulosis
	Secondary	Metastatic

Extradural tumours

As the name implies, these tumours lie outside the dura mater. Thus, neoplasia of the vertebral bodies and tumours lying in the extradural space of the vertebral canal fall into this category. Most vertebral body tumours are osteosarcomas. Fibrosarcoma, chondrosarcoma, haemangiosarcoma, and myeloma are less frequent. Pain is a predominant feature. Some vertebral tumours cause mild clinical signs in the initial stages, but show a dramatic worsening if a pathological fracture ensues (see **369**).

Extradural tumours may be metastatic in origin (most commonly carcinomas) and involve the vertebrae or extradural space. Thus, the discovery of an extradural tumour may indicate the possible presence of a primary focus elsewhere, particularly the mammary or thyroid glands, or the kidney.

In cats, the most common extradural tumour is lymphoma (Wheeler, 1989; Spodnick et al., 1992). Lymphoma also occurs in dogs. These tumours have the propensity to involve the dura mater and the spinal cord substance itself, but are included in this classification as the usual site is extradural. While neurological dysfunction may be the predominant sign, it should be remembered that systemic involvement of some sort is common with this disease.

Radiographic and ultrasonographic examination of the thorax and abdomen, and aspiration of lymph nodes and bone marrow are indicated to identify and stage the tumour (Gorman, 1991a).

Intradural–extramedullary

These tumours lie within the dura mater but outside the spinal cord parenchyma. The most common are meningiomas and nerve sheath tumours (neurofibroma, neurofibrosarcoma, schwannoma). Meningiomas are far less common in the spinal cord than in the brain. Nerve sheath tumours make up the majority of neoplasms in this location. Where they occur in the cervical (C_1–C_5) and thoracolumbar (T_3–L_3) spine, signs of spinal dysfunction are seen, as they cause spinal cord compression. The LMN dysfunction associated with these tumours makes electromyography useful, particularly in identifying which nerve roots are involved (see 'Electromyography,' page 54).

In young dogs, signs of thoracolumbar spinal disease may be caused by an unusual tumour - the neuroepithelioma, which typically occurs near the thoracolumbar junction in an intradural-extramedullary location (Summers *et al.*, 1988).

Intramedullary

Intramedullary tumours occur within the spinal cord substance and are the least common type. They are either gliomas or, very occasionally, metastatic tumours. Some cases of lymphoma in cats affect the spinal cord substance.

TREATMENT

Treatment is not possible in every animal with a spinal tumour, but an aggressive approach will prove rewarding in some patients. Vertebral body tumours are rarely good candidates for treatment, with the exception of myeloma.

Medical treatment

Medical treatment of spinal tumours is unlikely to provide curative therapy in most patients. Palliative therapy (analgesics, anti-inflammatory agents) may be used to alleviate peritumoural oedema, thus relieving clinical signs for relatively short periods. In lymphoma, chemotherapy alone may be employed if the diagnosis is reached without surgical intervention, and should be used following surgery (Gorman, 1991b).

Medical treatment also has a role in surgical patients. Spinal tumours are often painful and postoperative analgesia may be required (see Chapter 15). Medical management of paraneoplastic effects and metabolic derangements is also important.

Radiation treatment

Again, the value of radiation treatment is probably as an adjunct to surgery, although it may have a primary role in some tumours, particularly lymphoma (Dobson, 1991).

Surgical treatment

In the majority of cases where spinal tumours are diagnosed, surgical intervention may be considered. Surgery is directed toward two goals.
- To collect tissue for histopathological evaluation.
- To promote improved spinal cord function by a combination of tumour removal and decompression.

Surgical intervention is most appropriate where the mass is in the extradural space or in an intradural-extramedullary location. Surgical approaches must be tailored to the location of the tumour. Generally, wide exposure of the tumour and spinal cord is desirable.

Dorsal laminectomy is the approach of choice in most patients, although hemilaminectomy may be suitable in some. The 'ventral slot' approach is rarely useful for spinal tumour exploration as access to the spinal cord and nerve roots is severely limited.

Some general principles apply to the surgical removal of spinal tumours. Generally it is incorrect to think that a tumour has been completely removed. Because the spinal cord and the mass are often adjacent, it can be difficult to excise all neoplastic tissue and it is usually impossible to remove a wide enough border of tissue to prevent recurrence.

Removal of all visible neoplastic tissue could lead to the development of neurological deficits more severe than were present before surgery, which may or may not improve after surgery. Often the surgeon has to weigh the advantages of tumour removal against potential damage to the spinal cord and resulting neurological impairment. The use of surgical magnification (loupes or operating microscope) makes identification of tumour margins easier. Assuming that some neoplastic tissue is nearly always left behind, other therapies (chemotherapy or radiation) should be considered almost mandatory as follow up treatment. Their use before surgery may be considered to reduce tumour bulk.

Mass removal may lead to reperfusion injury of the spinal cord, and spinal cord manipulation can damage the nervous tissue. Use of methylprednisolone perioperatively may therefore be useful (see Chapter 6).

SURGERY

Dorsal laminectomy (370–381)

Cervical dorsal laminectomy is covered in **349–362**. Thoracolumbar dorsal laminectomy is covered below.

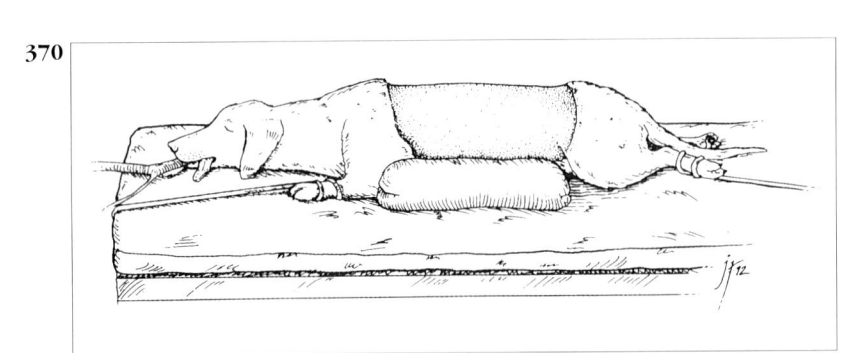

370 Positioning of dog for thoracolumbar dorsal laminectomy.

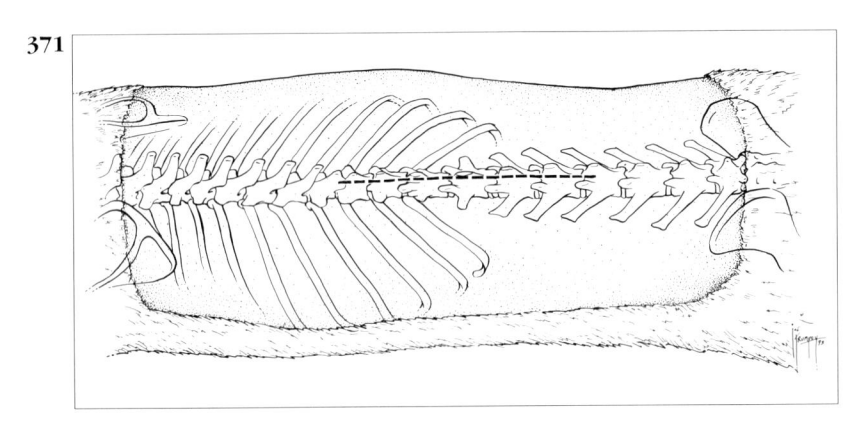

371 The skin incision is made 1 cm to one side of the midline. The precise site of the incision is governed by the location of the lesion.

12 NEOPLASIA

372 The skin is incised just off the midline, at least two vertebrae each side of the vertebra to be approached. The superficial fascia is mobilized and retracted to reveal the lumbodorsal fascia. Here the fascia has been incised, revealing the spinous processes.

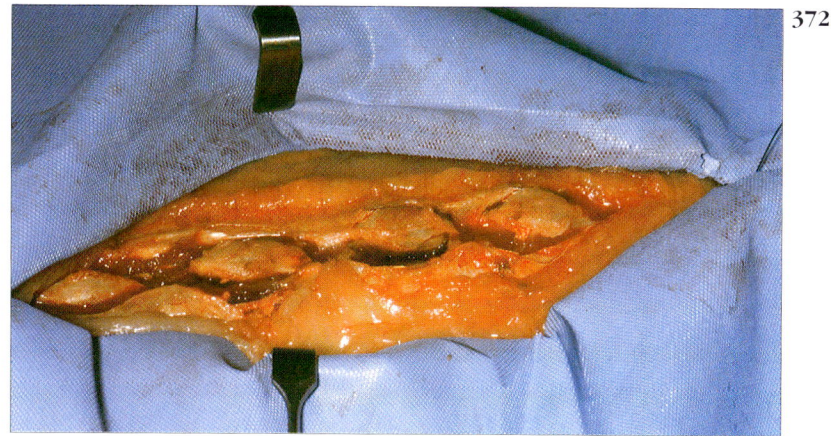

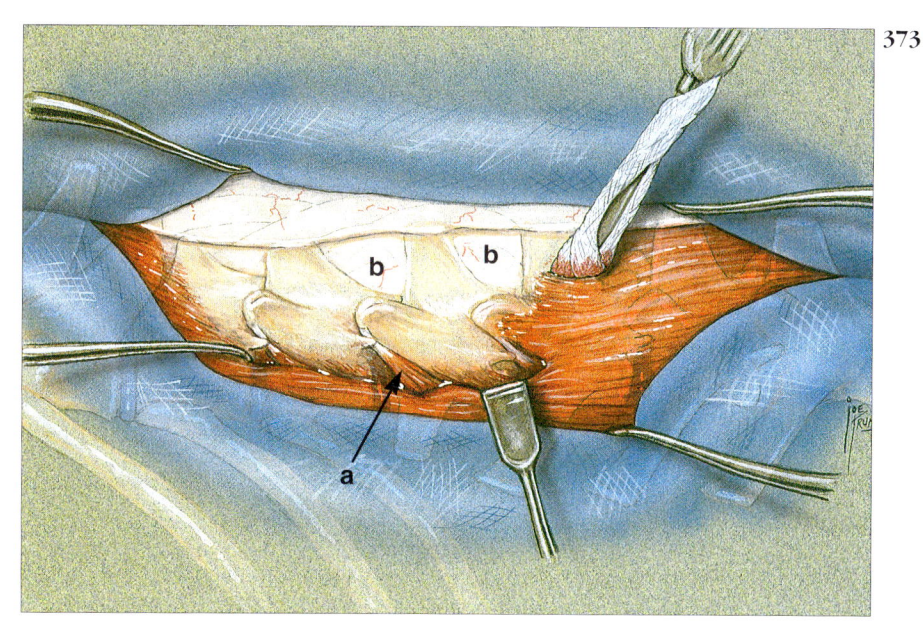

372

373

373 The lumbodorsal fascia is incised close to the spinous processes (arrows), revealing the epaxial muscles. These are elevated from the spinous processes and vertebral arch as in thoracolumbar hemilaminectomy (Chapter 8). There is a small muscular attachment to the accessory process (**a**). This tendon may be cut and the muscle belly retracted laterally. Care must be taken to avoid damaging the spinal nerve and vessels that lie under this muscle. The interspinous ligament (**b**) is removed from between the spinous processes.

161

DIAGNOSIS AND SURGERY OF SMALL ANIMAL SPINAL DISORDERS

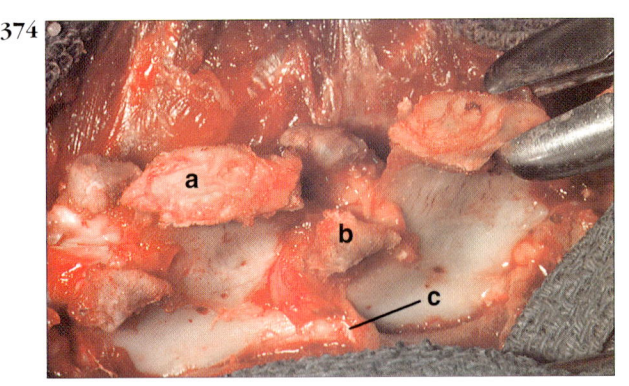

374 The multifidus muscles are elevated from the spinous processes (a) and the vertebral arch. This reveals the articular processes (**b**), and the tendinous attachment to the accessory process (**c**). The muscle retraction is maintained with Gelpi retractors. The dissection is completed on one side before starting the other side. The spinous processes are removed with rongeurs or bone cutters.

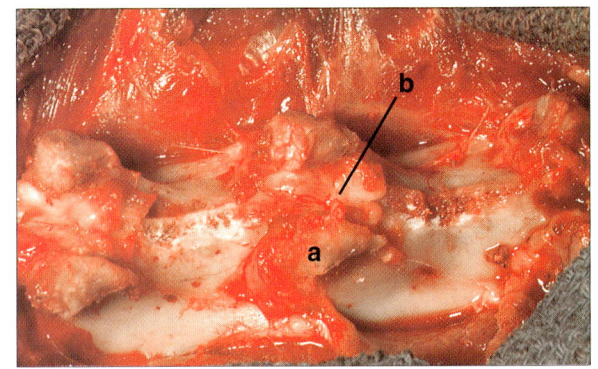

375 The spinous processes have been removed. The articular processes are still present (**a**) and the ligamentum flavum is visible (**b**).

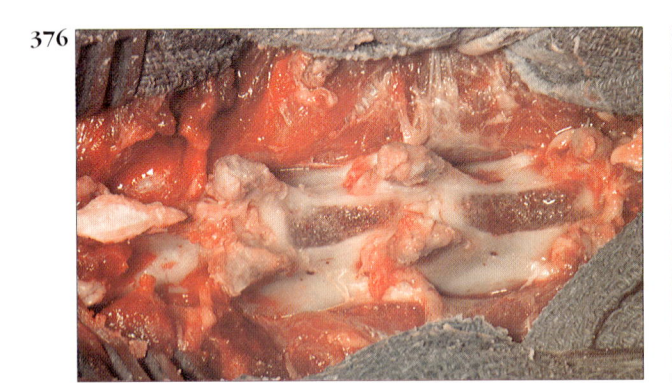

376 The laminectomy is commenced in the midline with a bur, preserving the articular processes at this stage. Here the cortical bone has been removed over two vertebrae, revealing the dark cancellous bone. See Chapter 10 for details on technique for using the bur.

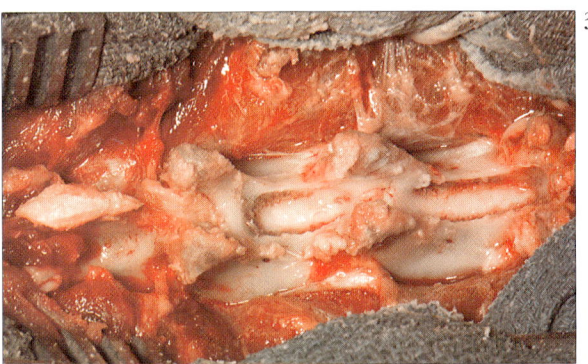

377 The cancellous bone has been removed with the bur to reveal the inner cortical bone. This is then thinned to eggshell thickness.

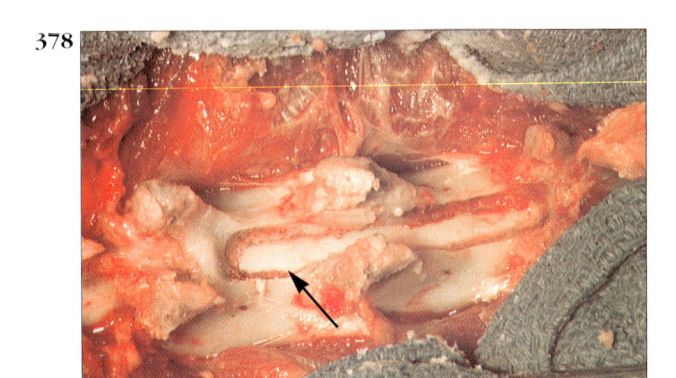

378 The final layer of bone is removed to reveal the spinal cord (arrow). This is achieved with fine rongeurs and a curette. This degree of exposure may be adequate for some circumstances.

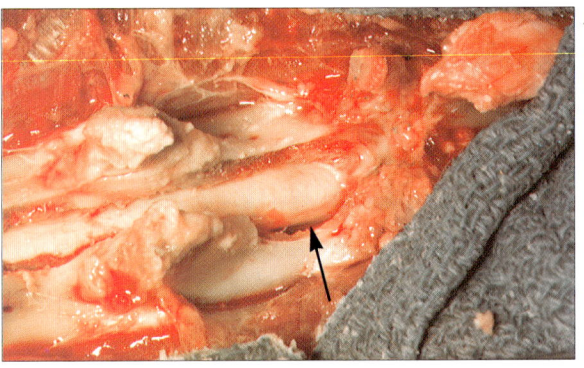

379 The approach can be modified depending on requirements. Here the pedicle is removed between the articular processes to expose the lateral aspect of the spinal cord (arrow).

12 NEOPLASIA

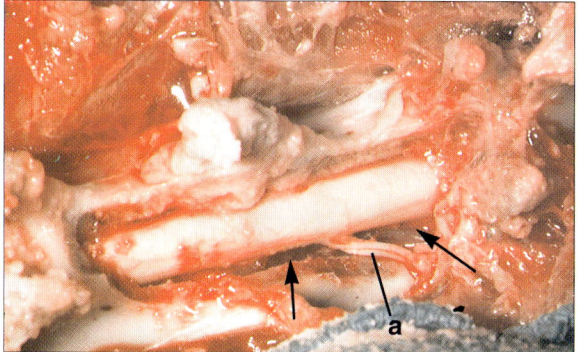

380 Here the left articular processes have been removed, as has the pedicle of the two vertebrae. This gives good access to the spinal nerve (**a**). Note the vertebral plexus lying on the floor of the vertebral canal (arrows); this should be avoided.

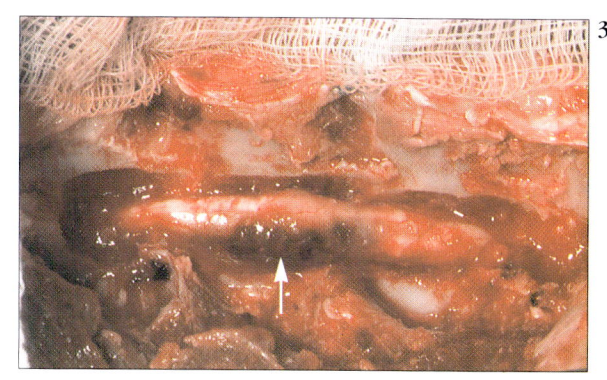

381 Spinal tumour surgically exposed (arrow). Histological diagnosis was a sarcoma.

Wound closure is routine. The laminectomy is covered with a fat graft or surgical cellulose. The muscles are apposed by continuous suture, and the lumbodorsal fascia closed with monofilament absorbable suture. (Dorsal laminectomy may be performed by the method shown here in traumatic injuries. If this is done, some type of spinal stabilisation is essential; see Chapter 13).

Hemilaminectomy (382–394)

Cervical hemilaminectomy is described below. Thoracolumbar hemilaminectomy is covered in **185–213**.

382 Patient positioning for cervical hemilaminectomy via a dorsolateral approach.

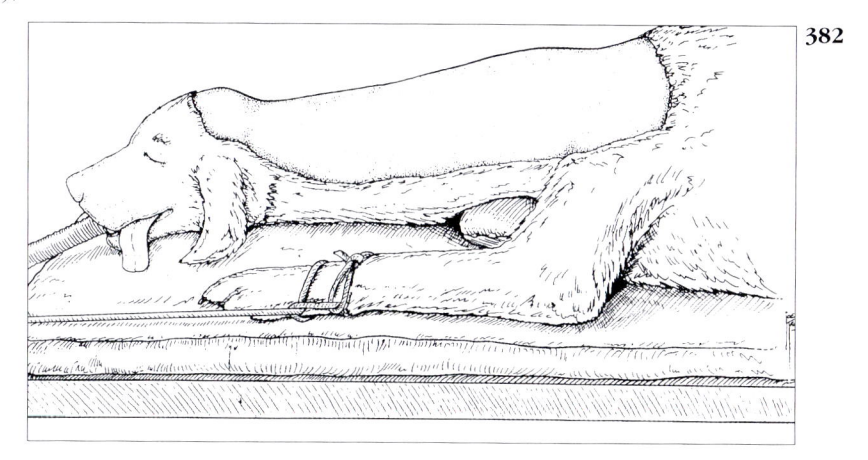

383 To approach the midcervical vertebrae, the incision extends from the occipital protuberance to the spinous process of T_2. The skin incision is to one side of the midline.

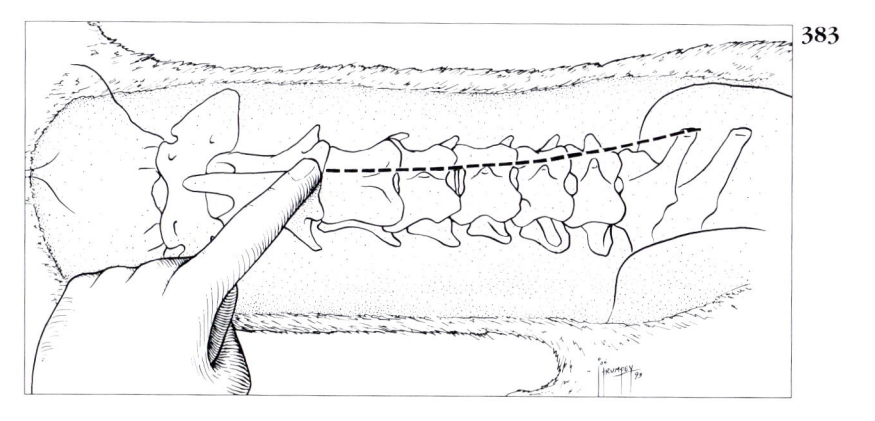

163

384

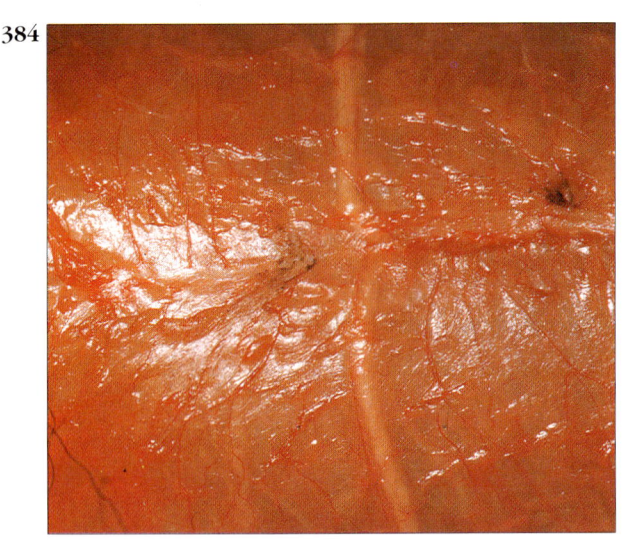

384 The skin and superficial fascia are incised to reveal the superficial muscles. Note the dorsal branches of the cervical nerves emerging in the midline and diverging laterally. The details of the anatomy are covered in Chapters 9 and 11.

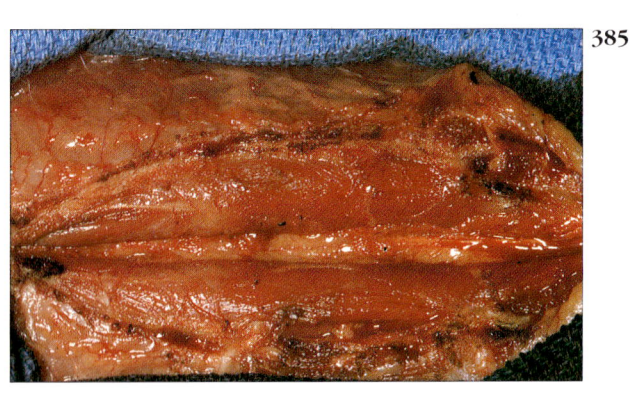

385

385 The incision is continued in the midline through the muscular aponeurosis. There are numerous blood vessels in the midline, which must be ligated or cauterized as necessary. The nuchal ligament is visible here and can be palpated.

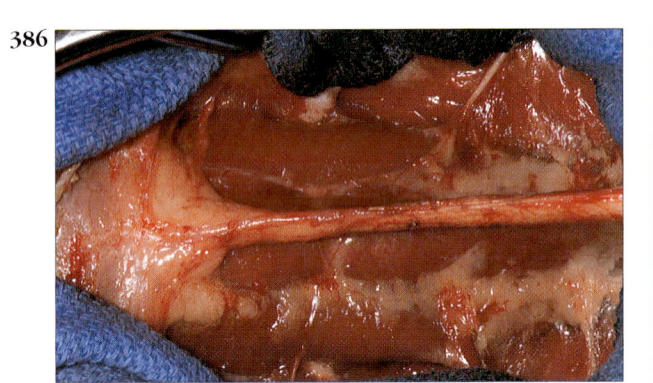

386

386 Nuchal ligament exposed. This may be retracted away from the surgeon or divided in the midline.

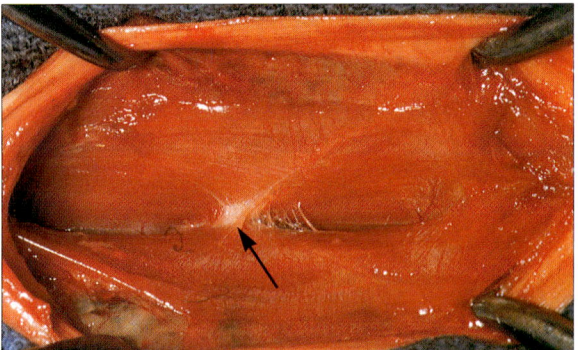

387

387 The nuchal ligament has been divided in the midline, as have the spinalis muscles. This reveals the muscular attachments to the spinous process of the cervical vertebra (arrow).

12 NEOPLASIA

388 The spinalis muscles have been elevated from the spinous processes (a) and vertebral laminae (b) on the side of the spine to be approached.

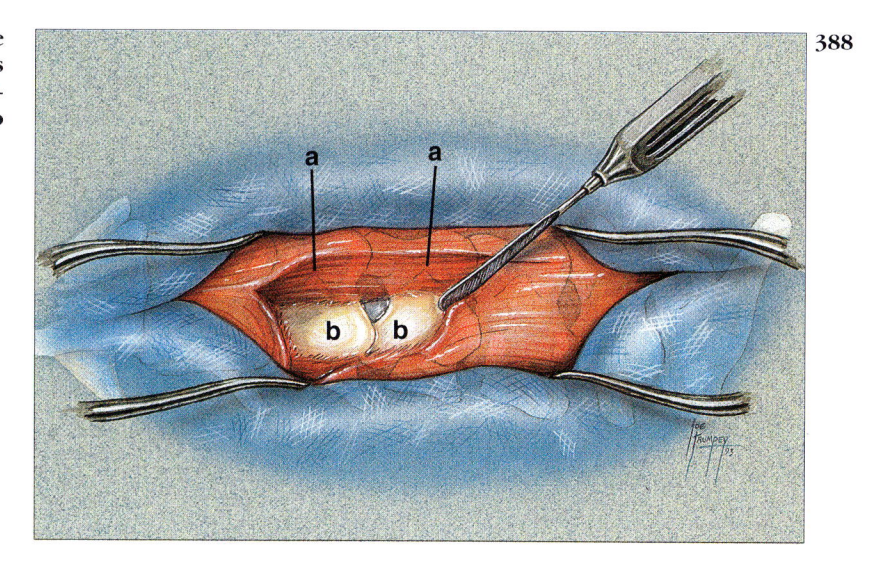

389 The paraspinal muscles are elevated from the articular process (a) and then further ventrally. Branches of the vertebral artery emerges here and must be ligated. The spinous process (**b**) and lamina (**c**) are seen here (see **9**).

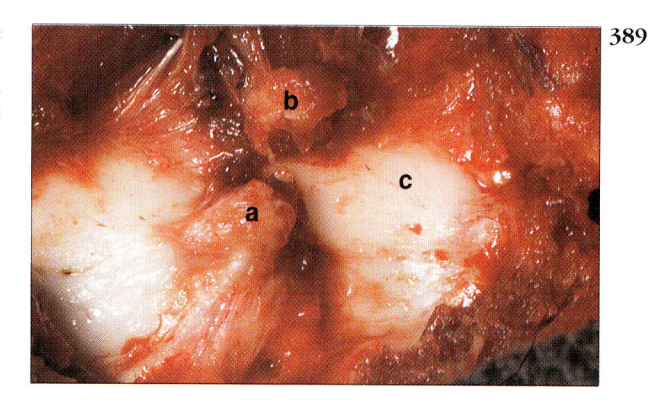

390 The articular process is removed with rongeurs. The laminectomy is commenced with a bur. Here the cartilage of the articular surfaces can be seen (arrow).

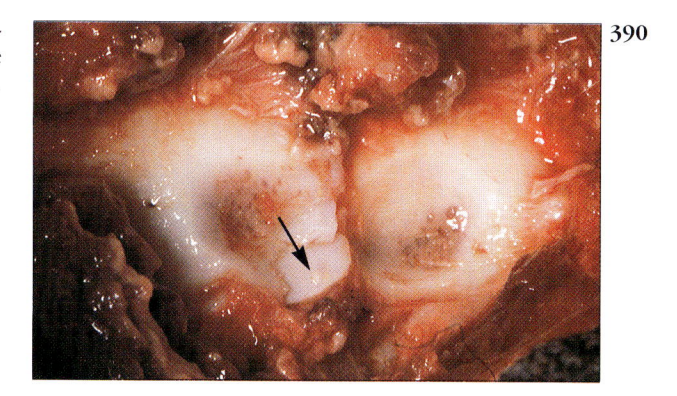

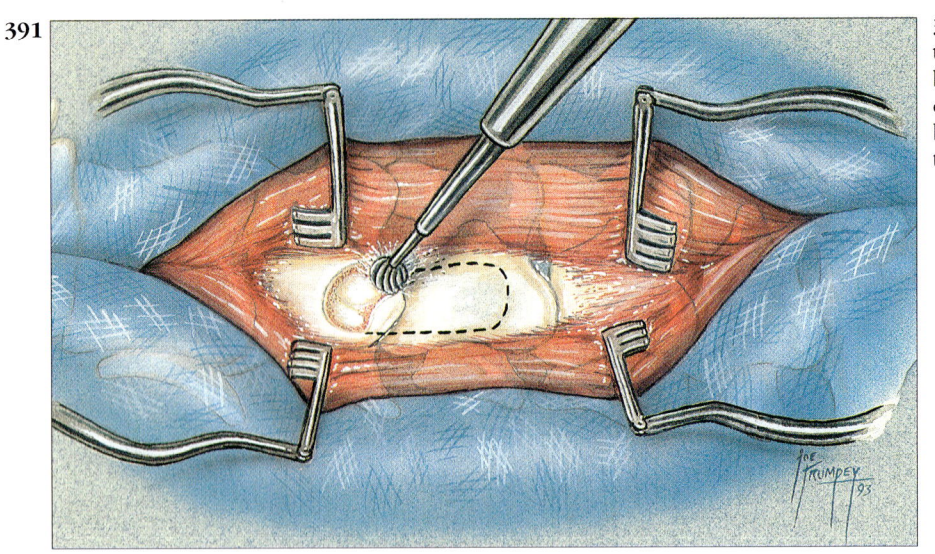

DIAGNOSIS AND SURGERY OF SMALL ANIMAL SPINAL DISORDERS

391 Site of hemilaminectomy. Here the bone has been removed in the most cranial vertebra. The site of bone removal is shown in the caudal vertebra.

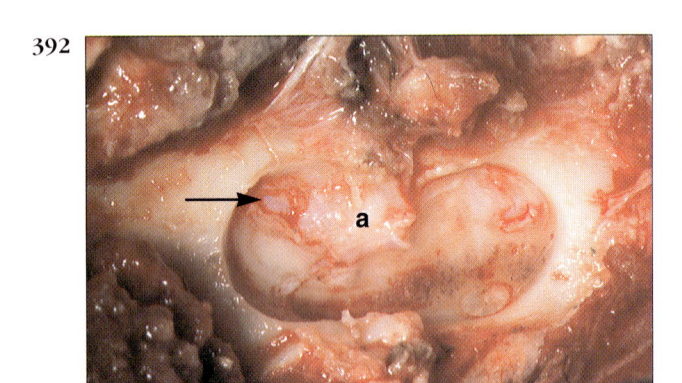

392 Bone is removed until the vertebral canal is entered. The bone is bured to eggshell thickness before the vertebral canal is entered. Here the inner cortical bone is visible, and the canal has been entered in the craniodorsal corner (arrow). The joint capsule is visible in the centre of the defect (**a**).

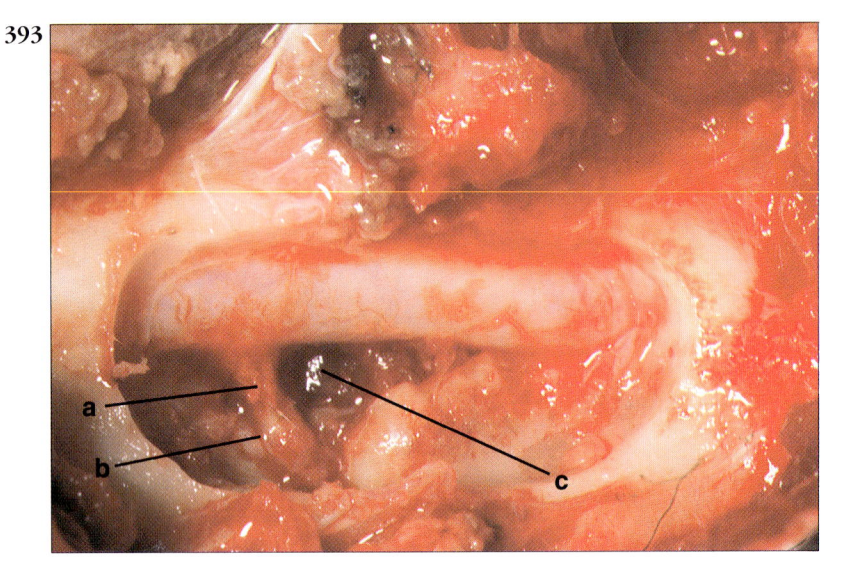

393 The laminectomy is continued to reveal the spinal cord. It may be extended into the intervertebral foramen to expose the nerve root (**a**) and spinal ganglion (**b**). Large branches of the vertebral artery and vein are present at this level. Haemorrhage may also occur from the internal vertebral venous plexus. This is best controlled with surgical cellulose or, as in this case, a piece of macerated muscle (**c**).

12 NEOPLASIA

394 The laminectomy is continued into the intervertebral foramen to reveal the nerve root and spinal ganglion. The laminectomy may be extended as appropriate for removal of neoplasms.

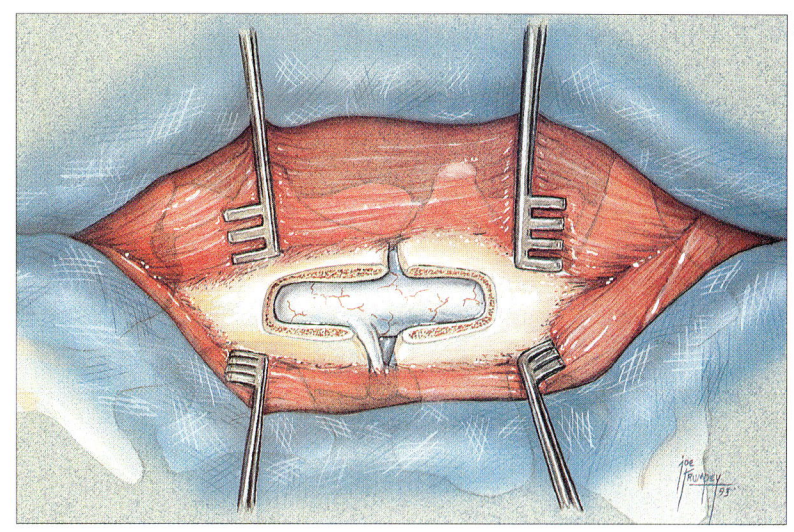

The defect is covered with a fat graft or surgical cellulose. Wound closure is routine.

Tumour dissection

Gentle tissue handling is vital in removal of spinal cord tumours. Manipulation of the spinal cord must be kept to a minimum to avoid iatrogenic spinal cord damage; it is preferable to avoid touching the spinal cord at all if possible. Performing an extensive laminectomy makes removal of extradural tumours easier. The use of keyhole approaches is not good practice.

Sacrificing a spinal nerve and vessels to improve access is useful if the tumour is difficult to remove, but this should be avoided if possible in the brachial and lumbosacral plexuses because of the LMN deficits that are caused. If the tumour is involving the dura mater, sharp dissection is used to avoid spinal cord manipulation.

Soft tumours can be removed by gentle suction, but it is important to retain a piece of the mass for histopathology. Intramedullary tumours are best approached via durotomy and dorsal myelotomy, followed by gentle dissection (see Chapter 6).

COMPLICATIONS

The neurological status of the patient may deteriorate, particularly after extensive spinal cord manipulations. Use of perioperative methylprednisolone may be useful in this regard (see Chapter 6). Making the incision away from the midline may reduce any tendency for wound breakdown by avoiding tension over the spinous processes. Good haemostasis is vital. Seroma or haematoma formation should be attended to carefully (see Chapters 6 and 15).

Dorsal laminectomy with removal of the articular processes reduces the stability of the spine (see Chapter 13). This should not be an important problem in animals with spinal tumours. Fat grafts are often used to cover dorsal laminectomies (**395** and 'Laminectomy healing,' page 64).

395 Fat graft reaction after dorsal laminectomy. The neurological status of this patient deteriorated significantly several days after the original surgery. Myelography revealed extradural compression. The graft was removed at a subsequent operation and the dog recovered. No bacteria were cultured from the fat graft. It is important not to make the graft too thick. See pages 64 and 65.

POSTOPERATIVE CARE (see Chapter 15)

Routine nursing considerations are discussed in Chapter 15. The use of analgesics is indicated in patients following radical spinal surgery. Some patients have a worse neurological status following surgery to remove tumours and, therefore, require a high standard of nursing care. If radiation treatment is planned, it is usual to delay this until the skin incision has healed.

PROGNOSIS

In some circumstances, where the tumour is not amenable to treatment because of its location, or where a fracture has occurred, euthanasia is indicated. Treatment may only lead to short term remission in some patients, but the quality of life during that period can be acceptable.

Longer term remission can often be achieved for lymphoma in both dogs and cats, leading to a significant degree of neurological recovery. Cats usually succumb eventually to systemic effects of the disease (Lane and Kornegay, 1991; Spodnick *et al.*, 1992). Some dogs that have resection of meningiomas have lengthy remission periods (Fingeroth *et al.*, 1987). Spinal tumours do tend to recur locally, usually because of incomplete resection. Widespread metastasis is rare. Radiation therapy may help reduce local recurrence following surgery and improve the prognosis in some patients.

FELINE SPINAL TUMOURS

Spinal tumours account for over half of all cases of feline spinal disease not associated with trauma (Wheeler, 1989).

A limited number of tumour types have been reported in the feline spine; lymphoma is the most common. Neurological signs were seen in 8% of cats with systemic lymphoma in one series (Meincke *et al.*, 1972) and 11% in another (Kornegay, 1981). While these figures cannot be regarded as absolute, they give an indication of the number of cats with lymphoma that have nervous system involvement.

Zaki and Hurvitz (1976) found that 82% of cats with lymphoma of the CNS had spinal involvement. In these cats, the tumours were situated extradurally with a low incidence of involvement of the vertebral bodies, dura mater or spinal cord itself. Other authors suggest that neoplastic infiltration of these structures is relatively common (Kornegay, 1981). In Zaki and Hurvitz's study, all cats had lymphoma in other organs, suggesting that the spine had become involved secondary to metastatic spread. The bone marrow is involved in approximately 50% of cats with extradural lymphoma (Cotter, 1986); thus aspiration of bone marrow will aid in the diagnosis in these cases. The vast majority of cats with spinal lymphoma are FeLV positive (Lane and Kornegay, 1991; Spodnick *et al.*, 1992).

396 Soft tissue mass in the thorax of a cat (a), ventral to extradural compression (arrow). The final diagnosis was lymphoma.

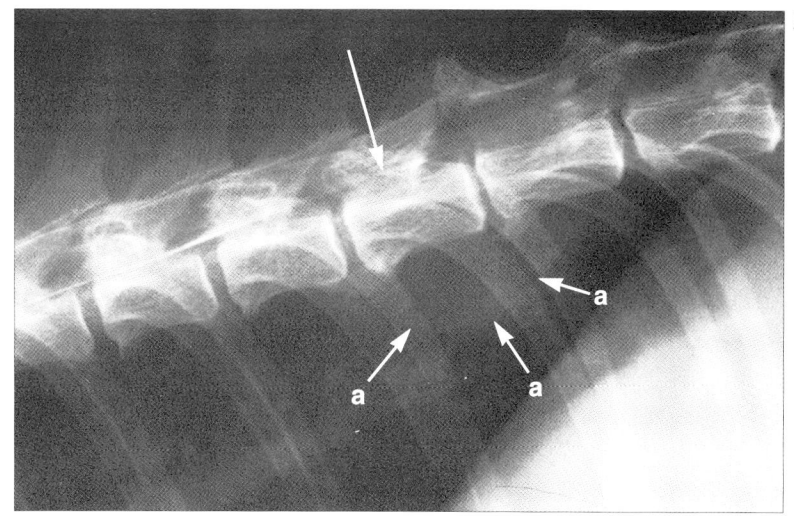

Other tumour types are far less commonly encountered. Vertebral osteosarcomas, myeloma, glioma, and neurofibrosarcoma have been reported (Wheeler, 1989). Meningiomas, while occurring commonly in the brain, are rarely seen in the spine (Luginbuhl et al., 1968).

Diagnosis

The diagnosis of feline spinal neoplasia is made largely by radiography. Some extradural tumours may affect the vertebral bodies, causing bony changes on survey radiographs, but this is not typical (see **368**). Myelography is required to confirm the diagnosis in most cats. In lymphoma, the myelogram usually reveals extradural compression although, occasionally, other patterns are seen, particularly if the nerve roots are involved. Other radiographic findings may indicate the possible presence of a spinal tumour (**396**). Soft tissue densities in the cranial thorax may be present with lymphoma affecting the mediastinum. Pulmonary metastases are rare.

Other diagnostic tests are indicated to confirm the presence of a tumour and to define its nature. Haematological evaluation, FeLV testing, bone marrow aspiration, and CSF analysis all contribute to the diagnosis. Lymphoma is one of the few CNS neoplasms where neoplastic cells may be seen in the CSF. Sometimes, fine needle aspiration (page 55) or biopsy at exploratory surgery may be the only means of making a histological diagnosis.

In an FeLV-positive cat with spinal disease related to an extradural soft tissue mass demonstrated by a myelogram, it may be reasonable to diagnose lymphoma and to treat the cat accordingly.

Treatment

In lymphoma, surgical debulking followed by chemotherapy may be performed, and should lead to a rapid improvement in neurological function. However, chemotherapy alone may lead to a similar rate of recovery (Cotter, 1986). Chemotherapeutic protocols are described elsewhere (Cotter, 1986; Gorman, 1991a). Clearly, surgical treatment alone in lymphoma is not appropriate, because of the multifocal nature of the disease. Radiotherapy may be of benefit in lymphoma, but also should be combined with chemotherapy (Lane and Kornegay, 1991; Dobson, 1991).

Where lymphoma has not been confirmed by other means, biopsy is required to make the diagnosis. Once the histological identity of the tumour is known, suitable therapy may be instituted. The ease with which dorsal laminectomy can be performed in the thoracolumbar spine of the cat makes surgical exploration a feasible proposition.

Prognosis

Initial improvement in the neurological status is likely following surgical excision, and this may be maintained for some time with appropriate chemotherapy. However, the long term prognosis is unfavourable because of the propensity for multifocal involvement, local recurrence or the development of systemic FeLV-related disease.

REFERENCES

Bagley, R.S., Kornegay, J.N., Page, R.L. and Thrall, D.E. (1993) Central nervous system. In *Textbook of Small Animal Surgery*, pp 2137–2166. (Ed. D. Slatter.) W.B. Saunders Co., Philadelphia.

Cotter, S.M. (1986) Clinical management of lymphoproliferative, myeloproliferative and plasma cell neoplasia. In *Oncology*, pp 169–194. (Ed. N.T. Gorman.) Churchill Livingstone, New York.

Dobson, J.M. (1991) Radiation therapy. In *Manual of Small Animal Oncology*, pp 161–173. (Ed. R.A.S. White.) BSAVA Publications, Cheltenham.

Fingeroth, J.M., Prata, R.G. and Patnaik, A.K. (1987) Spinal meningiomas in dogs: 13 cases (1972–1987). *Journal of the American Veterinary Medical Association* **191**, 720–726.

Gorman, N.T. (1991a) The haemolymphatic system. In *Manual of Small Animal Oncology*, pp 207–235. (Ed. R.A.S. White.) BSAVA Publications, Cheltenham.

Gorman, N.T. (1991b) Chemotherapy. In *Manual of Small Animal Oncology*, pp 127–159. (Ed. R.A.S. White.) BSAVA Publications, Cheltenham.

Irving, G. and McMillan, M.C. (1990) Fluoroscopically guided percutaneous fine needle aspiration biopsy of thoracolumbar spinal lesions in cats. *Progress in Veterinary Neurology* **1**, 473–475.

Kornegay, J.N. (1981) Feline neurology. *Compendium on Continuing Education for the Practicing Veterinarian* **3**, 203–213.

Kornegay, J.N. (1986) Central nervous system neoplasia. In *Neurologic Disorders: Contemporary Issues in Small Animal Practice* Vol. 5, pp 79–108. (Ed. J.N. Kornegay). Churchill Livingstone, New York.

Lane, S.B. and Kornegay, J.N. (1991) Spinal lymphosarcoma. In *Consultations in Feline Internal Medicine*. (Ed. J.R. August.) W.B. Saunders Co., Philadelphia.

Luginbuhl, H., Fankhauser, R. and McGrath, J.T. (1968) Spontaneous neoplasms of the nervous system of animals. *Progress in Neurological Surgery* **2**, 85.

Meincke, J.E., Hobbie, W.V. and Hardy, W.D. (1972) Lymphoreticular malignancies in the cat: clinical findings. *Journal of the American Veterinary Medical Association* **160**, 1093–1099.

Prata, R.G. (1977) Diagnosis of spinal cord tumours in the dog. *Veterinary Clinics of North America, Small Animal Practice* **7(1)**, 165–185.

Spodnick, G.J., Berg, J., Moore, F.M. and Cotter, S.M. (1992) Spinal lymphoma in cats: 21 cases (1976–1989). *Journal of the American Veterinary Medical Association* **200**, 373–376.

Summers, B.A., DeLahunta, A., McEntee, M. and Kuhajda, F.P. (1988) A novel intradural extramedullary spinal cord tumor in young dogs. *Acta Neuropathologica* (Berlin), **75**, 402–410.

Wheeler, S.J. (1989) Spinal tumours in cats. *Veterinary Annual* **29**, 270–277.

Wright J.A., Bell, D.A. and Clayton Jones, D.G. (1979) The clinical and radiological features associated with spinal tumours in thirty dogs. *Journal of Small Animal Practice* **20**, 461–472.

Zaki, F.A. (1977) Spontaneous central nervous system tumors in the dog. *Veterinary Clinics of North America, Small Animal Practice* **7(1)**, 153–163.

Zaki, F.A. and Hurvitz, A.L. (1976) Spontaneous neoplasms of the central nervous system of the cat. *Journal of Small Animal Practice* **17**, 773–782.

FURTHER READING

Cordy, D.R. (1990) Tumours of the nervous system and eye. In *Tumours in Domestic Animals*, pp 640–665. (Ed. J.E. Moulton.) University of California Press.

Hayes, H.M., Priester, W.A. and Pendergrass, T. (1975) Occurrence of nervous tissue tumours in cattle, horses, cats and dogs. *International Journal of Cancer* **15**, 39.

Luttgen, P.J., Braund, K.G., Brawner, W.R. and Vandevelde, M. (1980) A retrospective study of twenty-nine spinal tumours in the dog and the cat. *Journal of Small Animal Practice* **21**, 213–226.

13. TRAUMA

Trauma can result in a variety of spinal lesions (**Table 28**). Diagnosis should be straightforward from the history and physical findings in most dogs, but occasional cat owners are not aware of what has befallen their pet.

Table 28 Types of spinal injury

Vertebral fracture
Vertebral (sub)luxation
Vertebral fracture/luxation
Traumatic disc herniation
Spinal cord concussion

After the initial assessment and systemic stabilization of a spinal trauma patient, the general principles of treatment can be summarized as follows.
- Use methylprednisolone within 6–8 hours of the injury (see Chapter 6).
- Reduce vertebral malalignment and relieve spinal cord compression. Thoracolumbar fracture/luxations causing significant narrowing of the vertebral canal usually require surgical decompression. However decompression is not normally required if vertebral alignment is good or with concussive injuries.
- Provide stability by cage confinement, an external splint, or internal fixation.

INITIAL ASSESSMENT

Other injuries
The first priority is to treat shock and other life-threatening disorders (**397**). A thorough and meticulous physical examination is essential at this stage as many animals have additional non-neural injuries, which could be overlooked. **Table 29** lists some of the other disorders that may be associated with spinal trauma. In one study, 20% of dogs with injuries to the lumbar vertebrae had pelvic fractures, and 33% had cardiopulmonary lesions (Turner, 1987).

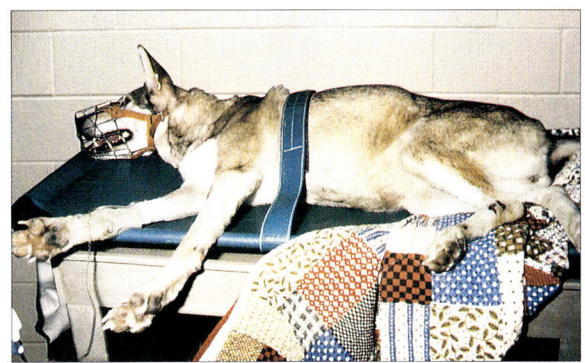

397 This dog is undergoing initial assessment for spinal trauma caused by a road traffic accident six hours earlier. The dog has been muzzled and strapped to a rigid board before being examined and radiographed. Aggressive intravenous fluid therapy is in progress and high-dose methylprednisolone will be given by slow intravenous injection.

Table 29 Other injuries associated with spinal trauma

Shock
Pulmonary or pleural lesions
Diaphragmatic rupture
Traumatic cardiomyopathy
Damaged urinary tract
Ruptured bile duct
Injury to other abdominal organs
Long bone or pelvic fractures
Brachial or lumbosacral plexus injury
Soft tissue injuries
Head injuries

Cardiovascular system

Post-traumatic cardiac arrhythmias are common and are easily overlooked as they can be delayed in onset by up to 48 hours. Periodic auscultation and ECG monitoring are required during this time. Arrhythmias can decrease cardiac output, reducing spinal cord perfusion and complicating anaesthesia, as well as being potentially fatal (Murtaugh and Ross, 1988).

Urinary tract

Bladder rupture usually causes discomfort on abdominal palpation, vomiting, depression, and haematuria within 24–48 hours. Damage to other parts of the urinary tract may take from 1–3 days to become clinically apparent, depending on the site and the degree of injury.

Other

Bile duct rupture, although rare, can result in unexplained patient deterioration 5–15 days after injury (Neer, 1992). As some injuries are not immediately apparent, the owner should be forewarned of possible further diagnostic evaluation and treatment.

After the initial assessment (including deep pain evaluation - see below) the patient is given analgesics. The narcotic agonists are preferred unless there is concomitant respiratory depression or head injury (see **Table 34,** page 204). Analgesia should be combined with some form of stabilization for the injury, so that the animal does not damage itself further. If presented within eight hours of injury, high-dose methylprednisolone should be given by slow intravenous injection (see Chapter 6). Sedatives should not be used routinely, because they do not address the problem of pain and may remove normal protective muscle tone. Adverse effects on the cardiovascular system may exacerbate shock and compromise spinal cord blood flow.

NEUROLOGICAL EXAMINATION

The neurological examination is essential to localize the deficit, to identify multiple spinal lesions, and to determine the prognosis. The single, most important prognostic factor following spinal trauma is the presence or absence of deep pain sensation (see **43**). If deep pain is absent caudal to a traumatic lesion, the prognosis for return of neurological function is very poor. Analgesics should only be given after deep pain has been assessed, as they could alter the findings.

RADIOGRAPHY

Survey radiography

Once a neuroanatomical diagnosis has been reached, survey radiographs are taken. The clinician must remember that radiographs are no substitute for the neurological examination; it is not possible to estimate the neurological status from the radiographs alone. Lateral views of the area of spine where the lesion is located are taken first. Oblique views to assess the articular processes may be taken with the animal in lateral recumbency and the beam angled (**398** and **408**).

Dorsoventral radiographs are best taken by the horizontal beam view. Failing that, extreme care must be taken when positioning the animal for ventrodorsal or dorsoventral radiographs. Anaesthesia

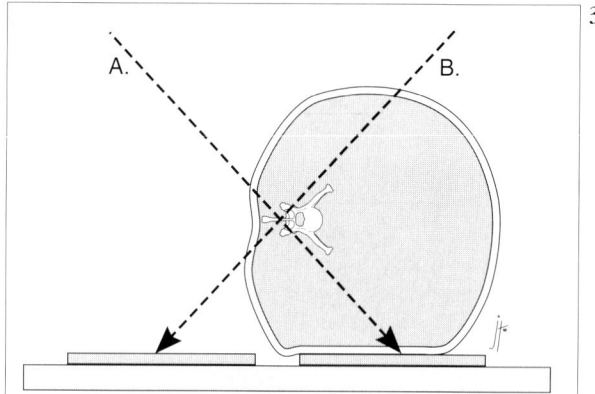

398 Diagram to illustrate assessment of the articular processes with the dog in lateral recumbency and with the X-ray beam angled. The process closest to the film is highlighted with the beam angled as in A; the other process by the beam angle B.

or heavy sedation is undesirable at this stage, as it will reduce the stabilizing effect of paravertebral muscle spasm. Some estimate of the stability of the fracture is gauged from its radiographic appearance (see below) and by careful palpation over the site. Multiple vertebral fractures are not common, and when they do occur, they are mostly restricted to the lumbar and sacral areas (Feeney and Oliver, 1980; Selcer et al., 1991).

Myelography

The next decision is whether to perform a myelogram. Advantages of myelography are as follows.
- Identification of other lesions when survey radiographs do not correlate with the neurological localization.
- Determining if there is persistent spinal cord compression, thus indicating if decompression is needed for extradural bone fragments, blood clots, or disc material.
- Identification of spinal cord transection. Even if there appears to be little displacement of the fracture at the time of presentation, there may have been a transient yet complete luxation at the time of the original trauma (**399**).

Myelography may also help to rule out the first three differential diagnoses listed in **Table 30**. Myelography is recommended for potential surgical candidates. An animal with good deep pain sensation that is to be managed by an external splint or cage rest does not need a myelogram. The advantages of myelography need to be weighed against the additional anaesthetic time, the expense and the potential complications.

Computed tomography may be useful in determining the presence of bone fragments compressing the spinal cord.

Table 30 Differential diagnosis of spinal trauma

Fibrocartilaginous embolus
Degenerative disc disease
Pathological fracture - neoplasia or bone disease
Bilateral pelvic/long bone fracture or cruciate rupture
Ischaemic neuromyopathy (cats)

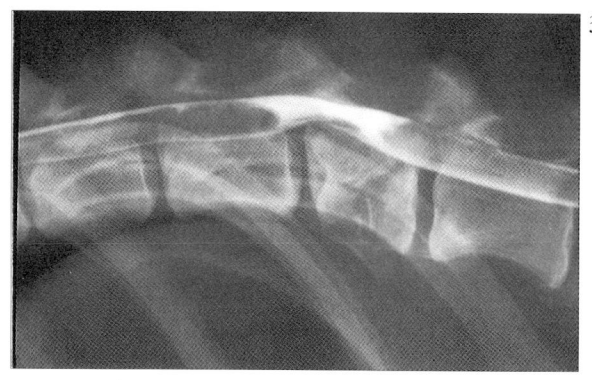

399 Myelographic appearance of a dog that has suffered an anatomical spinal cord transection following vertebral luxation. Note that there is minimal vertebral displacement at the time of radiography. The spinal cord was found to be completely transected at surgery.

BIOMECHANICS

Spinal fracture biomechanics

Fracture/luxations of the canine spine may be classified into three types, based on the anatomical compartment that has been compromised (**400**).
- **Damage to the dorsal compartment alone, including the vertebral arch or associated ligaments** (**401**). Injury to these structures is rare in isolation. Dorsal fixation by an external splint or modified segmental fixation is recommended.
- **Damage to the ventral compartment alone, including the vertebral body or intervertebral disc** (**402**). An external splint will also provide adequate stability for many fractures in this category. Metal implant and bone cement fixation or vertebral body plating provide the best methods of internal fixation.
- **Damage to both dorsal and ventral compartments** (**403**). Injuries of this type may necessitate fixation of both compartments, such as with a metal implant and bone cement or a dorsal spinal plate combined with a vertebral body plate.

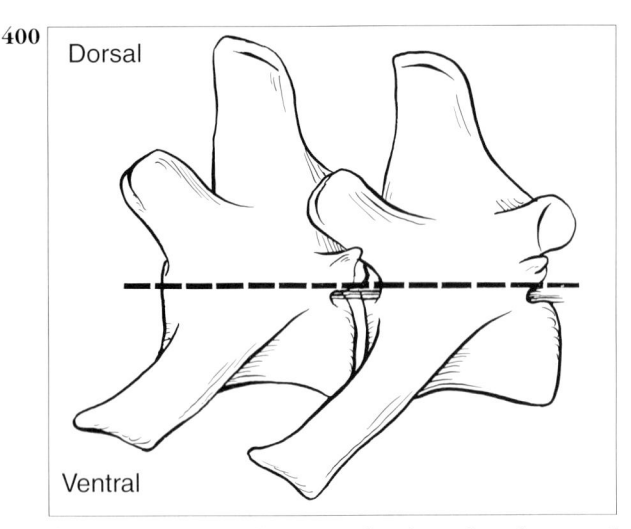

400 Diagram to illustrate the dorsal and ventral compartments of the vertebral column, as referred to in 401–403.

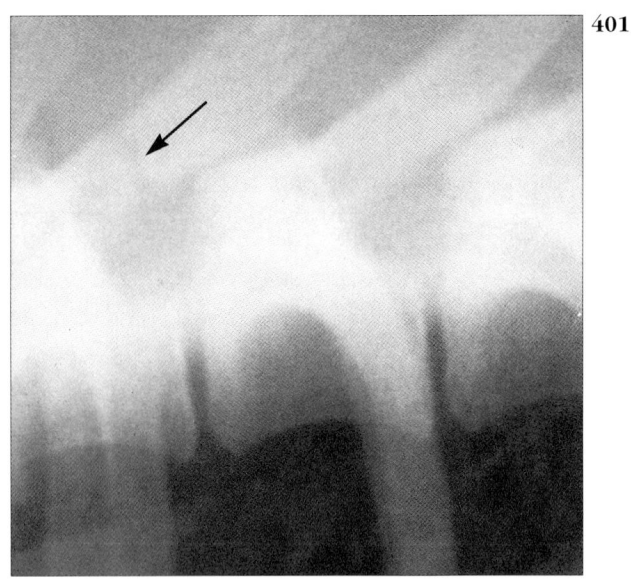

401 Radiograph of an isolated dorsal compartment injury. There is an oblique fracture through the vertebral arch of a mid-thoracic vertebra (arrow).

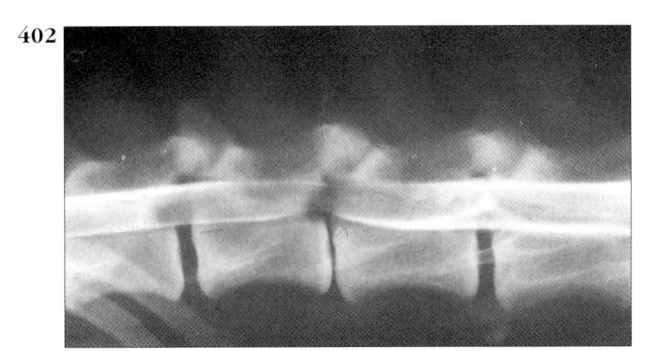

402 Radiograph of an isolated ventral compartment injury. This is consistent with rupture of the anulus fibrosus or a traumatic disc herniation, and is associated with sudden trauma that causes a previously healthy nucleus pulposus to rupture explosively into the vertebral canal. This causes an impact injury to the spinal cord without the usual mass effect associated with the mineralized material of degenerative disc disease.

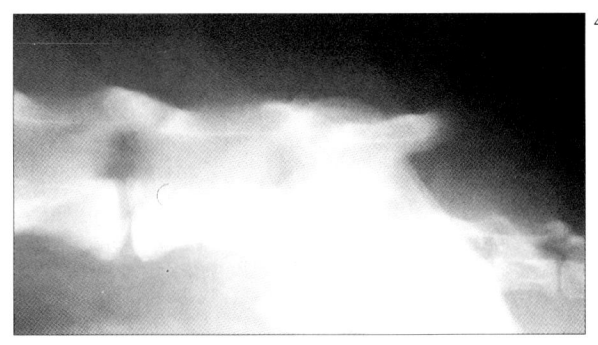

403 Radiograph of a dog with an L_7 fracture that demonstrates injury to both the dorsal and ventral compartments. Despite severe displacement at the fracture site, the dog could walk and had only mild neurological deficits. This relates both to the relatively spacious vertebral canal in this region and to the fact that only nerve roots are present caudal to the sixth lumbar vertebra.

13 TRAUMA

The major drawback of this method of classification is that the majority of injuries damage both dorsal and ventral compartments (Matthieson, 1983; Smith and Walter, 1985).

The main question for all spinal injuries is "How stable is the fracture/luxation site?" The main forces that act on the vertebral column are:
- Bending forces (dorsoventral and lateral).
- Rotational forces.
- Axial loading.
- Shear forces.

A second classification scheme is based on the ability of the vertebral column to resist these forces (**404–407**). It involves assessment of the vertebral body, which acts as a buttress to resist bending and axial loading, and of the articular processes, which resist all forces (Patterson and Smith, 1992). The articular processes are best assessed using lateral and oblique radiographs of the spine (**398** and **408**). The main advantage of the scheme is that it gives an indication of stability, and can serve as a guide to the best fixation procedure for each injury (see 'Biomechanics of fixation devices,' below).

404–407 Diagrams to illustrate a functional means of classifying vertebral fracture/luxations.

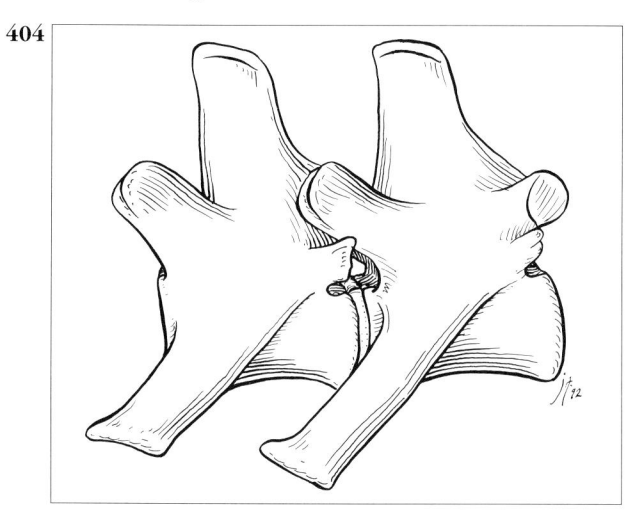

404 The vertebral buttress and articular processes are intact.

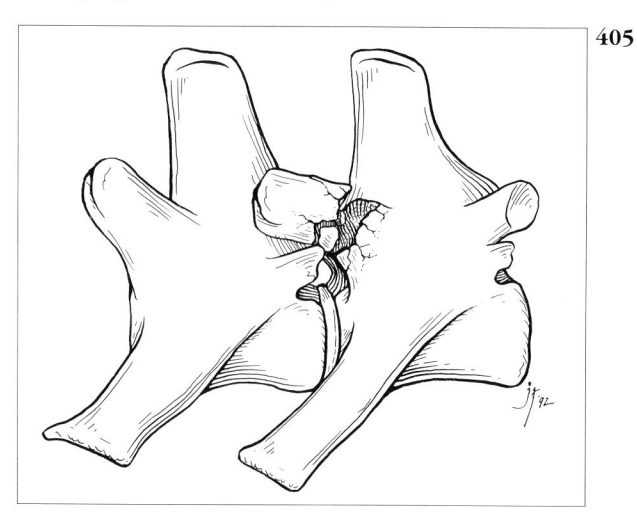

405 The vertebral buttress is intact; the articular processes are fractured.

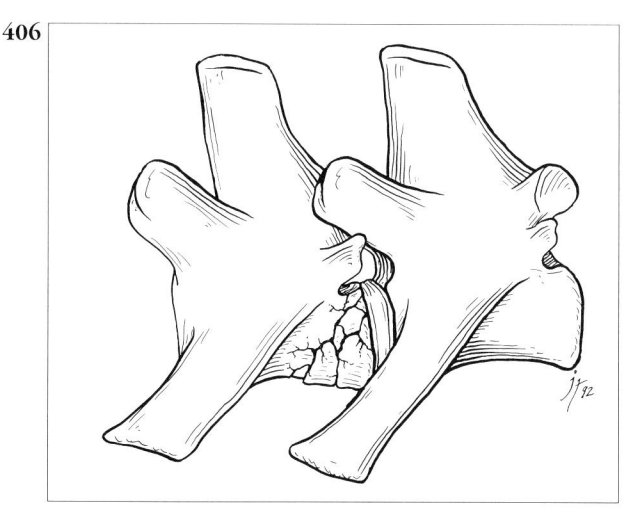

406 The vertebral buttress is fractured; the articular processes are intact.

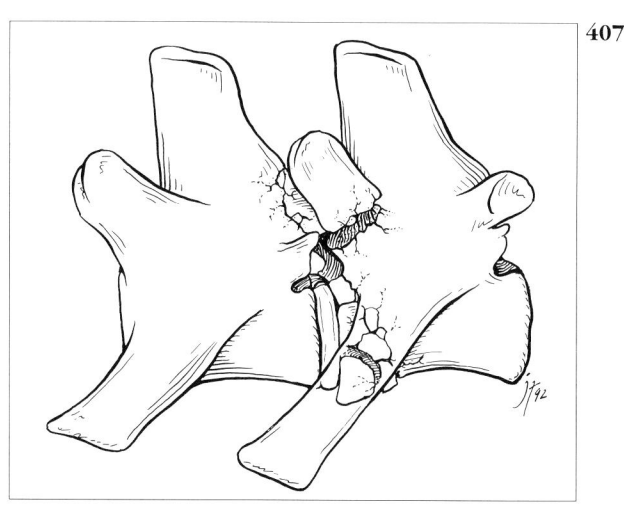

407 The vertebral buttress and articular processes are fractured.

- **Fractures that preserve both the ventral buttress and the articular processes are relatively stable**. They will usually respond favourably to almost any fixation technique (see **402**).
- **Fractures of the articular processes, which preserve the ventral buttress are most susceptible to rotation (409)**. The metal and bone cement technique best resists this force.
- **Fractures of the ventral buttress with intact articular processes are most susceptible to bending (410)**. A vertebral body plate combined with a dorsal spinal plate, best resists this force.
- **If the ventral buttress and articular processes are both fractured, the fixation technique must withstand almost all the forces that act on the vertebral column, including bending and rotation (411)**. No one technique is ideal, and the surgeon must choose between metal implants and bone cement, a dorsal spinal plate combined with a vertebral body plate, or possibly a body plate alone. An external splint does not resist axial compression and is generally not recommended for these types of fracture (Patterson and Smith, 1992). Our preference is for metal and cement fixation.

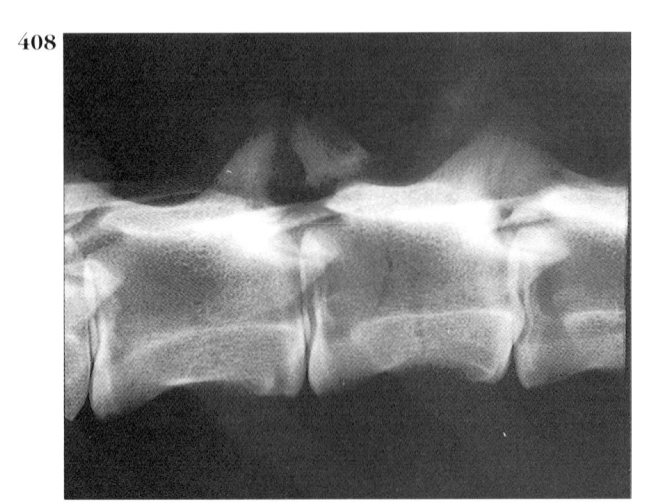

408 This oblique radiograph reveals a fracture of the articular processes.

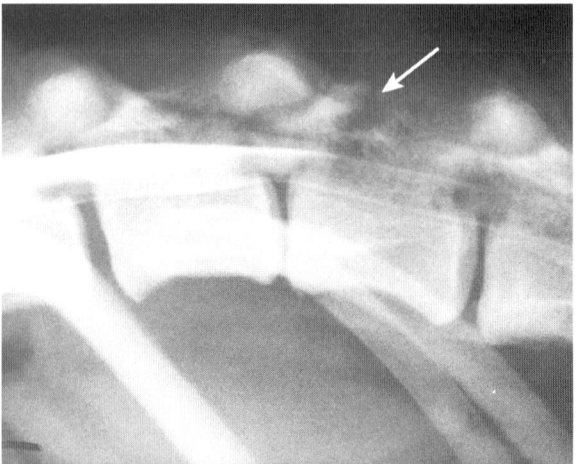

409 Radiograph of a dog with an intact vertebral buttress, but fracture of the articular processes and lamina (illustrated in 405).

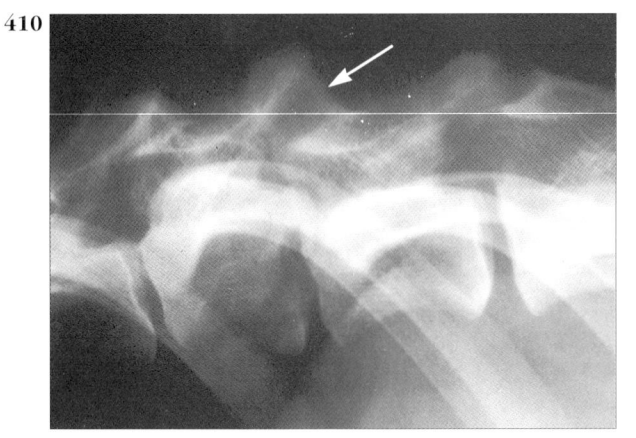

410 Radiograph of a dog with a fracture of the vertebral buttress and intact articular processes **(illustrated in 406)**. There is widening of the dorsal articular joint space (arrow) secondary to collapse of the buttress.

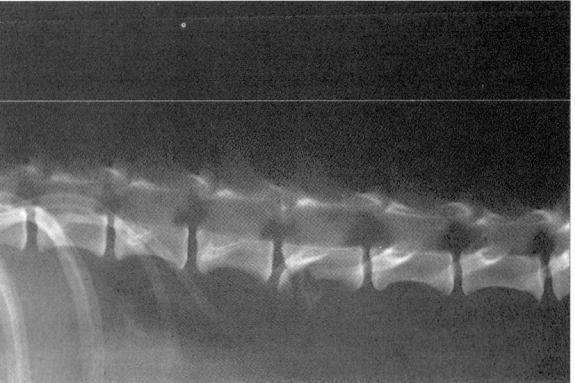

411 Radiograph of a dog with a fracture of both the vertebral buttress and articular processes (illustrated in 407).

The scheme described in **404–407** can only serve as a guide. The residual stability can only be estimated approximately from radiographs, and the implications of overestimating this stability could be disastrous. The relative contribution of the four main forces acting on the vertebral column is also unknown, and almost certainly varies between patients. For example, dorsoventral bending occurs when a paraplegic animal is lifted or as it attempts to raise its hindquarters. Rotation may occur as an animal rises from lateral recumbency, or as it moves with its pelvic limbs dragging to one side. Axial loading occurs from paravertebral muscle spasm. Only the effects of dorsoventral bending and rotational forces have been studied experimentally, which may not reflect the clinical situation.

Another way of assessing vertebral stability is by the use of stress radiography. This may reveal unstable vertebral segments, thus identifying subtle instability (**412, 413**). The risks are obvious and this is best done with caution under fluoroscopy.

Biomechanics of fixation devices

The biomechanics of some vertebral fixation devices have been studied experimentally.

One external splint design has been shown to prevent dorsoventral angulation of thoracolumbar spines subjected to large bending forces. These were in excess of those causing failure of five methods of internal fixation in a spinal fracture model, and were in the range of those experienced by a large paralysed dog undergoing routine nursing care. External splinting works best with injuries that largely preserve the ventral buttress, but has been used with success in patients with severe compromise of the ventral buttress (Patterson and Smith, 1992).

There are many methods of internal fixation. The technique that best resists dorsoventral bending forces is a combined dorsal spinal plate and vertebral body plate. The vertebral body plate alone is the strongest single fixation technique against bending, providing approximately twice the strength of vertebral body pins and bone cement (Walter *et al.*, 1986). The disadvantage of a vertebral body plate alone or in combination with a dorsal spinal plate is the vulnerability to rotational forces. Vertebral body pins and bone cement resist rotational forces best (Whaldron *et al.*, 1991).

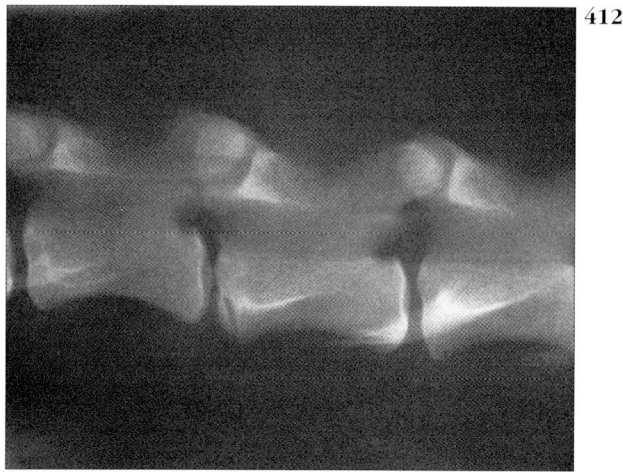

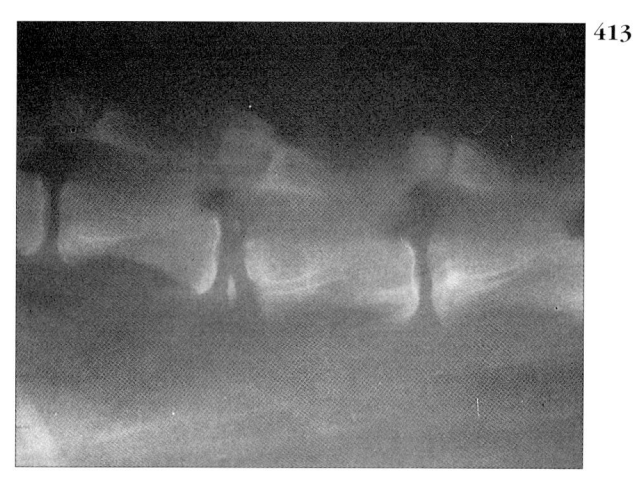

412, 413 Severe instability of a spinal fracture as demonstrated by a change in position between these two radiographs.

Failure of the pins and bone cement technique occurs mainly because of pin pull-out from the bone. Use of bone screws in place of intramedullary pins should improve the technique for the following reasons.
- Screws have greater resistance than pins to bone pullout.
- Screws are less likely to migrate than pins.
- Screws do not need to be cut, which could cause rocking and loosening of a pin.
- Screws do not need to be notched to provide anchorage for the cement, as pins do, because of the screw thread and head.
- Screws are interchangeable, so the optimum implant length can be selected.

The optimum configuration of pins or screws has yet to be determined by biomechanical testing.

Hemilaminectomy is the method of choice for decompression of the spinal cord, as dorsal laminectomy has been shown to result in much greater instability (Smith and Walter, 1988; Shires *et al.*, 1991).

TREATMENT

Choice of therapy

This decision depends initially on the prognosis suggested by the neurological examination (see Chapter 2). Severe shock and hypotension can exacerbate the neurological deficit, so it may be worth reassessing a

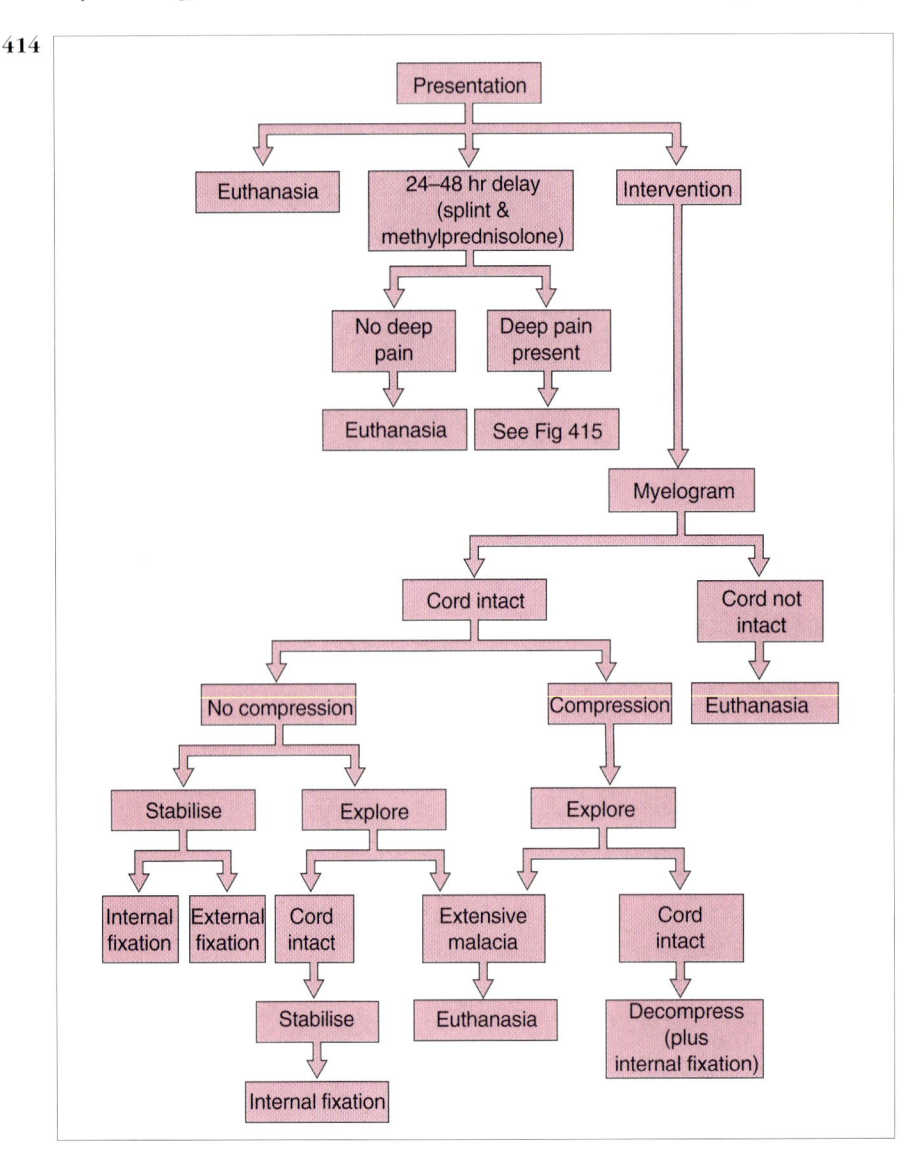

414 Management of animals with no deep pain sensation.

patient lacking deep pain sensation after allowing a 24–48 hour period of circulatory support. Any definitive treatment should only be undertaken once the owner has been made fully aware of the prognosis and the likely time course for recovery. The choice of therapy will vary with the neurological status.

Patients with no deep pain sensation
Here, the clinician has several options (**414**).
- Perform euthanasia because of the poor prognosis.
- Reassess after methylprednisolone therapy and 24–48 hours of circulatory and metabolic support, preferably combined with an external splint.
- Proceed with a myelogram to detect evidence of spinal cord transection (see **399**) or extensive necrosis, either of which indicate euthanasia.

If there is no obvious extradural compression of the spinal cord and the myelogram does not show evidence of spinal cord transection, the surgeon now has a choice.
- Perform a hemilaminectomy, with or without durotomy, in order to identify extensive spinal cord malacia. If the spinal cord is not malacic, proceed with internal fixation.
- Apply external support and reassess over 10–14 days. Deep pain sensation will usually have returned by then if recovery is going to occur.

Either approach is acceptable for animals with no deep pain perception, provided that the owner is aware the chances for a functional recovery are probably 10% at best.

Exploratory surgery can be an attractive option, but a severely compromised spinal cord may be less likely to survive when subjected to anaesthetic-induced hypotension and manipulation.

Patients with intact deep pain sensation
The decision between surgical and nonsurgical management is always difficult, and needs to be made on an individual patient basis. A suggested approach for animals that retain deep pain sensation is shown in **415**. The risks of implant failure or infection, overall hospitalisation time and cost are factors to be considered. A recent survey of over 200 animals with spinal fractures found that although surgical patients stayed in hospital for only half the time of medically treated patients, they incurred more than twice the expense. Furthermore, the final neurological status

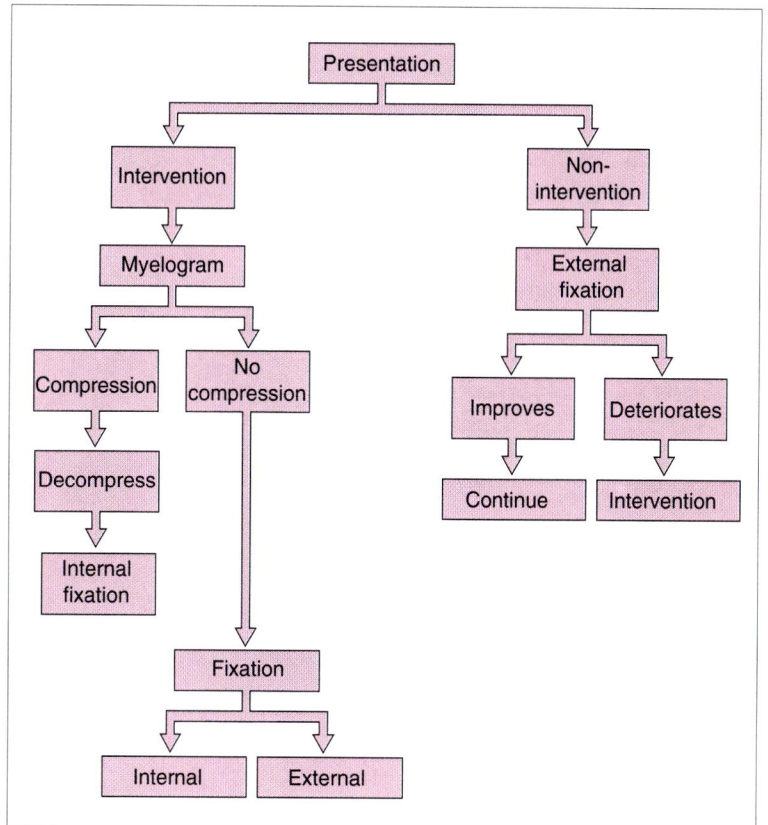

415 Management of animals with intact deep pain.

did not differ between animals treated medically and those treated by surgery (Selcer *et al.,* 1991).

We make the following general recommendations for these patients.
- Severe spinal cord compression or vertebral instability should be relieved surgically whenever possible. Reduction of malalignment and rigid fixation are the goals of surgery.
- Decompression should be performed if there is radiographic or myelographic evidence of marked spinal cord compression. Routine decompression of spinal trauma cases without compression is not indicated.
- If decompression is performed, the vertebral column must always be stabilized by internal fixation.

A final factor that may modify the decision regarding surgery is the anatomical location of the fracture or luxation.

Anatomical location of the fracture or luxation

Cervical spine
This region has the largest ratio of vertebral canal to spinal cord diameter compared to either the thoracic or lumbar regions. In general, if an animal with a cervical fracture does not die immediately from respiratory arrest, it has a good chance of a satisfactory recovery. Cage rest, with external support (**416**) in unstable or displaced fractures, provides sufficient stability for most fractures (Denny, 1983). This is not the easiest location to apply a splint, but one can be made from orthopaedic casting material.

Surgery is not without risk, but it may reduce recovery times and is recommended for:
- Traumatic atlantoaxial fracture/subluxations (see Chapter 9).
- Patients with severe tetraparesis or poor ventilatory function.
- Animals that remain painful after 48–72 hours, or those showing neurological deterioration.

Fractures involving the axis can be stabilized with a plate to the spinous process (**417**) or to the ventral aspect of the vertebral body, or with screws and bone cement.

For fracture/luxations caudal to C_2, the most useful technique is ventral placement of pins or screws and bone cement (**419**, see also Chapter 11 and **334**, **335**). The main disadvantage is that it is prone to failure if used to span more than one intervertebral space (see Chapter 11). Single interbody lag screw fixation (see **347**) or a ventrally positioned plate may also be useful (**418**). If dorsal stability is required, screws may be placed between the articular processes.

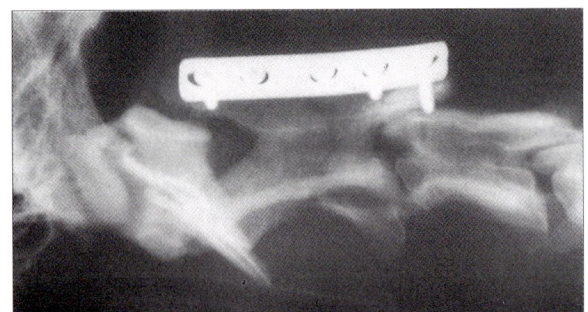

417 A dog with a fracture through the middle of the spinous process and body of C_2, which has been stabilized by a five-hole plate applied to the spinous process.

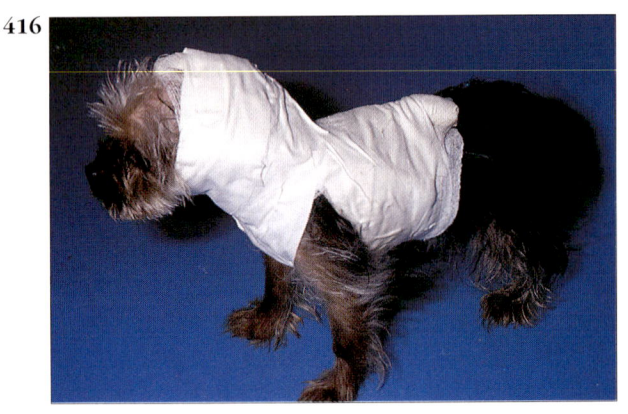

416 A dog with a fracture/luxation of C_2 which has been treated with an external splint. The splint should ideally extend from near the lateral canthus of the eyes to the mid-thoracic region.

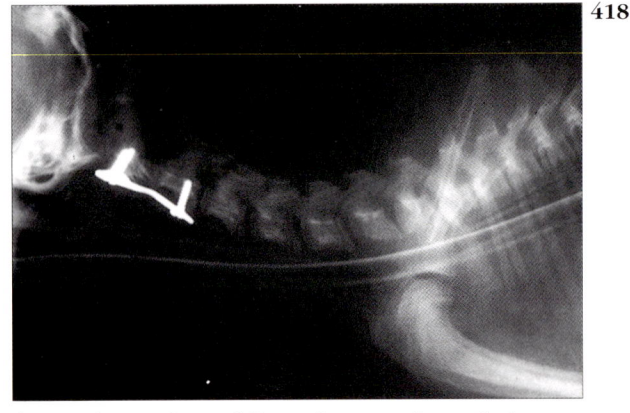

418 A dog with an oblique fracture through the cranial vertebral body of C_2, which has been stabilized by a plate applied to the ventral aspect of C_1 and C_2.

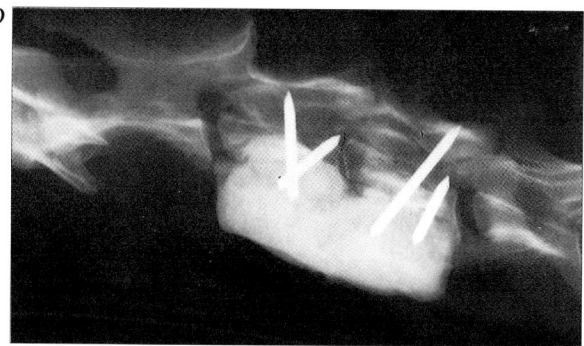

419 A dog with a fracture of $C_{3/4}$, which has been stabilized with pins and bone cement.

Thoracic and lumbar spine

This is the most commonly injured region of the vertebral column in dogs, and is also at most risk for devastating neurological consequences because of the relative lack of room in this part of the vertebral canal. A range of external and internal fixation techniques can be used to stabilize this region, the most useful being metal implants and bone cement.

L_6 and L_7 vertebrae and lumbosacral junction

The vertebral canal is relatively spacious in this region because the spinal cord ends at the sixth lumbar vertebra, and only nerve roots occupy the caudal part of the vertebral canal (see **3, 4**). For these reasons, injuries causing severe displacement may result in only mild neurological deficits (see **403**). In general, many of these fractures heal satisfactorily without surgical intervention. External support may be used or several surgical techniques are suitable. Animals with persistent pain or deteriorating neurological status are candidates for internal fixation. Our preferred technique is the use of screws and bone cement, with screws also being placed in the wing of the ilium if necessary (see **457, 458**).

Sacrocaudal fracture/luxations and tail avulsions

These occur most commonly in cats (Feeney and Oliver, 1980). Fractures of the caudal vertebrae are usually treated non-surgically or by tail amputation. The prognosis for return of urinary continence is good for cats with good anal tone and intact perineal sensation on initial examination. Cats that do not become continent within one month generally fail to regain urinary function (Moise and Flanders, 1983; Smeak and Olmstead, 1985).

Conservative management

Animals with fracture/luxations in the cervical or lumbosacral regions often respond well to cage confinement for 4–6 weeks. Analgesia is not usually required beyond 48 hours. Intractable pain or progressive neurological deficits warrant reassessment.

Advantages. It is inexpensive, there are no complications related to fixation devices, and the spinal cord is not subject to myelography, anaesthetic hypotension, or manipulation.

Disadvantages. Significant instability cannot be addressed, reduction is difficult, some animals suffer prolonged discomfort, and the neurological deficits may worsen or even become irreversible. Cage rest alone is not recommended for any but the most stable of fractures in the thoracolumbar region.

External splint (420–431)

Advantages include those of conservative management, but this technique provides far greater stability. It can be used as the sole means of fixation, or as a supplement to internal fixation. It is most applicable to midthoracic or lumbar fractures.

Disadvantages are development of complications such as urine scald or rub sores under the splint or straps, and the nursing care needed (**431**).

External fixation is a very useful nonsurgical technique for stabilizing spinal fracture/luxations, but one that requires careful patient selection, good splint management and a very high level of nursing care. When used as an adjunct to methods of internal fixation, the difficulty of observing the surgical wound should be borne in mind.

Good candidates for external fixation include paraparetic or paraplegic animals with intact deep pain sensation, intact articular processes or ventral buttress, no pelvic fractures, and no significant soft tissue wounds. Marginal candidates include animals with both fractured processes and a severely compromised ventral buttress, and those with pelvic, thoracic, or severe soft tissue injuries (Patterson and Smith, 1992).

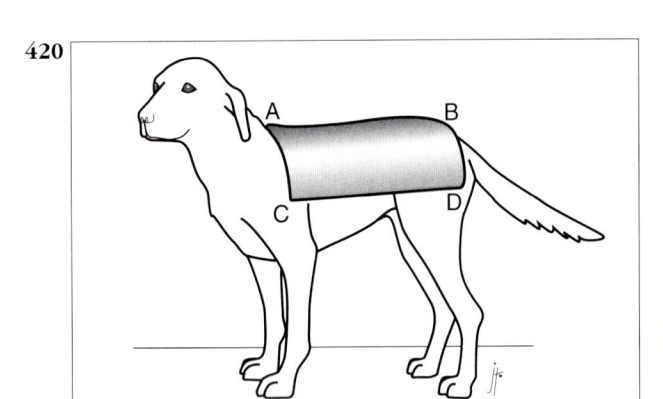

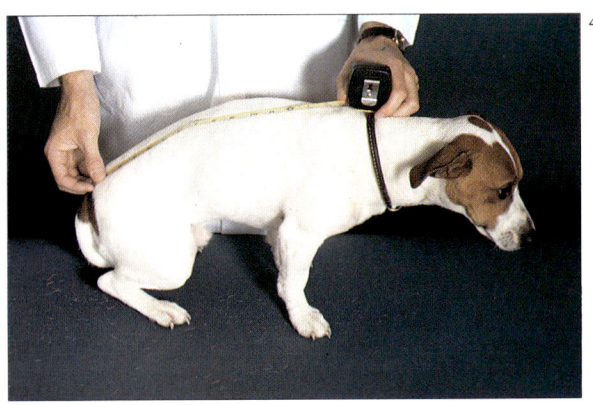

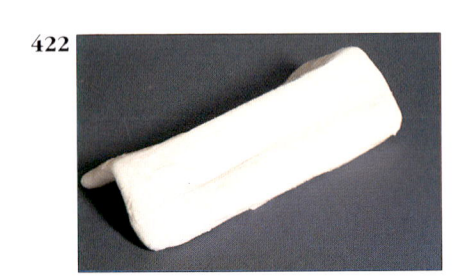

DIAGNOSIS AND SURGERY OF SMALL ANIMAL SPINAL DISORDERS

420 Diagram to illustrate the construction of an external splint that is to be applied to a dog with a spinal injury. The splint is made from sheet aluminium, 0.54 mm in thickness, double or triple layered if necessary for added rigidity. In animals under 10 kg, Orthoplast (Johnson and Johnson) may be substituted for aluminium. To make the splint, measure the dimensions A–B, A–C, and B–D, and cut the splint to these dimensions (from Patterson and Smith, 1992).

421 The splint extends from between the scapulae to the tail base, measured directly along the spine. (Note that most animals have marked kyphosis following spinal injury.).

422 The material is bent along its longitudinal axis into a ridge, which is made slightly flatter over the pelvic area. At the sides, the splint should extend laterally towards the shoulder and hip joints. The splint should be well padded with cotton secured by Elastoplast (Elasticon, Johnson & Johnson) especially at the edges of the material.

423 A better padding material is Elastogel (Southwest Technologies Inc., Kansas City, MO), which should reduce the likelihood of pressure or rub sores under the splint.

424 Some animals tolerate application of the splint while fully conscious, but most require sedation and a few will need general anaesthesia. With the animal on its side, the splint is slid under the dog with the dorsal ridge aligned along the animals dorsal midline.

425 The animal and splint are then rotated simultaneously until the animal is lying on its back in the splint. The dog usually relaxes in the splint, and the fracture will realign to some degree. The axillae and groin are then heavily padded with cotton wool, cast padding or gauze, prior to attaching the splint using Elastoplast. A superior means of preventing skin excoriation is to attach Elastogel to the inner surface of the Elastoplast in these regions. Elastoplast is the material of choice for the straps as it is light, porous and adhesive. Velcro straps are much easier to readjust but lack the elasticity of Elastoplast.

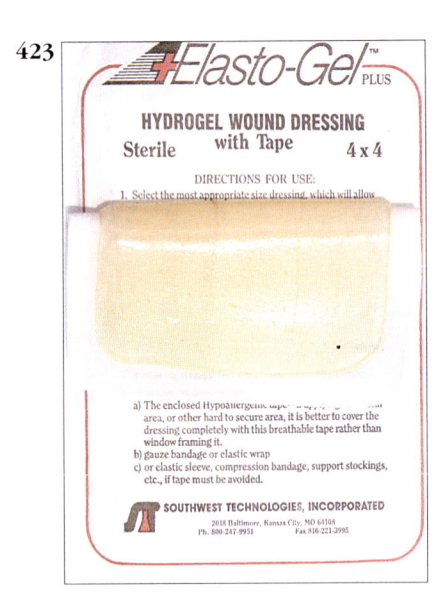

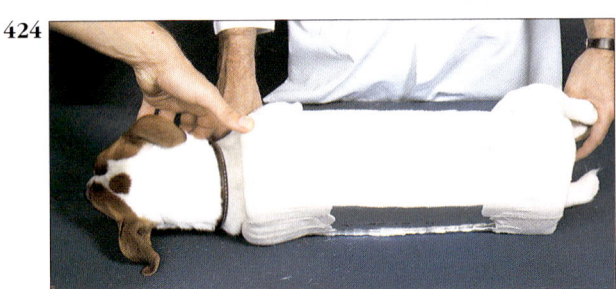

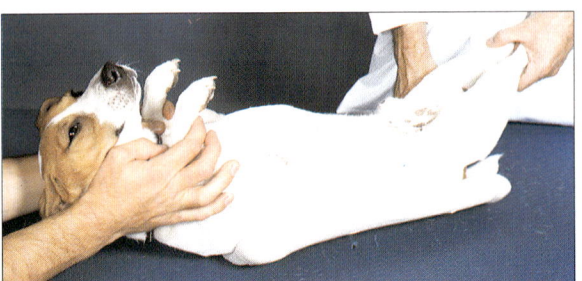

13 TRAUMA

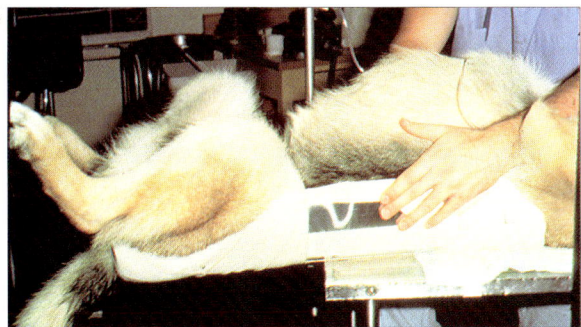

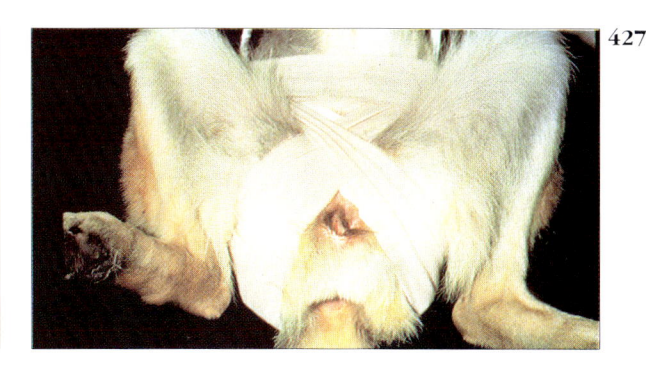

426 To secure the dog to the splint, first the caudal half of the animal is extended over the end of a table.

427 **Elastoplast is applied in a cruciate pattern over the pelvis, avoiding the anus and vulva**. In male animals, a large gap must be left to avoid the preputial opening. It is also important that any strap crossing the base of the penis is not too tight, or pressure necrosis of the urethra is possible.

428 **In male dogs, a cod-piece roughly the shape of a half flowerpot can be made from aluminium or Orthoplast to protect the base of the penis and to try to funnel urine away from the abdomen and inguinal straps**.

429 **In the pectoral region, the straps are applied as a figure of eight, extending in front of the shoulder and under the neck to act as a harness**. Post-splinting radiographs can be taken through the splint to check fracture alignment. The straps around the chest must not impede ventilation.

430 **The main advantages of an external splint are that it is inexpensive and strong**. It also facilitates lifting the animal, turning it from side to side, moving it to clean the kennel, or taking it out to void.

431 **The main disadvantage of an external splint is potential pressure sore formation, both along the edges or underneath the splint**. In addition, the straps often excoriate the skin in the axilla or inguinal region as shown here, and may hinder manual expression of the bladder. Prevention of urine scald in the groin area can prove a challenge. It is essential that as much of the area under the splint, and the skin of the groin and axilla, is examined daily. Urine-soiled straps must be replaced. Areas at risk from urine scalding or faecal soiling benefit from application of Desatin (Pfizer) ointment or corn starch powder. If there is any doubt about the development of sores, the straps or splint should be loosened sufficiently to allow proper inspection, and then reattached by additional Elastoplast. A useful indicator of potential problems is the animal's mental attitude; most animals are surprisingly comfortable in the splint unless decubitus develops. The splint should be maintained for a minimum of 4 weeks (3 for immature animals), and preferably then followed by 2–4 weeks of strict cage confinement.

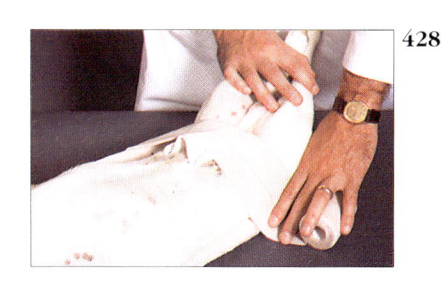

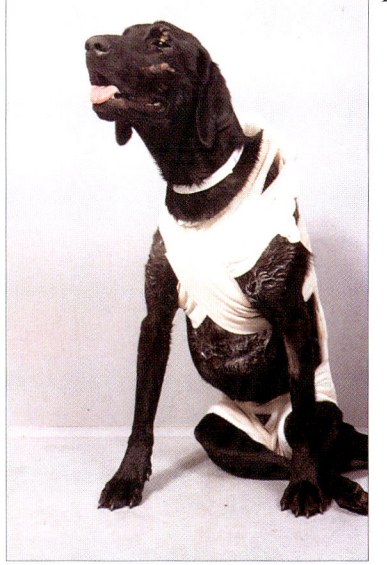

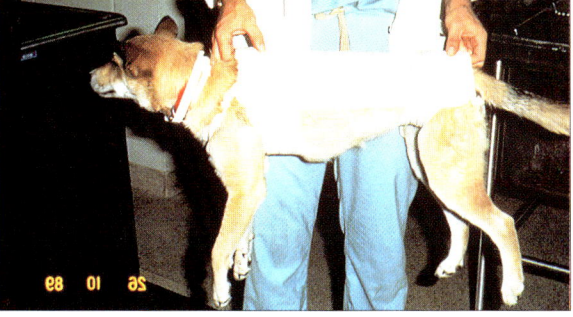

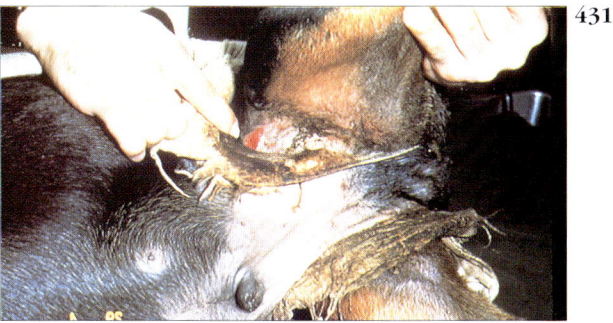

SURGERY

The procedures described are performed via a dorsal approach, as used for dorsal laminectomy (see **370-373**). Decompression is best achieved in the thoracolumbar spine by hemilaminectomy, if possible, as this has the least destabilising effect on the spine (see 'Biomechanics of fixation devices,' above).

Dorsal spinal plate (432, 433)

Disadvantages mainly relate to the lack of strength of the spinous processes, and their tendency to fracture and undergo pressure necrosis. These problems are greatest in the thoracic area and in small or young animals. This technique is one of the weakest against bending or rotational forces, and so cannot be recommended alone. The exception might be an isolated dorsal compartment injury, but even then an external splint or modified segmental fixation should prove superior.

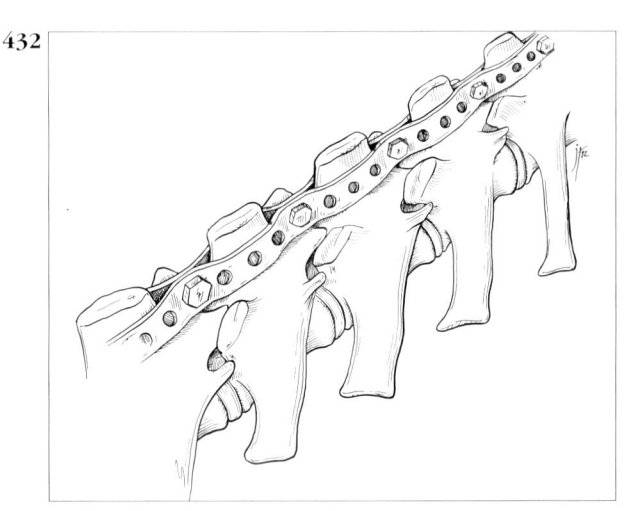

432 Diagram to show application of a plastic spinal plate (Lubra Co., Fort Collins, CO, USA) to the spinous processes.

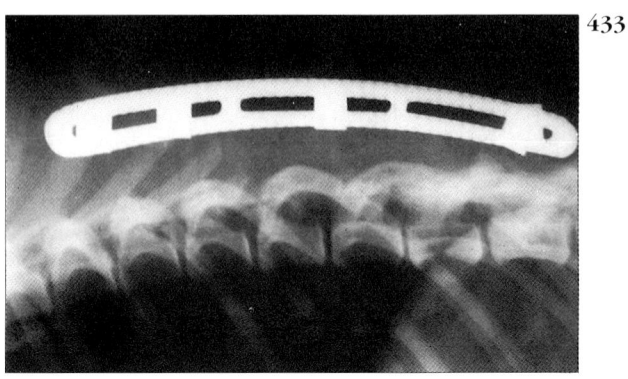

433 Radiograph of a metal plate applied to the spinous processes.

Vertebral body plate (434–437)

Advantages are that this is the strongest single technique to resist dorsoventral bending forces, and that it involves implants with which most clinicians are familiar. It immobilizes only a short segment of the vertebral column and can compensate for loss of the ventral buttress. Bilateral plating can be used if necessary.

Disadvantages are that it provides little resistance to rotational forces, and it is unsuitable in the caudal lumbar region because of the difficulty in avoiding the spinal nerves. In the caudal thoracic region, it is necessary to resect or disarticulate one or more rib heads to gain access to the vertebral bodies, which often causes pneumothorax.

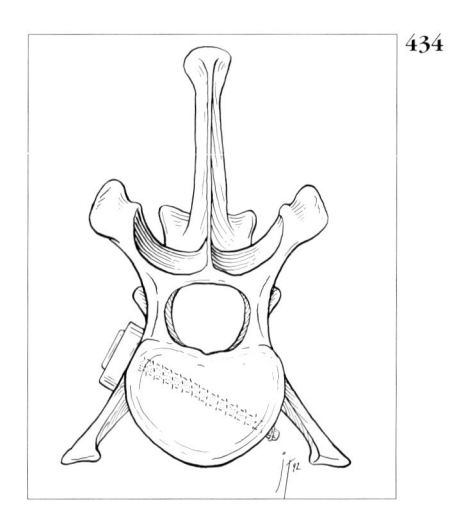

434 Position of a vertebral body plate and screws relative to the vertebral canal. A minimum of four cortices should be engaged by screws on either side of the fracture.

13 TRAUMA

435 In the thoracic region, the rib head(s) will usually require disarticulation, and then subsequent resection, or repositioning by orthopaedic wire through the articular processes as shown. Pneumothorax is a common sequel to this technique.

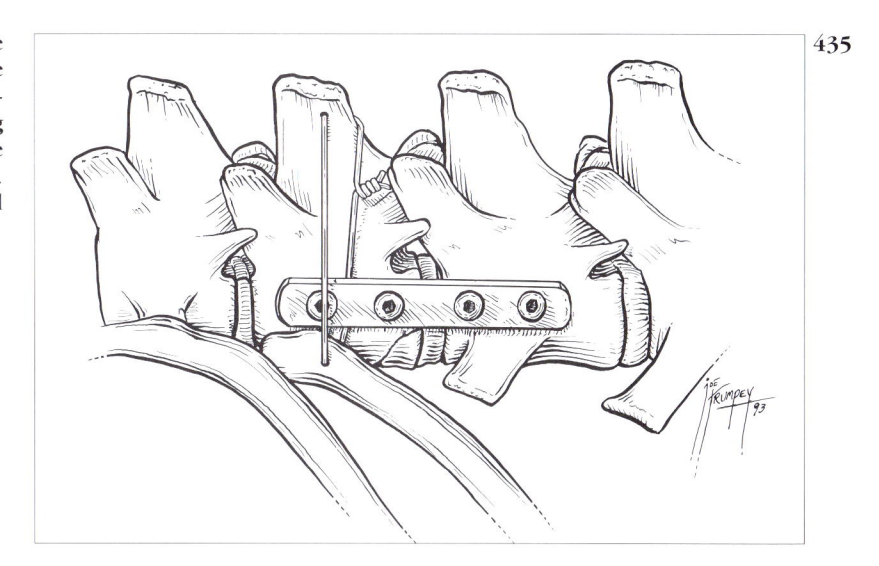

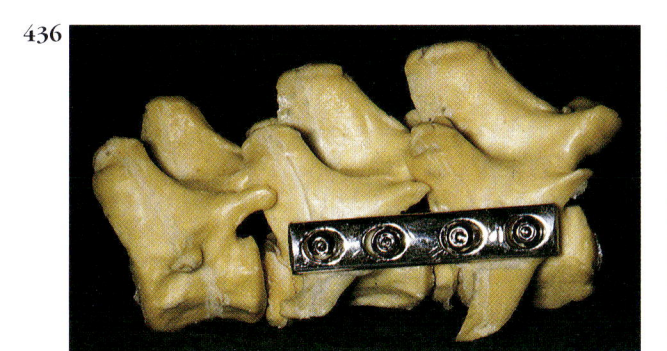

436 A four-hole plate applied to the vertebral bodies.

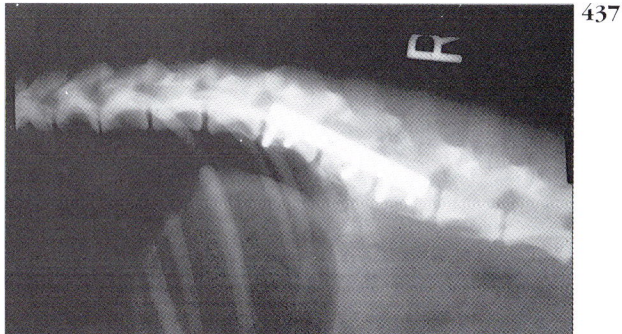

437 Radiograph of a vertebral body plate applied to a fracture in the lumbar region.

Dorsal spinal plate plus vertebral body plate

Advantages. This combination is the most resistant of all techniques against dorsoventral bending (Walter *et al.*, 1986).

Disadvantages are that the technique is unstable when subject to rotational forces, it requires considerable dissection of surrounding muscles, and is difficult to apply in the thoracic and caudal lumbar regions. An external splint may provide a stronger alternative to the dorsal spinal plate. In general, we prefer metal implants with bone cement.

Modified segmental fixation (438–440)

The original technique ('spinal stapling') was to wire four or five spinous processes to a Steinmann pin. Modifications include configuration of the pin in a 'U' shape, or the use of several pins in parallel. The technique is improved by wiring the articular processes to the pin and is termed modified segmental fixation (McAnulty *et al.*, 1986).

Advantages. It is economical, most clinics have the necessary orthopaedic implants, and it can work well when the vertebral buttress is intact.

Disadvantage is that it immobilizes a long segment of vertebral column, with the weak link being the orthopaedic wire, not the Steinmann pin. Also, the wire can fracture the articular processes, especially in small animals. It is not good for stabilising a compromised vertebral buttress, and though proposed for use in large breed dogs, results of biomechanical testing are poor (Shores *et al.*, 1988).

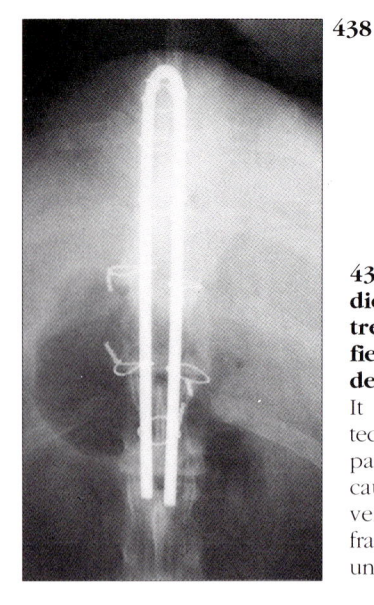

438 Dorsoventral radiograph of a fracture treated with a modified segmental fixation device (spinal staple). It is not the optimum technique to stabilise this particular fracture because of a defect in the vertebral buttress. The fracture, however, healed uneventfully.

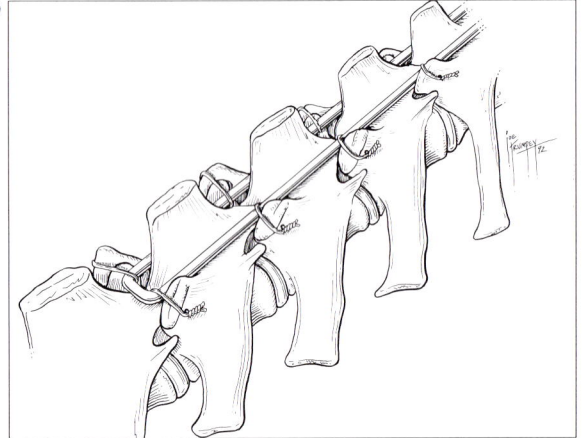

439 Diagram to show application of a spinal staple. The orthopaedic wire penetrates the articular processes and is twisted around the staple. Wires can also be placed through the spinous processes.

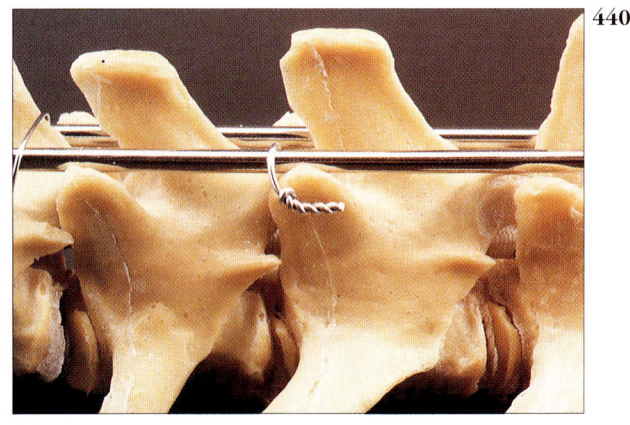

440 Close-up of an articular process to show the position of the wire in modified segmental fixation.

Transilial pin techniques (441, 442)

Advantage is the ready availability of the implants.

Disadvantages are that the transilial pin tends to migrate, and may not provide adequate stability if used on its own. The main disadvantage of the Kirschner–Ehmer is the potential for infection to enter the surgical site along the pin tracts, and the problems with maintenance of the external frame in this region (Shores *et al.*, 1989).

13 TRAUMA

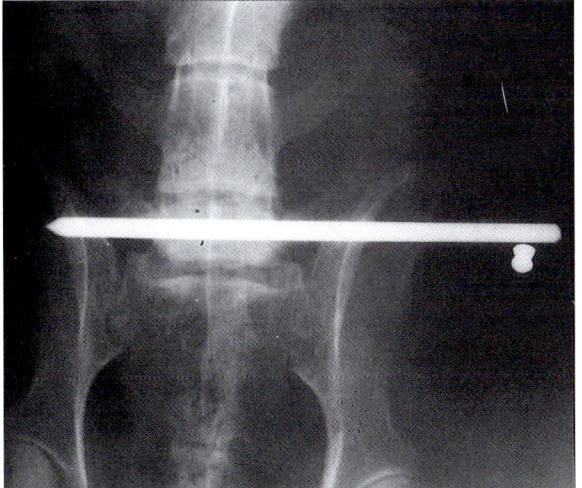

441 A transilial pin has been used to treat this L₇ fracture, but it migrated before the fracture healed. Following implant removal, the dog made a satisfactory recovery after four weeks strict cage confinement.

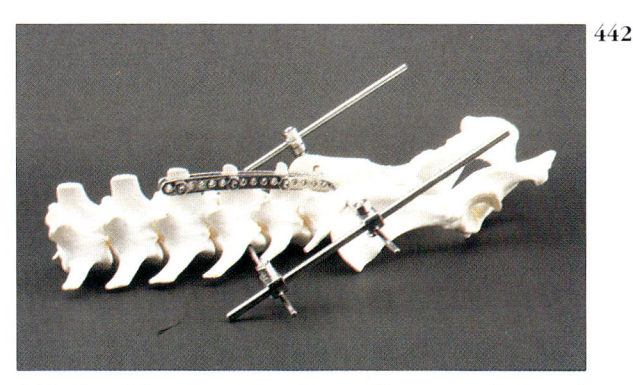

442 Combination Kirschner–Ehmer and dorsal spinal plate. The transilial portion of the fixator passes through the caudal hole in the dorsal spinal plate.

Metal and bone cement (443–458)

This technique was first described using Steinmann pins placed through the vertebral bodies (Rouse and Miller, 1975; Blass and Seim, 1984). We prefer bone screws rather than pins for the reasons described under 'Biomechanics of fixation devices' above.

Advantages are that this requires less soft tissue dissection than the other procedures, it immobilises a short segment of the vertebral column, and it is suitable for thoracic and caudal lumbar areas because the ribs and spinal nerves can easily be avoided. Pins and bone cement provide the greatest rotational stability and strength of all techniques tested (Whaldron *et al.*, 1991), and these biomechanical properties are probably improved by using screws instead of pins. Screws and bone cement is our preferred technique for most types of spinal fracture/luxation, and has been used in dogs of all sizes and breeds with good results, including those with significant compromise of the ventral buttress.

Disadvantages (459, 460) include the poor resistance to dorsoventral bending, potential for pin migration or implant failure, difficulty in closing soft tissues over the implants, and the risk of infection of the bone cement. The bone cement renders revision of a failure difficult.

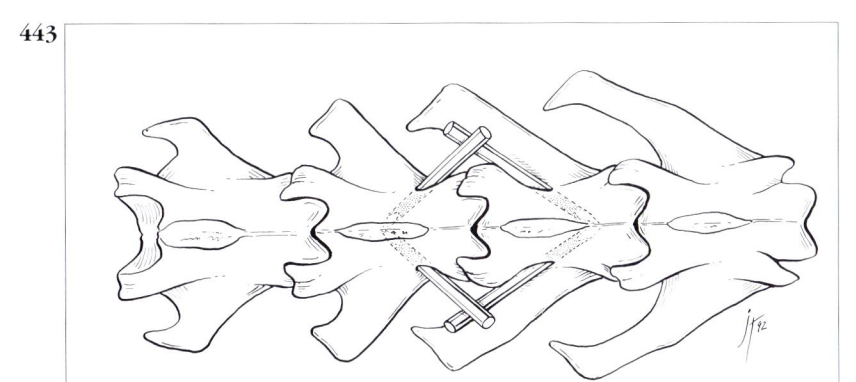

443, 444 Diagrams to illustrate the position of Steinmann pins for methylmethacrylate fixation. The pins are driven into the vertebral bodies in a diverging manner.

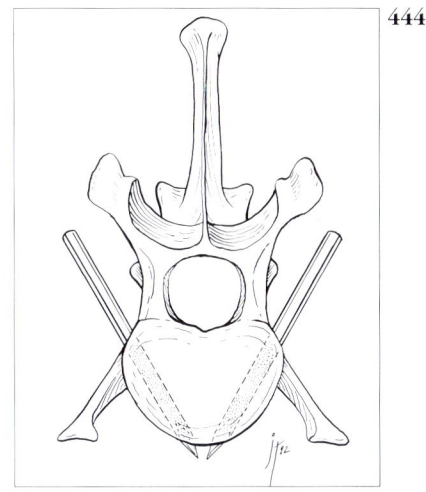

187

445 The pins are cut, notched, and the ends bent to provide purchase for the bone cement. Before bone cement application, intravenous antibiotic effective against staphylococci (such as cephazolin 20 mg/kg) is given and repeated every one to two hours during surgery. The same antibiotic is added to the methylmethacrylate powder (1 g to 40 g of powder) before adding the liquid catalyst. The bone cement is placed over the fracture and pins in a doughnut fashion.

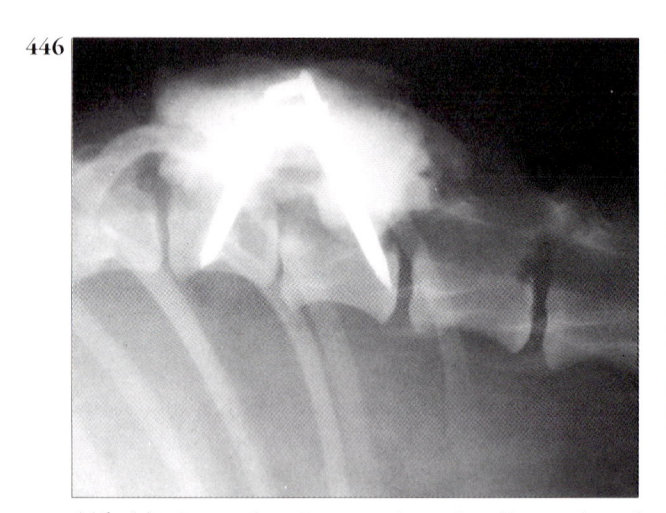

446, 447 Lateral and ventrodorsal radiographs of pins and bone cement fixation.

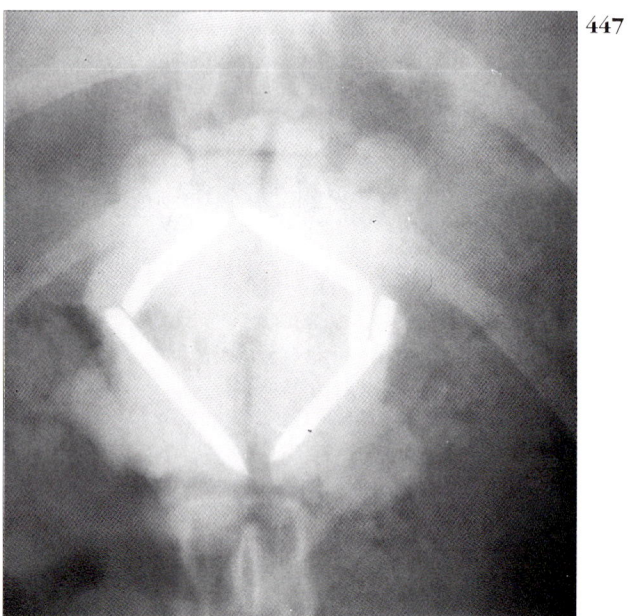

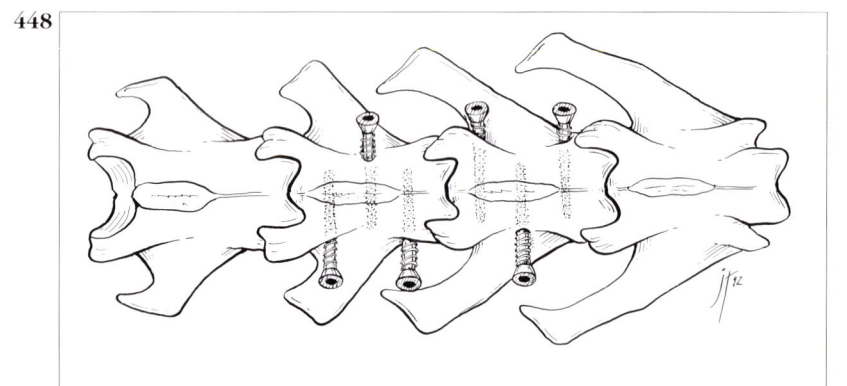

448, 449 Diagram to show screw placement for screw and bone cement fixation.

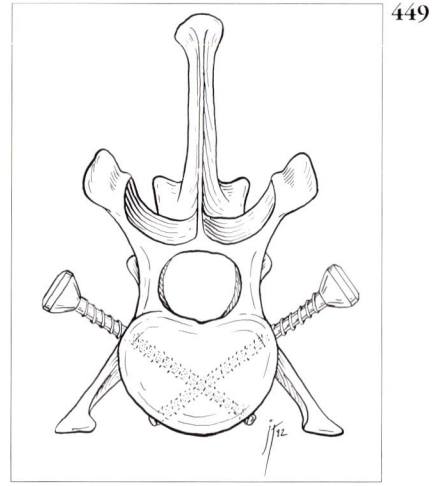

13 TRAUMA

450 Screw placement in the vertebral body before bone cement application.

450

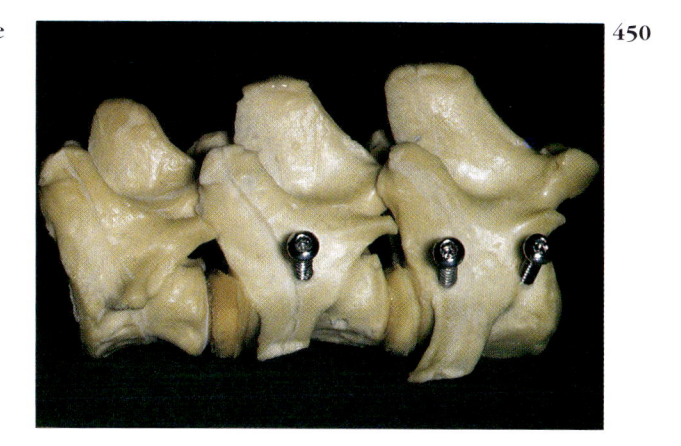

451

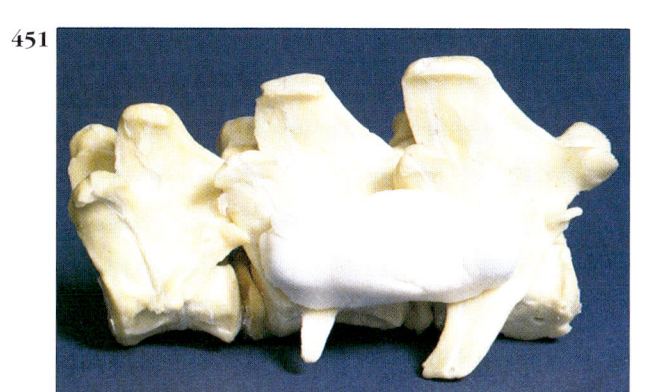

452

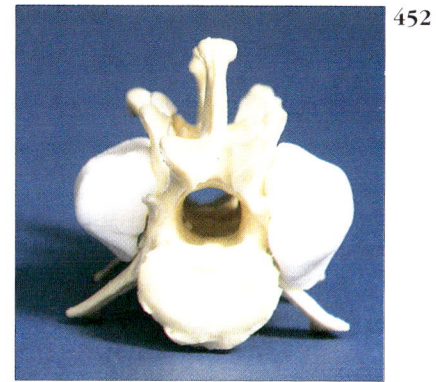

451, 452 Vertebral bodies after bone cement has been applied.

453

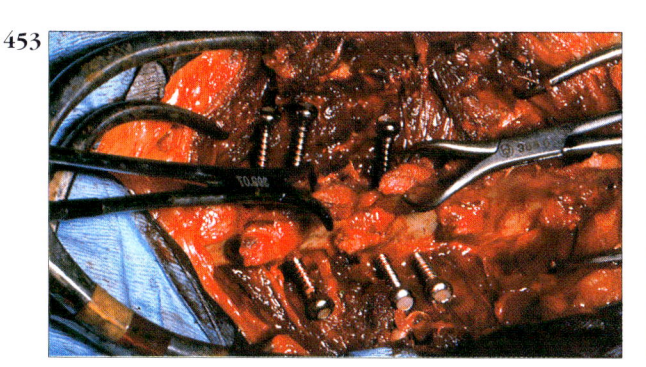

454

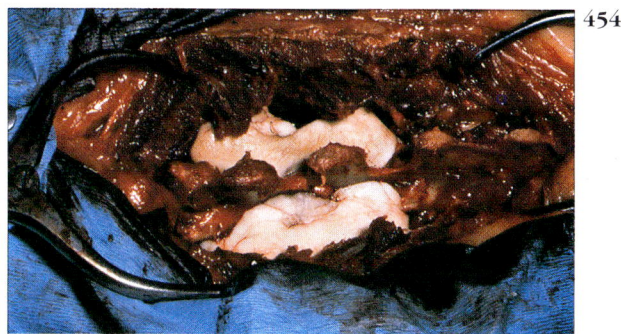

453, 454 Intraoperative view of screw and bone cement technique. Note that bone wax has been used to fill the screw heads (which will be covered in cement) to facilitate implant removal at a later date if necessary. Note also that the luxation is being held in reduction by the use of bone holding forceps applied to each spinous process. Kirschner wires can be placed through the articular processes once the fracture has been apposed to maintain alignment. Bone cement is applied in a cylindrical pattern on each side of the vertebrae. Wound closure is easier here than when cement is applied in a doughnut pattern. The wound is irrigated with saline to dissipate heat generated by the curing of the cement. The spinal nerves are protected by tongue depressors caudal to L_5.

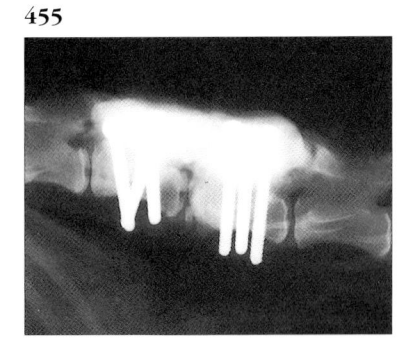

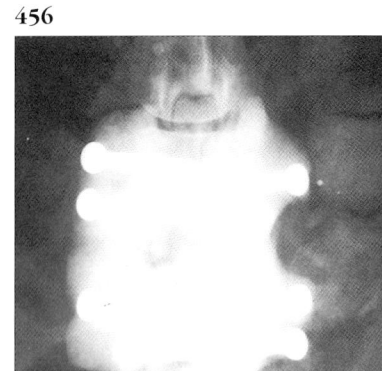

DIAGNOSIS AND SURGERY OF SMALL ANIMAL SPINAL DISORDERS

455, 456 Radiographs of screws and bone cement.

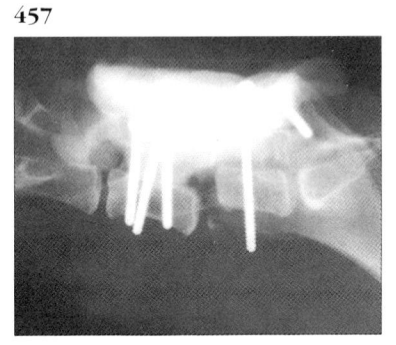

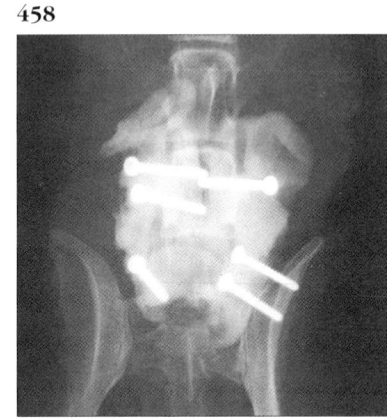

457, 458 Radiographs of a dog with a fracture of L_7, which has been stabilized with screws and bone cement. Note that two of the screws on one side have been inserted into the wing of the ilium to provide additional purchase for the implant.

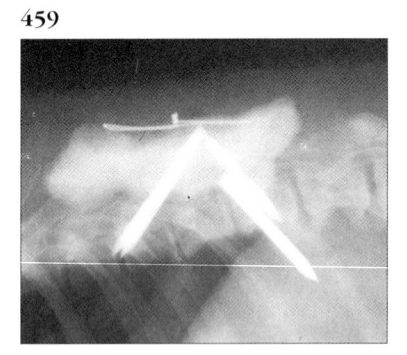

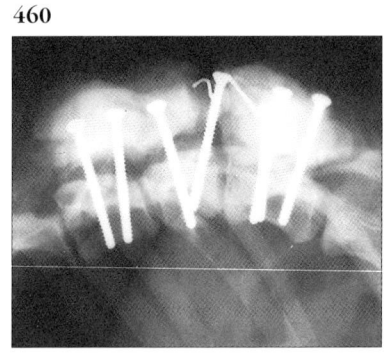

459 Migration of one pin.

460 Dog with failure of the bone cement after screw and cement fixation. The cement was applied too thinly near one of the screws. A resistant *Streptococcus faecalis* was also isolated from a draining tract over the surgical wound.

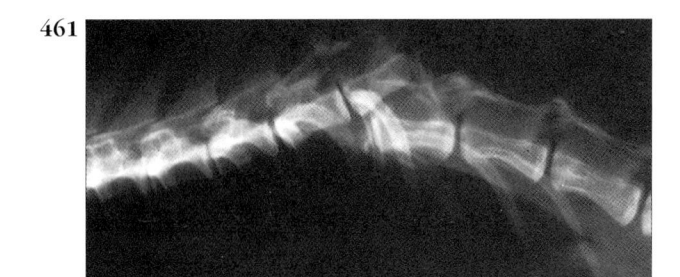

FELINE SPINAL INJURIES

Feline spinal injuries are often more devastating than those in dogs (**461**). Nonsurgical therapy is useful, but some cats tolerate splints poorly. In theory any internal fixation technique can be applied.

461 Example of the devastating type of spinal injury commonly encountered in cats.

PROGNOSIS

The prognosis is similar to that given for thoracolumbar disc disease, although grade 5 deficits rarely recover after trauma. If the patient is to make a functional recovery, improvement by at least one neurological grade should be seen within four weeks of the injury. Although methylprednisolone may improve the recovery rate, adequate fixation of an unstable vertebral column by internal or external means is essential.

REFERENCES

Blass C.E. and Seim, H.B. (1984) Spinal fixation in dogs using Steinmann pins and methylmethacrylate. *Veterinary Surgery* **13**, 203–210.

Denny, H.R. (1983) Fractures of the cervical vertebrae in the dog. *Veterinary Annual* **23**, 236–240.

Feeney, D.A. and Oliver, J.E. (1980) Blunt spinal trauma in the dog and cat: Insight into radiographic lesions. *Journal of the American Animal Hospital Association* **16**, 885–890.

Matthieson, D.T. (1983) Thoracolumbar spinal fractures/luxations: surgical management. *Compendium on Continuing Education for the Practicing Veterinarian* **10**, 867–878.

McAnulty, J.F., Lenehan, T.M. and Maletz, L.M. (1986) Modified segmental spinal instrumentation in repair of spinal fractures and luxations in dogs. *Veterinary Surgery* **15**, 143–149.

Moise, N.S. and Flanders, J.A. (1983) Micturition disorders in cats with sacrocaudal vertebral lesions. *Current Veterinary Therapy* VIII, pp 772–776. (Ed. R.W. Kirk). W.B. Saunders Co., Philadelphia.

Murtaugh, R.J. and Ross, J.N. (1988) Cardiac arrhythmias: pathogenesis and treatment in the trauma patient. *Compendium on Continuing Education for the Practicing Veterinarian* **10**, 332–339.

Neer, M.T. (1992) A review of disorders of the gallbladder and extrahepatic biliary tract in the dog and cat. *Journal of Veterinary Internal Medicine* **6**, 186–192.

Patterson, R.H. and Smith, G.K. (1992) Backsplinting for treatment of thoracic and lumbar fracture/luxation in the dog: principles of application and case series. *Veterinary Comparative Orthopaedics and Traumatology* **5**, 179–187.

Rouse, G.P. and Miller, J.I. (1975) The use of methylmethacrylate for spinal stabilization. *Journal of the American Animal Hospital Association* **11**, 418–425.

Selcer, R.R., Bubb, W.J. and Walker T.L. (1991). Management of vertebral column fractures in dogs and cats: 211 cases (1977–1985). *Journal of the American Veterinary Medical Association* **198**, 1965–1968.

Shires, P.K., Waldron, D.R., Hedlund, C.S., Blass, C.E. and Massoudi, L. (1991) A biomechanical study of rotational stability in unaltered and surgically altered canine thoracolumbar vertebral motion units. *Progress in Veterinary Neurology* **2**, 6–14.

Shores, A., Nichols, C., Koelling, H.A. and Fox, W.R. (1988) Combined Kirschner–Ehmer apparatus for dorsal spinal plate fixation of caudal lumbar fractures in dogs: Biomechanical properties. *American Journal of Veterinary Research* **49**, 1979–1982.

Shores, A., Nichols, C., Rochat, M., Fox, S.M., Burt, G.J. and Fox W.R. (1989) Combined Kirschner–Ehmer device and dorsal spinal plate fixation technique for caudal lumbar vertebral fractures in dogs. *Journal of the American Veterinary Medical Association* **195**, 335–339.

Smeak, D.D. and Olmstead, M.L. (1985) Fracture/luxations of the sacrococcygeal area in the cat. A retrospective study of 51 cases. *Veterinary Surgery* **14**, 319–324.

Smith, G.K. and Walter, M.C. (1985) Fractures and luxations of the spine. In *Textbook of Small Animal Orthopaedics*, pp 307–332. (Ed. C.D. Newton.) J.B. Lippincott Company, Philadelphia.

Smith, G.K. and Walter M.C. (1988) Spinal decompressive procedures and dorsal compartment injuries: comparative biomechanical study in canine cadavers. *American Journal of Veterinary Research* **49**, 266–273.

Turner, D.W. (1987) Fractures and fracture/luxations of the lumbar spine: A retrospective study in the dog. *Journal of the American Animal Hospital Association* **23**, 460–464.

Walter, M.C., Smith, G.K. and Newton, C.D. (1986) Canine lumbar spinal internal fixation techniques. A comparative biomechanical study. *Veterinary Surgery* **15**, 191–198.

Waldron, D.R., Shires, P.K., McCain, W., Hedlund, C. and Blass, C.E. (1991) The rotational stabilizing effect of spinal fixation techniques in an unstable vertebral model. *Progress in Veterinary Neurology* **2**, 105–110.

14. MISCELLANEOUS CONDITIONS

This chapter covers various other important conditions of the spine that are likely to be encountered but are not specifically covered elsewhere in this book. Surgical treatment is not indicated in many of these conditions, thus they must be correctly diagnosed to avoid unneccessary operations. Key references are given, but the list is not intended to be encyclopaedic. For a full listing, see Braund (1992) and LeCouteur and Child (1989), both of which are comprehensive and have excellent bibliographies. The diseases are listed here alphabetically.

ARACHNOID CYSTS

In an arachnoid cyst there is a focal accumulation of CSF in the subarachnoid space, which compresses the spinal cord. (Parker *et al.*, 1983; Dyce *et al.*, 1991). The condition should be suspected in a young dog with progressive signs of myelopathy, but which is pain free (**462**). Diagnosis is by myelography.

Surgical decompression may be effective. Trauma has been suggested as a cause, as has dysraphism in view of the reports of the condition in Weimaraners and Rhodesian ridgebacks.

462 Cisternal myelogram in an eight-month-old Jack Russell terrier with grade 3 T_3–L_3 signs. Note the accumulations of contrast medium and the subsequent arrest of the columns. The diagnosis of arachnoid cyst was confirmed at postmortem examination.

ASCENDING/DESCENDING MYELOMALACIA

This is discussed in Chapter 8.

CALCINOSIS CIRCUMSCRIPTA

Calcinosis circumscripta has been described as a cause of compressive spinal cord dysfunction in young dogs (Dukes McEwan *et al.*, 1992). Diagnosis is by radiography, a mineralized mass being visible at the site of cord compression. The cause is not known. Surgical decompression may be successful.

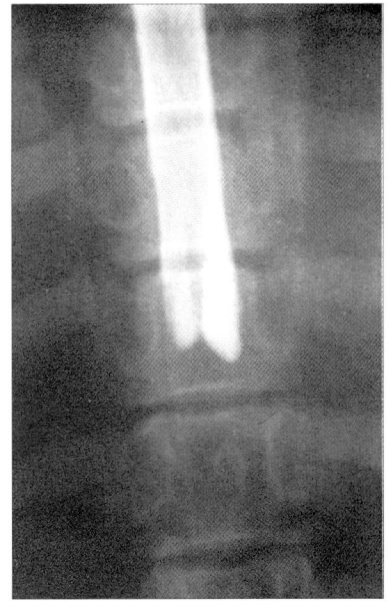

CONGENITAL VERTEBRAL ANOMALIES

Vertebral malformations are common findings in dogs and are occasionally seen in cats. However, they are often clinically insignificant, causing no neurological deficits. Some do cause compressive myelopathy, or may be associated with anomalies of the spinal cord (Bailey, 1975; Bailey and Morgan, 1992).

Hemivertebrae are the most common defects seen in dogs, usually in Pugs, Bulldogs, and Boston terriers. They are wedge-shaped and may cause spinal deviation in the lateral or dorsoventral plane depending on the orientation of the wedge. They are the result of failure of formation of part of the

14 MISCELLANEOUS CONDITIONS

vertebral body (**463**). Some dogs have butterfly vertebrae which result from failure of formation of the central part of the vertebra (**464**). A skeletal abnormality is often apparent on physical examination. Hemivertebrae may result in a chronic progressive myelopathy, but the site of spinal cord compression should be confirmed by myelography if decompressive surgery is proposed. It may be necessary to stabilise the vertebral column following decompressive surgery. Block vertebrae (**465**) result from a failure of division of the segments; they rarely cause clinical signs. Many cases of atlantoaxial subluxation have an underlying congenital vertebral malformation — see Chapter 9.

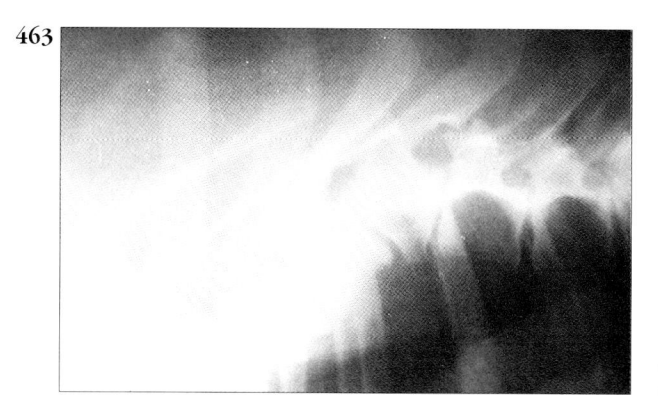

463 Wedge vertebra causing spinal deformity.

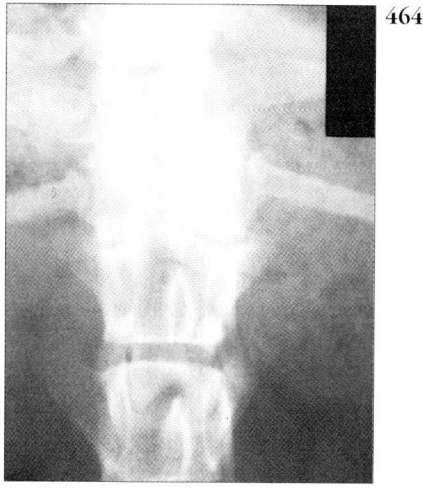

464 Butterfly vertebra. This was an incidental finding in an English bulldog.

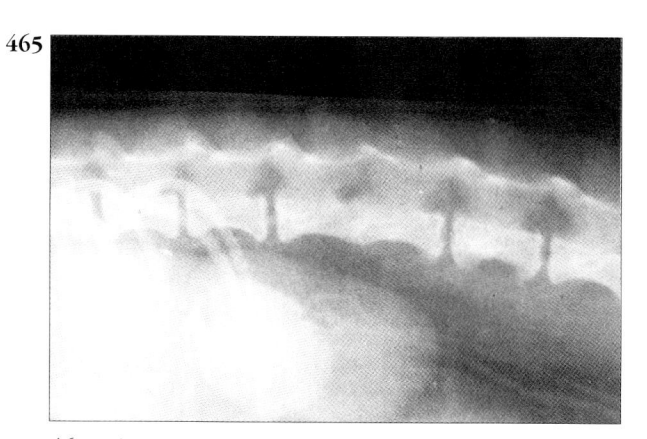

465 Block vertebrae. Again an incidental finding.

DEGENERATIVE MYELOPATHY (CHRONIC DEGENERATIVE RADICULOMYELOPATHY, CDRM)

This is a degenerative condition of the spinal cord of dogs, mostly seen in large breeds and particularly German shepherds (**466**). Onset of signs is from five years of age. Degenerative changes are found in the spinal cord and nerve roots, mainly affecting the thoracolumbar spinal cord. There is a loss of myelin and axons, and cellular infiltration in the most severely affected regions. The aetiology is not clear.

Progressive pelvic limb ataxia, loss of conscious proprioception, and paraparesis occur. The neurological examination indicates a T_3–L_3 lesion in most dogs, but some lose the patellar reflex because of the dorsal nerve root involvement. Urinary and faecal function is normal. Spinal pain is not seen. Signs in affected dogs progress over several months, and eventually the thoracic limbs will be involved.

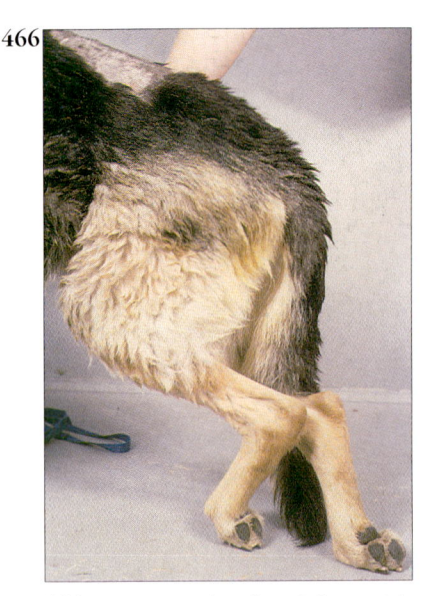

DIAGNOSIS AND SURGERY OF SMALL ANIMAL SPINAL DISORDERS

466 German shepherd dog with degenerative myelopathy. Note the knuckling of the feet.

Table 31 Suggested treatment protocol for degenerative myelopathy (from Clemmons, 1992)

Exercise	Alternate day periods including walking, running, and swimming, to 30 minutes twice a week and 1 hour once a week
Vitamin B	High potency complex q12 hours
Vitamin E	2000 IU/day
Aminocaproic acid	500 mg q8 hours. If no improvement within 8 weeks, do not continue. Make up 192 ml aminocaproic acid (250 mg/ml for injection) with 96 ml hematinic compound. This provides 500 mg animocaproic acid in 3 ml of solution
Corticosteroids	Use only during periods of worsening. Prednisone 1 mg/kg/day in three divided doses for 3 days, 0.33 mg/kg q12 hours for two days, 0.5 mg/kg alternate days for two weeks

The diagnosis is confirmed by the absence of structural spinal cord disease evident on myelography. Even if other lesions are found, for example, a mild disc protrusion, the possibility of degenerative myelopathy also being present should be considered. Analysis of lumbar CSF may reveal a moderately raised protein. Depressed cell-mediated immunity has been shown in this condition and its demonstration may be useful as a diagnostic test (Clemmons, 1989, 1992).

A treatment protocol of exercise, vitamins, occasional corticosteroids, and aminocaproic acid has been suggested (**Table 31**). The variable natural history of the disease makes the success of any treatment difficult to judge.

DISCOSPONDYLITIS

Discospondylitis is an inflammatory condition centred on the intervertebral disc and involving the vertebral end plates and adjacent bone of the vertebral body, usually caused by bacteria. *Staphylococcus intermedius* is the most common agent, but *Brucella canis*, *Streptococcus* spp., and *Escherichia coli* are also found. Fungal infections are rare (Kornegay, 1986).

Usually the bacteria gain access to the vertebra by haematogenous spread from other foci in the body, of which the bladder is most common. Occasional cases associated with foreign body migration are seen, usually grass seeds (awns). Iatrogenic cases following spinal surgery have also been recognised. Immunosuppression may be a predisposing factor in this disease. Large breeds of dogs are most often affected. The condition is rare in cats, most of which have external evidence of an infectious focus (Malik *et al.*, 1990).

14 MISCELLANEOUS CONDITIONS

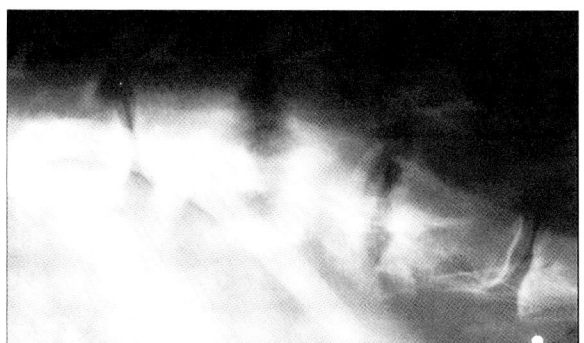

467 Discospondylitis in three-year-old Rottweiler. Note lesions at L_1/L_2 and L_2/L_3. There is widening of the intervertebral space, loss of the vertebral endplates and ventral new bone formation.

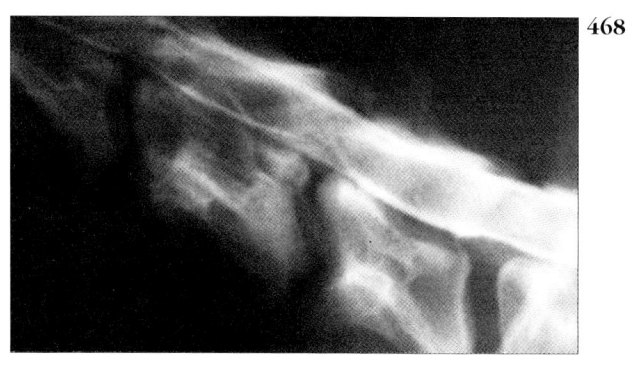

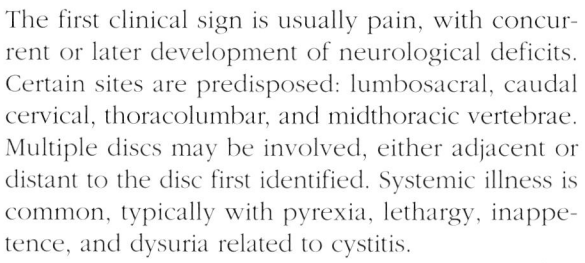

468 Discospondylitis in a Dobermann that developed following a ventral slot. Note split myelogram column indicating asymmetrical spinal cord compression over the affected disc space.

The first clinical sign is usually pain, with concurrent or later development of neurological deficits. Certain sites are predisposed: lumbosacral, caudal cervical, thoracolumbar, and midthoracic vertebrae. Multiple discs may be involved, either adjacent or distant to the disc first identified. Systemic illness is common, typically with pyrexia, lethargy, inappetence, and dysuria related to cystitis.

Diagnosis is by radiography (**467, 468**). Generally the radiographic changes are clearly seen, but occasionally the radiographs will be normal even though infection is present. Here bone scanning may reveal the lesion (Chapter 4) (Stefanacci and Wheeler, 1991). Blood or urine cultures, or both, are positive in about two thirds of patients. *Brucella canis* titres should be analysed in endemic areas.

Treatment of bacterial discospondylitis is initially by use of appropriate antibiotics. In view of the predominance of *Staph. intermedius*, use of cephradine or cloxacillin are the best initial choices. Ampicillin and amoxycillin are not suitable because the organism is resistant to these drugs through the mechanism of β–lactamase production. Further treatment is governed by clinical progression and results of bacteriological testing. Treatment must be continued for six weeks, even when the response is good. The prognosis is generally favourable.

Surgical curettage of solitary lesions is possible, often leading to rapid resolution of signs. It provides material for culture and promotes blood supply to the affected disc. Surgical intervention is largely a matter of personal preference, but should be considered in patients with unsatisfactory response to antibiotics.

Occasional patients will suffer severe collapse of the intervertebral space or vertebrae, causing marked spinal deformity with pain and significant neurological deficits. Surgical decompression and stabilization should only be embarked upon in carefully considered circumstances, in view of the difficulty in providing rigid fixation of the spine. Decompression of discospondylitis lesions by laminectomy without stabilisation can be dangerous as it may lead to marked instability and is not recommended.

If *B. canis* is diagnosed, minocycline (25 mg/kg PO q24 hours for two weeks) and streptomycin (5 mg/kg IM or SQ q12 hours for one week) or gentamycin (2 mg/kg IM or SQ q12 hours for one week) is recommended (Carmichael and Greene, 1990). There is potential for zoonotic spread, and recurrence is common. It may be wise to castrate male dogs with *B. canis* infection as the testes can act as a reservoir of infection.

FIBROCARTILAGINOUS EMBOLISM (ISCHAEMIC MYELOPATHY)

Fibrocartilaginous embolism (FCE) is a syndrome of acute, severe neurological dysfunction of dogs. It is an important differential diagnosis in cases of disc disease, trauma, and other acute spinal conditions (Griffiths, 1973; Zaki and Prata, 1976; Neer, 1992). The emboli have been identified as being composed of fibrocartilage, identical to the nucleus pulposus of the disc. In pathological studies of cases of FCE, emboli may be found in the vasculature of the spinal cord substance or nerve roots. The exact mechanism by which the FCE gain access to these areas is not clear.

Adult dogs of large and giant breeds are most often affected, but other breeds are seen with the condition, particularly the Miniature schnauzer. FCE occurs in any age of dog, although most are adults between three and seven years. The condition appears to be very rare in cats (Zaki *et al.*, 1976).

Acute, severe neurological presentations occur, often following vigorous exercise or mild trauma. Owners may note a progression of the signs over a period of several hours, perhaps from an initial lameness to eventual paralysis. Pain is not seen on clinical examination, but owners may report that the patient appeared uncomfortable during the development of the condition. Any part of the spinal cord may be affected, and often the signs are markedly asymmetrical. Involvement of the cervical and lumbar intumescences produces combinations of UMN- and LMN-type deficits.

Confirmation of the diagnosis is by elimination of other causes of these signs. Myelography should be performed to rule out compressive spinal cord lesions. Generally, the myelogram will be normal, but in some cases of FCE, it will show an intramedullary pattern of spinal cord swelling. Changes in CSF are nonspecific.

Treatment is by supportive care of the patient. Use of methylprednisolone, as in spinal trauma, may be useful in the first few hours following onset (see Chapter 6). Prolonged use of corticosteroids is not indicated.

The prognosis is guarded: UMN deficits often improve, but LMN deficits carry a worse prognosis, because of the involvement of the ventral horn cells in the ischaemic area of spinal cord.

HAEMORRHAGE

Haemorrhage and haematoma formation may occur within the spinal cord, in the subarachnoid space or in the epidural space. However, they are rare causes of spinal dysfunction, usually related to trauma or clotting disorders. If spinal haemorrhage is suspected in the absence of trauma, tests for clotting function should be performed. Analysis of CSF may reveal xanthochromia (see **62**). If fresh blood is seen in a CSF sample, it is most likely to be caused by puncture of a dural vessel rather than a reflection of the underlying disease.

Surgical decompression may be indicated in compressive lesions not associated with clotting disorders. Coagulopathy should be attended to, if present, and conservative therapy directed at the spinal lesion.

HYPERVITAMINOSIS A

Cats fed a diet with excessive vitamin A may suffer from a skeletal condition characterised by severe exostosis of the vertebrae, particularly in the cervical spine. Other parts of the spine and the limbs may also be involved (Clark, 1971). Clinical signs related to nerve root and spinal cord compression are seen. Neck pain and rigidity, ataxia, paresis of the thoracic limbs, and lameness are seen. The diagnosis is suspected in a cat fed exclusively on liver, and is confirmed by radiography (**469**).

Treatment is difficult. Stopping vitamin A intake can arrest the development of further exostoses, and anti-inflammatory drugs may relieve clinical signs.

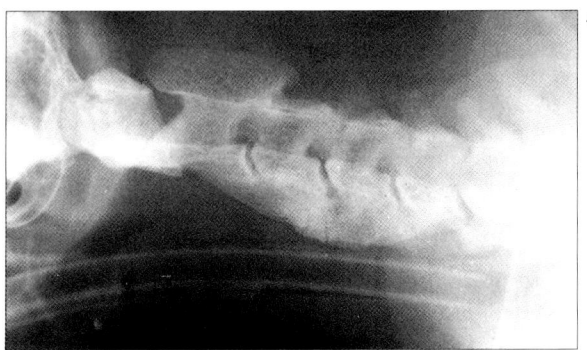

469 Hypervitaminosis A in a cat, with massive vertebral proliferation.

14 MISCELLANEOUS CONDITIONS

INFLAMMATORY CNS DISEASES

Aseptic meningitis (steroid-responsive meningitis, breed-specific meningitis)

Several aseptic meningitis syndromes have been described in dogs (Meric, 1993). Meningitis and polyarteritis has been described in a colony of young research Beagles (Harcourt, 1978). Bernese mountain dogs also suffer from a similar syndrome (Presthus, 1989).

The clinical signs are typical of meningitis, with depression, cervical pain, stiff gait, and pyrexia. The disease may be acute or have a relapsing pattern. Analysis of CSF reveals marked pleocytosis (with CSF white blood cell counts in the hundreds or even thousands per ml), mainly comprised of neutrophils and increased protein concentrations. Infectious agents are not seen in the CSF and culture is negative. The CSF may be relatively normal between bouts of the disease. An immune-mediated mechanism is suspected. The disease is similar to necrotizing vasculitis of the meningeal arteries (Meric *et al.*, 1986).

Treatment is with corticosteroids (prednisolone 1-2 mg/kg/day initially, later reducing) until clinical signs are controlled. Treatment is continued for several weeks and cessation of treatment may see relapse in some dogs, requiring further steroid administration. The prognosis is generally good, although some dogs experience relapses.

Canine distemper virus infection

Canine distemper virus infection is the most common infectious cause of neurological disease in dogs. Demyelination and inflammation occur in certain sites in the CNS. The virulence of the virus strain and the immunocompetence of the dog are important factors in determining the severity of the disease. Other CNS infections may be seen in association with the immunosuppression related to CDV. Systemic signs of disease may occur, although this is not a consistent feature (Tipold *et al.*, 1992). The neurological signs may be multifocal or specifically suggestive of a focal lesion, and may be acute in onset (Raw *et al.*, 1992).

Confirmation of a diagnosis of CDV infection ante mortem is difficult. Analysis of CSF is the most useful test (see Chapter 4) (Sorjonen, 1992).

Treatment is restricted to managing the clinical signs and providing supportive care. Corticosteroids may be useful in some patients, but the prognosis is poor.

Feline infectious peritonitis virus infection (FIP)

Neurological signs, including spinal cord syndromes, may be seen in cats with FIP virus infection. Multisystemic signs, particularly ocular involvement, are seen in most affected cats. Neurological signs are most often associated with the dry form of the disease (Kornegay, 1978). CSF is usually abnormal with increased protein and a mixed, predominantly neutrophilic pleocytosis (see Chapter 4). There is no definitive treatment and the prognosis is poor.

Granulomatous meningoencephalomyelitis reticulosis (GME)

This is an inflammatory disease of the CNS of unknown aetiology. Any part of the CNS may be involved, either in a focal or diffuse form. Perivascular accumulations of mononuclear cells are present throughout the CNS, which can lead to the formation of large granulomas (Cordy, 1979; Thomas and Eger, 1989).

Clinical signs are typical of meningoencephalomyelitis; onset is usually between three and seven years of age. Spinal cord syndromes may be seen alone or as part of a multifocal presentation. The signs of spinal disease may include neurological deficits or may be restricted to spinal hyperaesthesia. The course is usually chronic, but some cases show a rapid decline.

Analysis of CSF reveals moderate, mainly mononuclear pleocytosis with increased protein, but the findings are nonspecific. Some dogs with spinal cord involvement have myelographic patterns suggestive of intramedullary lesions (see **84** and **92–94**) Treatment with immunosuppressive doses of corticosteroids may lead to improvement (prednisolone 1–2 mg/kg/day). The long term prognosis is poor.

Other infectious agents

Infection of the spinal cord by organisms other than viruses, leading to meningitis and myelitis, is rare in dogs and cats. Spinal infections are often associated with brain involvement, causing multifocal neurological signs. Many organisms have been implicated, including bacteria, fungi, rickettsia, and *Prototheca* species; the distribution of many of these organisms is regional. Organisms reportedly isolated from spinal cords of dogs and cats are given in **Table 32**.

The signs are typical of inflammatory CNS disease as described above. Some infections show mainly signs of intracranial disease, typically rickettsial infections when seizures, dullness, depression, and vestibular signs occur. Pelvic limb hyperextension is often seen in toxoplasmosis. Systemic signs of infection may be apparent, for example, gastrointestinal disturbance or respiratory signs, which may indicate the means of entry into the CNS. Patients may be pyrexic, but this is variable.

Table 32 Non-viral organisms implicated in inflammatory CNS disease in dogs and cats

Bacteria	*Actinomyces*
	Nocardia
	Pasteurella spp.
	Staph. aureus, intermedius, epidermidis, albus
Fungi	*Blastomyces dermatitidis*
	Coccidioides imitis
	Cryptococcus neoformans
	Histoplasma capsulatum
Protozoa	*Toxoplasma gondii*
	Neospora caninum
Rickettsia	*Ehrlichia canis*
	Rickettsia rickettsii
Prototheca	*Prototheca* spp.

Confirmation of the diagnosis is usually by CSF analysis. Pleocytosis is variable, but very high cell counts (in the thousands per µl) may be seen, mostly composed of neutrophils, and eosinophils may also be present. Organisms may be seen in the CSF. Culture may be attempted but is often unrewarding. Serological testing may be useful in some infections, for example, in rickettsial infections or cryptococcosis (Greene, 1990).

Those rare patients where bacterial infections are identified should be treated with antibiotics. The bacterial sensitivity and CNS penetration of the drug must be considered in choosing an antibiotic (Keen, 1989). Fungal infections are difficult to treat, but amphotericin B, itraconazole, and fluconazole have been suggested. Rickettsial infections are treated with tetracyclines, preferably doxycycline, or chloramphenicol (Greene and Breitschwerdt, 1990). Protozoal infections may be treated with clindamycin.

The use of corticosteroids in meningomyelitis is controversial. They are contraindicated in fungal infection, but may have a role in bacterial infections. The potential consequences of corticosteroid use must be considered before their administration.

ISCHAEMIC NEUROMYOPATHY (AORTIC EMBOLISM, ILIAC THROMBOSIS)

Ischaemic neuromyopathy is a common cause of acute paraplegia in cats. Areflexia, absent deep pain sensation, cold limbs, absent femoral pulses, and swollen painful gastrocnemius muscles are the common features. Affected cats have cyanotic nail beds and toes that do not bleed with needle prick. Occasional cats have signs referable to renal, gastrointestinal, or other dysfunction. Diagnosis is based on the clinical signs (Griffiths and Duncan, 1979). Preexisting cardiomyopathy underlies the thromboembolic episode, but the presence of a thrombus does not entirely explain the clinical signs. There appears to be a failure of collateral circulation because of release of vasoactive substances from the area of the thrombus.

Treatment is aimed at stabilizing the circulation, with suitable fluid therapy and cardiac medications. Drug therapy aimed at promoting reperfusion has been recommended: acepromazine for vasodilation, heparin to inhibit coagulation, and aspirin for antiplatelet activity. All these medications have potentially severe side-effects. Thrombolytic therapy has been advocated, but this also may be hazardous (Pion and Kittleson, 1989). Surgical removal of the thrombus has also been described.

Whatever method of treatment is chosen, the prognosis is guarded. The neurological status will improve in approximately 50% of cats, but the underlying cardiac disease may be difficult to resolve and recurrences can occur.

LEUKOENCEPHALOMALACIA

Leukoencephalomalacia is a degenerative CNS disease, reported only in Rottweilers in the USA, The Netherlands, and Australia. There is malacia throughout the spinal cord, particularly in the cervical region, due to demyelination and cavitation. The aetiology is unclear (Chrisman, 1992).

Affected dogs show clinical signs from one–four years of age. There is pelvic limb ataxia and hypermetria, progressing through paraparesis to tetraparesis over a period of months. Conscious proprioceptive deficits are marked. Limb reflexes are intact or even hyperactive.

Differentiation from neuroaxonal dystrophy and other CNS conditions is important. All routine diagnostic tests are normal in leukoencephalomalacia. The major differential features are the presence of conscious proprioceptive deficits in leukoencephalomalacia, and tremor seen in neuroaxonal dystrophy.

There is no treatment and the prognosis is poor, most dogs with leukoencephalomalacia being euthanatised within one year of presentation.

MULTIPLE CARTILAGINOUS EXOSTOSES (OSTEOCHONDROMATOSIS)

Cartilaginous exostoses may cause spinal cord compression at any site of the vertebral column of dogs and cats. Lesions may also occur on the ribs and limb bones. There is abnormal differentiation of cartilage cells in bones that develop by endochondral ossification, leading to the production of large masses composed of a thin cortex lined by cartilage, and a core of cancellous bone. The aetiology is unclear (Gambardella et al., 1975). The masses continue to grow until skeletal maturity is reached. Diagnosis is by radiography (**470**).

Surgical decompression of compressive lesions may be necessary.

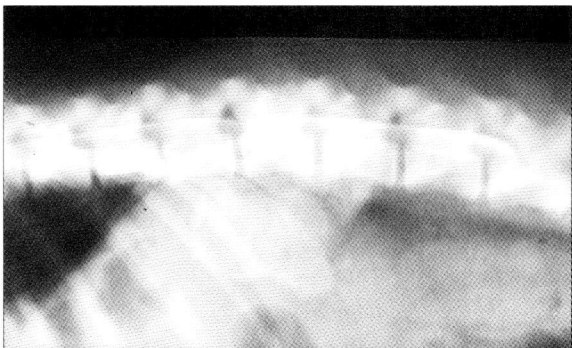

470 Multiple cartilaginous exostoses.

NEUROAXONAL DYSTROPHY

Neuroaxonal dystrophy is a degenerative CNS disease seen mainly in Rottweilers, but also occasionally reported in cats. It is thought to be an autosomal recessive condition in the Rottweiler. Axonal dystrophy with axonal spheroids is seen in parts of the CNS, including the dorsal horn grey matter of the spinal cord, and the gracile, cuneate, and dorsal spinocerebellar tract nuclei. Cerebellar atrophy may also be seen. The aetiology is unknown (Chrisman, 1992).

Affected dogs show clinical signs from puppyhood, but they may not be noticed until the dog is adult. There is pelvic limb ataxia and hypermetria of the thoracic limbs. Conscious proprioception is normal. Limb reflexes are intact or even hyperactive. Head incoordination, tremor, positional nystagmus, and loss of menace response (due to cerebellar involvement) develop later, often after several years. Weakness is not seen.

Differentiation from leukoencephalomalacia and other CNS conditions is important. Routine diagnostic tests are normal.

There is no treatment and the prognosis is poor, although affected dogs may survive as active pets for several years.

PILONIDAL SINUS (DERMOID SINUS, EPIDERMOID CYST)

In pilonidal sinus the skin over the dorsal midline is inverted and, in some dogs, communicates with the dura mater. Rhodesian ridgebacks and Shih tzus have a high incidence. Infection from the cyst may extend to the spinal cord, causing meningitis and myelitis with associated clinical signs.

Diagnosis is based on the clinical signs. If a cyst is suspected to be in communication with the vertebral canal, fistulography may be performed but it is important to use a non-ionic contrast medium. Infected lesions are treated by antibiotics and surgical excision; it may be necessary to perform a laminectomy to retrieve all the tissue. Careless exploration of this type of lesion, without a full appreciation of its extent, can lead to the development of marked neurological deficits.

SACROCAUDAL DYSGENESIS

Cats and dogs with congenital tail defects often have vertebral abnormalities of the sacrum and caudal vertebrae. Manx cats, Pugs, and Bulldogs are most often affected. The vertebral abnormalities may themselves result in neurological signs of the pelvic limbs and viscera (urinary tract and anus). There may be malformations of the spinal cord, for example, spina bifida with associated skin lesions. This condition is inherited in the Manx cat.

Diagnosis is suspected from the clinical signs. Radiography will demonstrate vertebral abnormalities and myelography may reveal spinal cord malformations. Treatment is not possible and the prognosis is poor.

SPINA BIFIDA

This is a developmental defect resulting from failure of fusion of the embryonic vertebral arch. There may be protrusion of the meninges or spinal cord into a meningocoele, a myelocoele, or a meningomyelocoele; this is termed spina bifida aperta. Alternatively, there may be no protrusion of nervous tissue termed spina bifida occulta (Wilson, 1982). The aetiology is unknown, but there is a high incidence in English bulldogs.

The condition most often involves the caudal lumbar spine. Clinical signs indicative of L_4–S_3 spinal cord dysfunction occur. Radiography may reveal defects in the dorsal vertebral arch, for example, paired spinous processes, and myelography may demonstrate a meningocoele. Treatment is not possible.

SPINAL DYSRAPHISM (MYELODYSPLASIA)

Malformations of the spinal cord have been described in several breeds of dogs, particularly Weimaraners (Van den Broek et al., 1991). Various lesions of the central canal, grey matter, dorsal sulcus, and ventral fissure have been described. The condition is inherited in Weimaraners. Signs indicative of T_3–L_3 spinal cord disease are seen in puppies. A bunnyhopping pelvic limb gait is often seen. Abnormalities of the hair coat, a depression of the sternum and head tilt may be seen. The signs may or may not be progressive, and there is no treatment.

14 MISCELLANEOUS CONDITIONS

SPONDYLOSIS DEFORMANS

Spondylosis deformans is a common radiographic finding in older dogs, but rarely is it associated with clinical signs. Generally osteophytes develop ventrally and laterally on the vertebral body, and may grow to the point that they cross the intervertebral space (**471**) (Larsen and Selby, 1981). The anticlinal region, thoracolumbar junction, and lumbosacral joint are particularly affected. Where these changes are seen at the lumbosacral joint they may be related to clinical signs of lumbosacral disease. However, this diagnosis should not be reached on the basis of survey radiographs alone, as such changes are seen in many normal dogs (see Chapter 10).

It is important to differentiate spondylosis deformans from the changes seen in discospondylitis (see **467**, **468**).

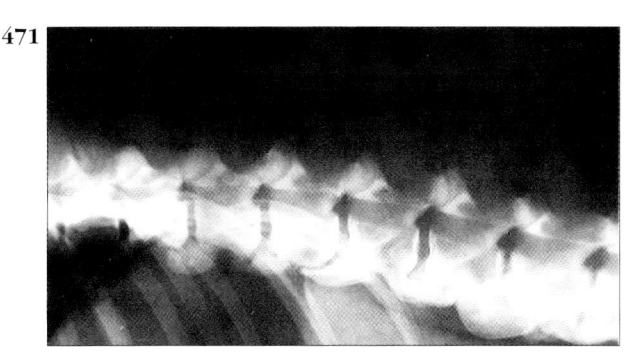

471 Spondylosis deformans. This was an incidental finding in a seven-year-old Boxer.

STORAGE DISEASES

Lysosomal storage diseases occur where there is a defect of metabolism because of a dysfunction in a specific enzyme pathway. They are relatively common in dogs and cats, and frequently cause neurological signs, which are seen from early in life and are progressive. The majority are inherited in an autosomal recessive pattern (Evans, 1989). Diagnosis is based on various biopsies, depending on the nature of the disease. There is no treatment, and the prognosis is poor.

SYRINGOMYELIA

Syringomyelia and hydromyelia are fluid-filled cavitations of the spinal cord and central canal. Syringomyelia may be associated with any type of acquired spinal cord lesion, although the cause is not known. Hydromyelia is often associated with congenital spinal malformations, and may be the result of altered CSF pressures. Syringomyelia is seen in Weimaraners with dysraphism. Cavitation of the spinal cord in both conditions may be progressive. Clinical differentiation is not possible. Clinical signs of spinal cord dysfunction depend on the location of the lesion in the vertebral column. Associated skeletal changes including torticollis or scoliosis may be seen (Child *et al.*, 1986). Diagnosis may be aided by MRI.

REFERENCES

Bailey, C.S. (1975) An embryological approach to the clinical significance of congenital vertebral and spinal cord abnormalities. *Journal of the American Animal Hospital Association* **11**, 426–434.

Bailey, C.S. and Morgan, J.P. (1992) Congenital spinal malformations. *Veterinary Clinics of North America, Small Animal Practice* **22**(**4**), 985–1015.

Braund, K.G. (1992) *Clinical Syndromes in Veterinary Neurology*. 2nd Edn., Mosby, St Louis.

Breitschwerdt, E.B. and Greene, C.E. (1990) Rocky Mountain spotted fever and Q fever. In *Infectious diseases of the dog and cat*, pp. 419–433. (Ed. C.E. Greene.) W.B. Saunders Co., Philadelphia.

Carmichael, L.E. and Greene, C.E. (1990) Canine brucellosis. In *Infectious diseases of the dog and cat*, pp. 573–584. (Ed. C.E. Greene.) W.B. Saunders Co., Philadelphia, .

Child, G., Higgins, R.J. and Cuddon, P.A. (1986) Acquired scoliosis associated with hydromyelia and syringomyelia in two dogs. *Journal of the American Veterinary Medical Association* **189**, 909–912.

Chrisman, C.L. (1992) Neurological diseases of Rottweilers; Neuroaxonal dystrophy and leukoencephalomalacia. *Journal of Small Animal Practice* **33**, 500–504.

Clark, L. (1971) Hypervitaminosis A: a review. *Australian Veterinary Journal* **47**, 568–571.

Clemmons, R.M. (1989) Degenerative myelopathy. *Current Veterinary Therapy X*, pp 830–834. (Ed. R.W. Kirk.) W.B. Saunders Co., Philadelphia.

Clemmons, R.M. (1992) Degenerative myelopathy. *Veterinary Clinics of North America, Small Animal Practice* **22**(**4**), 965–971.

Cordy, D.R. (1979) Canine granulomatous meningoencephalomyelitis. *Veterinary Pathology* **16**, 325–333.

Dukes McEwan, J., Thomson, C.E., Sullivan, M., Callanan, S. and Park, M. (1992) Thoracic spinal calcinosis circumscripta causing cord compression in two German shepherd dog littermates. *Veterinary Record* **130**, 575–578.

Dyce, J., Herrtage, M.E., Houlton, J.E.F. and Palmer, A.C. (1991) Canine spinal arachnoid cysts. *Journal of Small Animal Practice* **32**, 433–437.

Evans, R.J. (1989) Lysosomal storage disease in dogs and cats. *Journal of Small Animal Practice* **30**, 144–150.

Gambardella, P.C., Osborne, C.A. and Stevens, J.B. (1975) Multiple cartilaginous exostoses in the dog. *Journal of the American Veterinary Medical Association* **166**, 761–768.

Greene, C.E. (1990) *Infectious Diseases of the Dog and Cat.* W.B. Saunders Co., Philadelphia.

Greene, C.E. and Breitschwerdt, E.B. (1990) Rocky Mountain Spotted Fever and Q Fever. In *Infectious Diseases of the Dog and Cat.* (Ed. C.E. Greene) W.B. Saunders Co., Philadelphia, pp427–429.

Griffiths, I.R. (1973) Spinal cord infarction due to emboli arising from the intervertebral discs in the dog. *Journal of Comparative Pathology* **83**, 225–232.

Griffiths, I.R. and Duncan, I.D. (1979) Ischaemic neuromyopathy in cats. *Veterinary Record* **104**, 518–522.

Harcourt, R.A. (1978) Polyarteritis in a colony of Beagles. *Veterinary Record* **102**, 519–522.

Keen, P.M. (1989) Clinical pharmacology and therapeutics of the nervous system. In *Manual of Small Animal Neurology*, pp 107–117. (Ed. S.J. Wheeler.) BSAVA Publications, Cheltenham.

Kornegay, J.N. (1978) Feline infectious peritonitis: the central nervous system form. *Journal of the American Animal Hospital Association* **14**, 580–584.

Kornegay, J.N. (1986) Discospondylitis. In *Current Veterinary Therapy IX*, pp 810–814. W.B. Saunders Co., Philadelphia.

Larsen, J.S. and Selby, L.A (1981) Spondylosis deformans in large dogs relative risk by breed, age and sex. *Journal of the American Animal Hospital Association* **17**, 623–625.

LeCouteur, R.A. and Child, G. (1989) Diseases of the spinal cord. In *Textbook of Veterinary Internal Medicine*, 3rd edn, pp 624–701 (Ed. S.J. Ettinger.) W.B. Saunders Co., Philadelphia.

Malik, R., Latter, M. and Love, D.N. (1990) Bacterial discospondylitis in a cat. *Journal of Small Animal Practice* **31**, 404–406.

Meric, S. (1988) Canine meningitis: a changing emphasis. *Journal of Veterinary Internal Medicine* **2**, 26–35.

Meric, S.M. (1993) Breedspecific meningitis in dogs. *Current Veterinary Therapy XI*, pp 1007–1009. (Eds. R.W. Kirk and J.D. Bonagura.) W.B. Saunders Co., Philadelphia.

Meric, S.M., Child, G. and Higgins, R.J. (1986) Necrotizing vasculitis of the spinal pachymeningeal arteries in three Bernese mountain littermates. *Journal of the American Animal Hospital Association* **22**, 459–465.

Morgan, J.P. (1969) Spinal dural ossification in the dog: Incidence and distribution based on a radiographic study. *Journal of the American Veterinary Radiology Society* **10**, 43–48.

Neer, T.M. (1992) Fibrocartilaginous emboli. *Veterinary Clinics of North America, Small Animal Practice* **22**(4), 1017–1026.

Parker, A.J., Adams, W.M. and Zachary, J.F. (1983) Spinal arachnoid cysts in the dog. *Journal of the American Animal Hospital Association* **19**, 1001–1008.

Pion, P.D. and Kittleson, M.D. (1989) Therapy for feline aortic thromboembolism. *Current Veterinary Therapy X*, pp 295–302. W.B. Saunders Co., Philadelphia.

Presthus, J. (1989) Aseptic suppurative meningitis in Bernese Mountain Dogs. *Norsk Veterinaertidsskrift* **101**, 169–175.

Raw, M.E., Pearson, G.R., Brown, P.J. and Baumgartner, W. (1992) Canine distemper infection associated with acute nervous signs in dogs. *Veterinary Record* **130**, 291–293.

Sorjonen, D.C. (1992) Myelitis and meningitis. *Veterinary Clinics of North America, Small Animal Practice* **22**, 951–964.

Stefanacci, J.D. and Wheeler, S.J. (1991) Skeletal scintigraphy in canine discospondylitis. *Proceedings, American College of Veterinary Radiology Annual Scientific Meeting*, p. 66.

Thomas, J.B. and Eger, C. (1989) Granulomatous meningoencephalomyelitis in 21 dogs. *Journal of Small Animal Practice* **30**, 287–293.

Tipold, A., Vandevelde, M. and Jaggy, A. (1992) Neurological manifestations of canine distemper virus infection. *Journal of Small Animal Practice* **33**, 466–470.

van den Broek, A.H.M., Else, R.W., Abercromby, R. and France, M. (1991) Spinal dysraphism in the Weimaraner. *Journal of Small Animal Practice* **32**, 258–260.

Wilson, J.W. (1982) Spina bifida in the dog and cat. *Compendium on Continuing Education for the Practicing Veterinarian* **4**, 626–633.

Zaki, F.A. and Prata, R.G. (1976) Necrotizing myelopathy secondary to embolization of herniated intervertebral disk material in the dog. *Journal of the American Veterinary Medical Association* **169**, 222–228.

Zaki, F.A., Prata, R.G. and Werner. L.L. (1976) Necrotizing myelopathy in a cat. *Journal of the American Veterinary Medical Association* **169**, 228–229.

15. POSTOPERATIVE CARE

The surgeon should accept that some form of postoperative complication will develop in many neurosurgical patients. This may range from a simple urinary tract infection to less common but life threatening conditions such as pneumonia or pancreatitis. If complications are viewed as something to be expected, the surgeon is more likely to have the patient monitored appropriately (**Table 33**).

Table 33 Important clinical signs to recognize in the postoperative neurosurgical patient

Post-myelographic seizures
Inappetance
Depression
Fever
Diarrhoea or vomiting
Melaena or 'coffee ground' vomit
Change in ability to void, or the ease of manual expression
Blood or floccular material in urine
Urine scald
Decubital ulcers
Pain

Care of neurosurgical patients is often very labour intensive. It is important that hospital nursing staff have a high standard of training and are properly informed about what parameters to monitor, how often to monitor them, and what the most likely complications are going to be in each individual patient. Clear written instructions should be given to the client at the time of discharge.

ANALGESIA

Neurosurgical procedures often cause a great deal of pain for human patients. It is likely that veterinary surgeons have tended to overlook the degree of pain suffered by our patients. Doubt as to whether an animal really is in pain often causes a clinician to withhold analgesics, yet the same clinician will administer antibiotics without documented evidence of infection (Crane, 1987). When in doubt, a dose of narcotic should be tested for effect.

Opioid analgesics

It is preferable to use one of the relatively long-acting opioid analgesics in the first 12–24 hours after surgery. The approximate duration of action of these drugs, together with their advantages and disadvantages, are outlined in **Table 34**. Preoperative or intraoperative narcotic administration reduces the requirement for postoperative analgesia.

Pure opioid agonists are the most potent analgesics, but have more potential side-effects. Dose-dependent respiratory depression means that they must be used with great care in animals with potentially decreased ventilatory function, such as those with cranial cervical spinal cord lesions or thoracic injuries, as may be seen in trauma patients. Opioid agonists increase intracranial pressure and should not be used in any animal that has suffered head trauma.

Epidural morphine has been used extensively in veterinary medicine and may prove of value in neurosurgical patients. No complications have been reported and respiratory depression has not been a problem (Valverde et al., 1989; Dodman et al., 1992). It should be given preoperatively as it has an onset lag time of 20–60 minutes and it is difficult to give during surgery. Analgesia lasts for 10–24 hours and can be effective as far cranial as the thoracic limbs. It is not associated with sensory, sympathetic, or motor blockade, so the patient can walk without impairment, in contrast to the spinal administration of local anaesthetics. The dose for morphine (preferably preservative-free) is 0.1 mg/kg, diluted in warm saline to a volume of 1 ml per 5 kg, injected into the lumbosacral epidural space. Urinary retention is a potentially troublesome side-effect of epidural morphine.

Table 34 Narcotic analgesis agents[1,2,3]

Drug	Dose	Frequency	Advantages	Disadvantages
Morphine (pure agonist)	**Dog:** 0.1–0.8 mg/kg IM, or IV infusion 0.1–0.2 mg/kg/hr **Cat:** 0.1 mg/kg IM	4 hrs	Inexpensive Sedative	Respiratory depression Bradycardia** Emesis Increased intracranial pressure Caution IV Controlled drug
Oxymorphone (pure agonist)	**Dog:** 0.02–0.08 mg/kg IM or IV **Cat:** 0.02 mg/kg IM	4–6 hrs	Less respiratory and GI effects than morphine	As for morphine Auditory hypersensitivity Expense
Butorphanol (agonist/ antagonist)	**Dog:** 0.2–0.6 mg/kg IM or SQ **Cat:** 0.2–0.4 mg/kg IM	2–4 hrs	Reduced respiratory or cardiovascular effects	Less potent analgesic in severe pain
Buprenorphine (agonist/ antagonist)	**Dog:** 0.005–0.02mg/kg IM or SQ **Cat:** 0.005–0.01 mg/kg IM	4–8 hrs (up to 14 hrs)	Reduced respiratory or cardiovascular effects	Bradycardia** (If respiratory depression does occur it can be difficult to reverse)
Naloxone* (pure antagonist)	**Dog and cat:** 0.04 mg/kg IV or IM	1–2 hrs	Reversal agent especially for respiratory depression	Shorter acting than agonists so animal may become re-narcotized

* It is possible to antagonize respiratory depression selectively by titrating with the pure narcotic antagonist naloxone (1 ml vial diluted to 10 ml in saline), and yet preserve some analgesia. Titration may need to be repeated as frequently as every hour to prevent renarcotization as the naloxone wears off. Buprenorphine is only poorly antagonized by naloxone, and one of the newer reversal agents such as naltrexone may be needed.

** Concomitant administration of atropine may be required to overcome bradycardia.

[1] Haskins, 1990; [2] Sackman, 1991; [3] Haskins, 1992.

Non-steroidal anti-inflammatory drug analgesia

NSAIDs only relieve pain of low to moderate intensity, but may prove useful in cases where narcotics are not suitable (**Table 35**). Because of the tendency for neurosurgical patients to develop gastrointestinal disturbances, NSAIDs should probably be used for no more than 24 hours. A major contraindication is if the dog has recently had corticosteroids, including high-dose methylprednisolone, because of the high risk of gastrointestinal bleeding and perforation (Strombeck and Guilford, 1990). Misoprostol, a synthetic prostaglandin E, protects the gastrointestinal tract and can be used prophylactically to counter the gastrointestinal side-effects of the NSAIDs. Carprofen, a new NSAID is also of special interest because it does not reduce PgE levels in the gut (McKellar et al., 1991), and no significant gastrointestinal problems were observed in over 100 dogs with degenerative joint disease in which it was used (Holtsinger et al., 1992). Care in the use of NSAIDs is needed in animals with renal, hepatic or cardiac dysfunction. Aspirin may decrease platelet aggregation and so cause significantly increased bleeding times (**472**). Thus, it should not be used preoperatively.

15. POSTOPERATIVE CARE

472

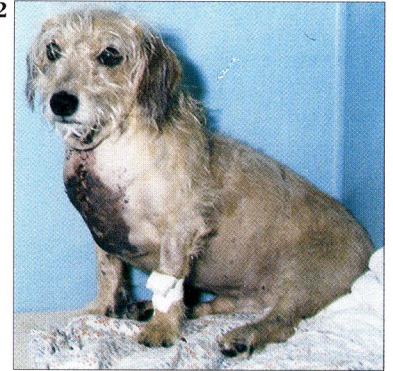

472 Postoperative appearance of a dog that was given 120 mg of aspirin 24 hours before surgery for a cervical disc. The severe bruising of the skin was presumed to be caused by poor platelet aggregation resulting from the effects of aspirin.

Table 35 Non-steroidal anti-inflammatory drug analgesia [1,2,3,4,5]

Drug	Dose (dog)	Dose (cat)
Aspirin (not large enteric-coated tablets)	10–25 mg/kg PO q12 hours	10 mg/kg PO q36–48 hours
Phenylbutazone	10–25 mg/kg PO q8 hours	Not recommended
Meclofenamic acid	1.1 mg/kg PO q24 hours	Not recommended
Flunixin	0.5–1.0 mg/kg PO q24 hours	Not recommended
Carprofen	2.2 mg/kg PO q12 hours	?

[1] Haskins, 1990; [2] Sackman, 1991; [3] Strombeck and Guilford, 1990; [4] Holtsinger et al., 1992; [5] McKellar et al., 1991.

Other drugs
The skeletal muscle relaxant methocarbamol (55–132 mg/kg PO in divided doses) can be very useful to relieve muscle spasm after thoracolumbar disc fenestration and many other types of surgery.

Analgesia in cats
Selected opioids can be used in cats. High doses cause CNS excitation, but otherwise the side-effects are as described in **Table 34**. Of the NSAIDs, only aspirin is generally recommended in cats, and because metabolism is different in cats than in dogs, it is important to give it at much reduced frequencies. Acetaminophen should not be used in cats.

NURSING CARE

Moving patients
When moving an animal with a spinal lesion, especially an anaesthetized patient, proper support should be provided for the spine. Use of a board or stretcher is useful (see **397**).

Myelography
Following the injection of contrast agent into the subarachnoid space, it is very important that the animal's head is kept elevated, both during the myelographic examination and during recovery from anaesthesia. In our experience, this simple precaution is frequently overlooked as a means of preventing postmyelographic seizures.

Treatment plans
The best way to nurse a neurological patient, especially one with multiple problems, is to make a plan for each day as illustrated in **Tables 36 and 37**. In this manner, voiding requirements, physiotherapy needs, medications, laboratory work and routine tasks are planned out and not forgotten.

Cleanliness
Animals that soil themselves repeatedly may be much easier to manage if their entire hindquarters are shaved.

Urinalysis
If urinary incontinence is present, a urinalysis should be done every two or three days, regardless of whether the patient is on antibiotics.

Table 36 Example of a plan for nursing neurological patients: taken from the hospital record of a four-year-old male Dachshund that had undergone a hemilaminectomy for thoracolumbar disc extrusion four days previously. The dog was paraplegic and incontinent, with reduced deep pain sensation. An *E.coli*, sensitive to trimethoprim/sulpha, had been cultured from his urine on admission. X = task completed.

Task	8 a.m.	12 p.m	4 p.m.	8 p.m.
TPR	X		☐	
Express bladder	X	☐	☐	☐
Feed 1/4 can	X	☐		
Check drinking water	X	☐	☐	☐
Phenoxybenzamine 5 mg PO	X		☐	
Diazepam 2.5 mg PO	X	☐	☐	
Trimethoprim–sulpha 160 mg PO	X		☐	
Urinalysis				☐

Recumbency

Recumbent tetraparetic animals need to be turned regularly, ideally every 2–4 hours, because sustained hypostatic congestion predisposes the patient to pneumonia. They should also be kept on a water bed if possible.

Hydration and nutrition

Tetraparetic animals dehydrate very easily and should be offered water from a sternal position every four hours, or be given intravenous fluids. Total protein, haematocrit, and serum electrolyte concentrations should be monitored regularly in these patients.

Nutritional support for the neurosurgical patient should also be evaluated carefully. Stress, particularly from trauma or surgery increases metabolic rate, so enhanced nutritional intake is important to minimize the tendency to deplete body protein. The patient should be given palatable, high quality meals several times daily to cope with the increased requirement. Conversely, an inactive, paraplegic dog may need a slight reduction in its nutritional intake (Donoghue, 1989).

Table 37 Example of a plan for nursing neurological patients: taken from the hospital record of a six-year-old male Dobermann (same dog as shown in 477) with caudal cervical spondylomyelopathy that had undergone a ventral decompression one week previously. The dog was recumbent, tetraparetic, and although continent, he needed manual expression of his bladder to initiate voiding. Food was being withheld as he had suffered severe bloody diarrhoea the previous day, for which he was being treated with sucralfate. The dog also tended to chew his feet if they were left unbandaged. The chest radiograph was being performed because the dog appeared depressed and auscultation of the lungs suggested early pneumonia. The dog was already being turned every four hours. The nursing care for this patient is particularly complex, and illustrates the support needed for certain types of neurosurgical patient.

Task	8 a.m.	12 p.m.	4 p.m.	8 p.m.	12 a.m
TPR	X		☐		
Express bladder and take outside by day	X	☐	☐	☐	☐
Nil per os except water; prop up to drink	X	☐	☐	☐	☐
Sucralfate 500 mg PO	X		☐	☐	☐
Rebandage feet	X				
Turn	X	☐	☐	☐	☐
Chest radiograph	☐				
Place in sling for 30 minutes	X	☐	☐		

FLOORING FOR RECUMBENT PATIENTS

Different flooring materials and their indications are illustrated in **473–477**.

In general, a raised grate is best for most small paraparetic or paraplegic patients. The advantage of a grate is the reduced tendency for an animal to lie in its own urine and faeces, particularly if non-retentive bedding is also provided. A grate does not, however, provide padding and is not suitable for larger recumbent patients or those with established decubitus. In such cases, a variety of padded

15. POSTOPERATIVE CARE

flooring materials can be used; each has advantages and disadvantages. Nursing staff must be made aware that patients with disturbed pain perception are at extreme risk for developing thermal burns (**478**). A thermostatically controlled circulating water blanket is the only safe way to warm a neurological patient (**479**). Electric heating blankets can be dangerously unreliable (Swaim *et al.*, 1989).

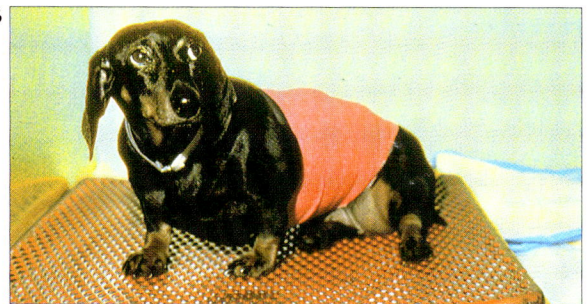

473 Paraplegic dog sitting on a raised grate. This flooring allows urine, and to some extent faeces, to pass through it and so keeps the dog cleaner and drier. This flooring is suitable for most small patients, and for larger patients with minimal neurological deficits.

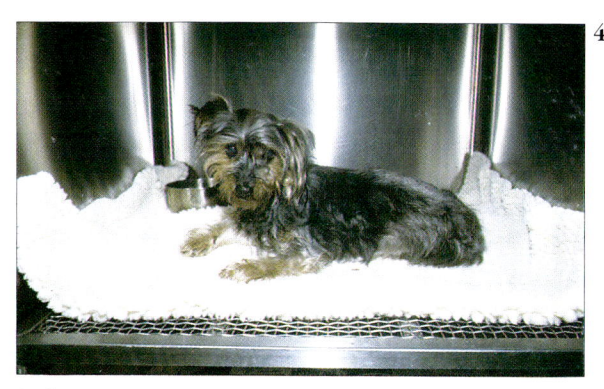

474 Non-retentive bedding. This is an excellent material to use with a raised grate, as it stays dry yet allows liquids to pass rapidly through to the cage floor beneath.

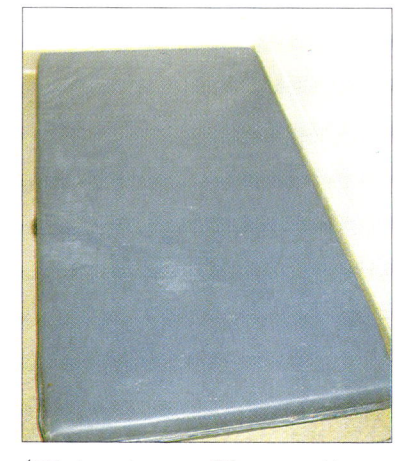

475 A waterproof foam mattress. This can be of varying thickness for different sized patients. In general, as thick a depth of foam as possible should be used. Non-retentive bedding is again recommended, particularly as urine tends to pool in the depression made by the patient. This can be a useful surface, but long term, it probably gives no more protection against decubitus than a bed protects humans from bedsores. Although soft, the foam tends to compress under the weight of the patient to give a relatively firm and unyielding surface.

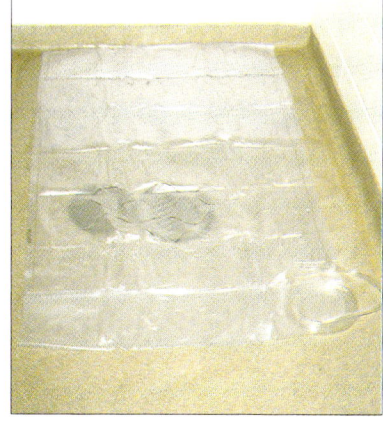

476 An inflatable air bed. This probably provides better protection against decubitus than foam sheets, as it is less prone to compression. With large patients, the air bed may need to be maximally inflated to prevent contact with the floor, but then the bed is so tense that it tends to compress the patient's skin. Use of several moderately inflated air beds stacked on top of each other may help overcome this problem. A very useful, cheap, and disposable alternative is provided by plastic bubble packing material. The largest sized bubbles seem to work best.

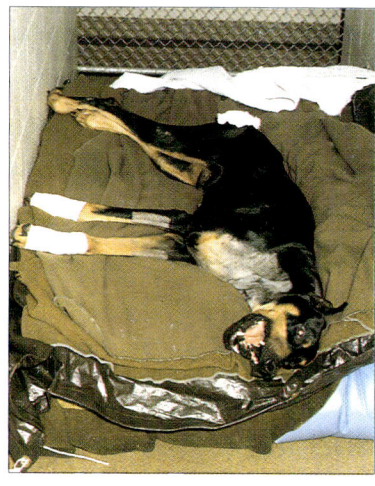

477 A waterbed. This is in many respects the ideal surface for a large recumbent patient. Problems include the cost and the fact that unless heated, there may be a significant danger of cooling the animal. With both the air bed and waterbed, there are the problems of punctures, and the tendency for the patient to roll off the edge unless the bed is surrounded by some sort of barrier. Non-retentive bedding should also be used.

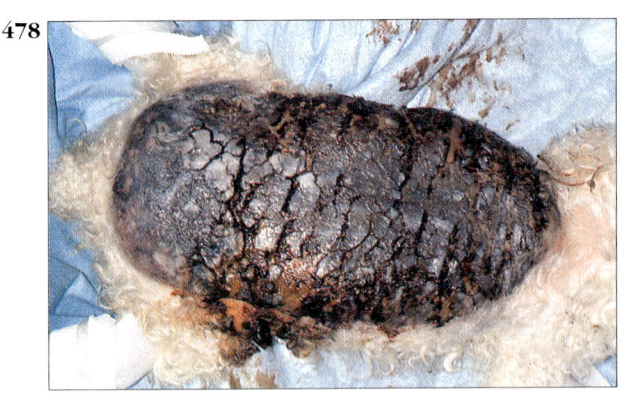

DIAGNOSIS AND SURGERY OF SMALL ANIMAL SPINAL DISORDERS

478 Thermal burn in a patient that was placed on a hot water bottle. Neurological patients are particularly susceptible to thermal burns because not only can they have disturbed nociception, but they may be unable to move away from the heat source.

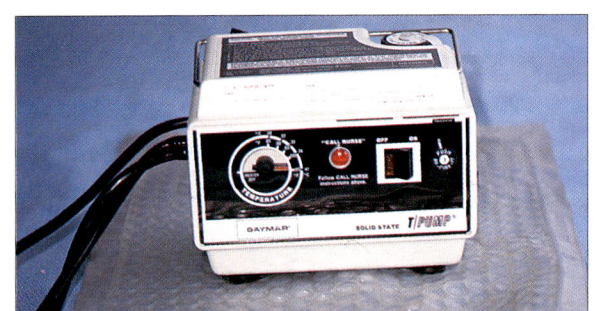

479 Neurological patients are also susceptible to cooling excessively. This is because they may have difficulty avoiding drafts or generating their own heat. Heat can only be safely supplied by warming the surrounding air, or by providing direct heat using a thermostatically controlled water blanket.

PHYSIOTHERAPY

However good the flooring material, the aim is to minimize the recumbency period because this is when the animal is most susceptible to complications. This period can be shortened to some extent by early and effective physiotherapy. Massage or passive limb flexion can usually begin almost immediately after recovery from surgery. Massage should be performed in a distal to proximal direction in order to promote venous return (Berry and Reyers, 1990). Towel walking of paraplegic dogs or supporting a tetraparetic patient in a sling are often possible within 24 or 48 hours of surgery (**480, 481**). Tetraparetic animals with good motor function can be walked with assistance using a tracking harness (**482**).

An external splint (see **430**) makes physiotherapy safer for an animal with an unstable thoracolumbar lesion.

Swimming in a whirlpool bath or a bathtub is invaluable. The animal must be thoroughly dried afterwards (**483–485**).

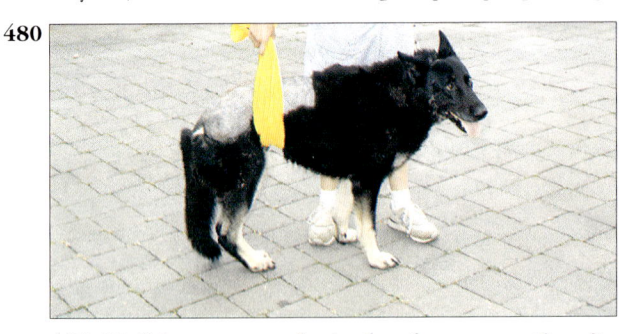

480 Walking a paraplegic dog by supporting its hindquarters with a towel placed under the abdomen, just in front of the pelvic limbs. This is an excellent form of physiotherapy for a paraparetic or paraplegic animal. The tail can also be used for support, as long as it is held at the base to avoid injury.

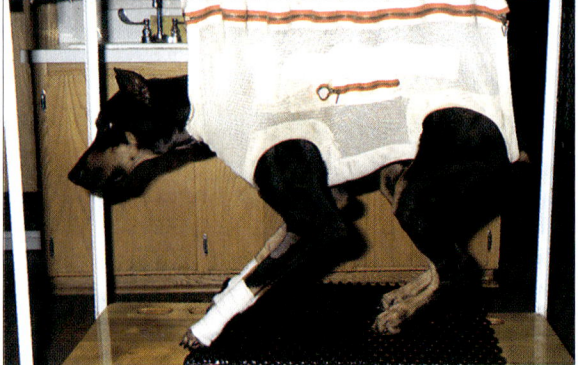

481 Although more difficult to provide than towel walking, this sling and homemade frame is a very useful way of rehabilitating tetraparetic or tetraplegic patients. It has the added advantages of improving the patients mental attitude, reducing the risks of thrombotic disease, and allowing the animal to be safely placed in a whirlpool bath (see **483**).

15. POSTOPERATIVE CARE

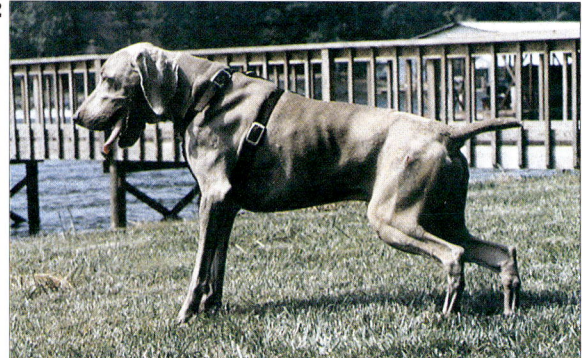

482 This dog is wearing a tracking harness, which can be a very effective way to support an ataxic, tetraparetic dog with reasonably good motor function. This is the same dog as illustrated in **502** and **503**, four months after undergoing surgery for caudal cervical spondylomyelopathy. Note that the decubital ulcer visible in **502** has contracted considerably, but is still not completely healed and eventually required surgical closure. This is the same dog illustrated in **332–4** and **365**.

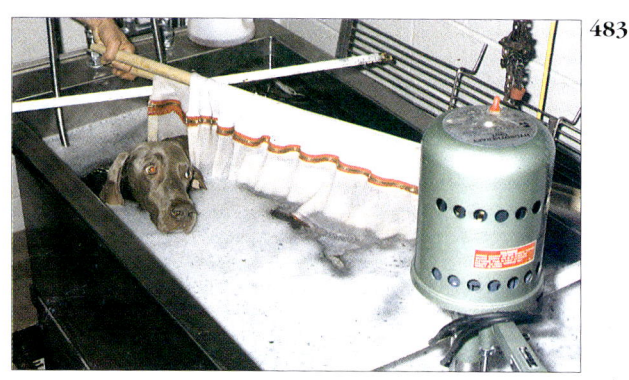

483 The same sling as shown in 481 has been used to support this dog inside a whirlpool bath. There is a person at the end of each supporting pole, which should be positioned so that one end of a pole does not inadvertently slip. While in the pool, the patient's limbs should be flexed and the animal encouraged to swim. Chlorhexidine has been added to the water, which should be at 38–40°C, and the tank must be drained daily. It is not recommended that patients with surgical wounds be bathed until a minimum of five days after surgery. At the end of the session, the patient's coat must be dried, first with towels and then with a warm air drier (see **485**) to prevent hypothermia.

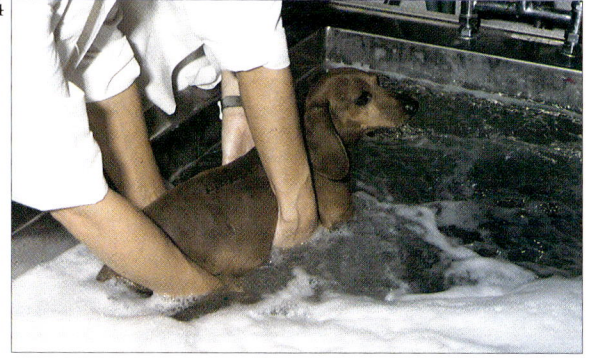

484 A small patient such as this Dachshund can be suspended by hand in a bathtub. It is preferable to have two people available if the water is deeper than the height of the dog. It is surprisingly easy to drop a struggling wet dog which, if paralysed, is then unable to keep itself afloat. The handlers should wear waterproof clothing.

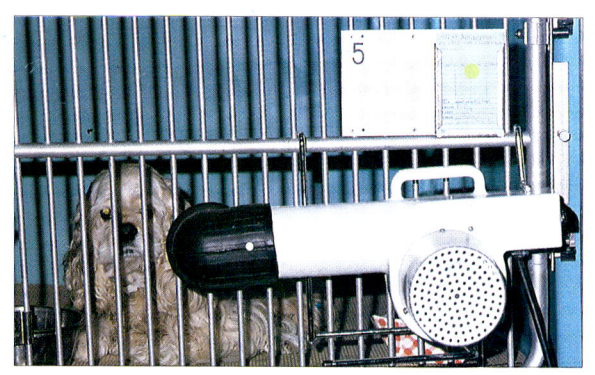

485 This patient is being dried using a warm air blower. Neurological patients are often inefficient at shaking and licking themselves dry. They may also be unable to generate their own heat, or even simply avoid drafts as well as normal animals. The drier must not be too hot, as the patient may be unable to move away or may not even feel the heat on denervated areas.

DIAGNOSIS AND SURGERY OF SMALL ANIMAL SPINAL DISORDERS

In addition to the physical wellbeing of the patient, the mental attitude of the animal often has a significant effect on the outcome of the case, particularly when recovery is delayed (see **503**). For dogs facing protracted recovery periods, temporary use of a paraplegic cart can serve a role in rehabilitation. In special circumstances, some dogs will do well in a cart long term (**486, 487**).

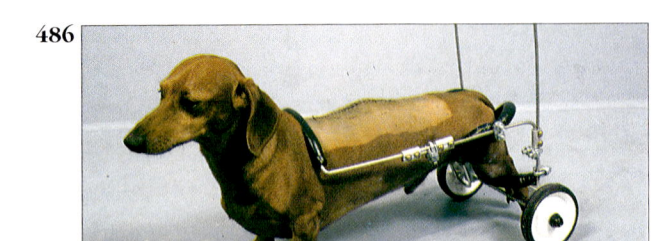

486 A cart designed for use in paraplegic dogs. These are made in a variety of sizes to suit different types of dog. In general, the risk of the dog coming to rely on the cart is probably outweighed by the stimulus provided by the enhanced mobility (K9 Carts).

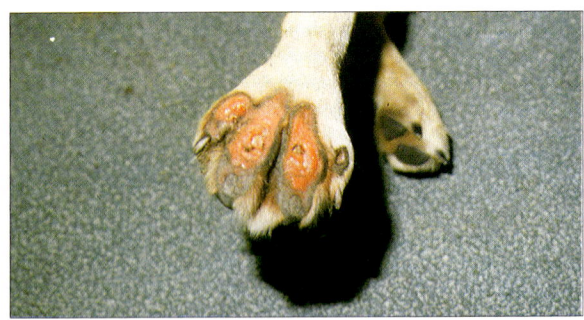

487 Self mutilation, dramatically illustrated here, would make this dog an unsuitable candidate to use a cart permanently. The permanent use of carts is suitable for selected patients in which there is no hope for return of neurological function. It is important, however, that the owner is informed of the final prognosis, is able to cope with the physical demands of getting the dog into and out of the cart, can be with the dog while it is in the cart, and can manage the incontinence and tendency for urine scald. Furthermore, the owner must ensure that the bladder is emptied at least three times daily, and must monitor the urine regularly by dipstick at home and veterinary visit. The dog must also be of a suitable temperament. Provided that these criteria are satisfied, many dogs can have an excellent quality of life and can live for years in this way.

CONTROL OF URINARY FUNCTION

The clinician should be aware of the animal's preoperative urinary status, but it can change as a result of surgery.

Anatomy and physiology (488, 489)

The detrusor muscle normally contracts in a coordinated fashion to empty the bladder. Each individual smooth muscle cell in the bladder wall is joined to its neighbours by so-called 'tight junctions'. These junctions have low electrical resistance so that the wave of membrane depolarization spreads rapidly from cell to cell over the whole detrusor muscle. Overdistension of the bladder can disrupt the 'tight junctions,' so preventing (in some patients permanently) the normal coordinated contraction of the detrusor muscle fibres. This should be prevented at all costs by strict attention to assisted emptying of the bladder (see below). Both the smooth and the skeletal muscle tone of the urethra contribute to maintaining a functional urethral sphincter mechanism. (These will be referred to collectively as the urethral sphincter unless stated otherwise.)

Disorders of micturition

Micturition disorders are broadly divisible into either UMN deficits affecting the spinal cord proximal to the sacral segments, or LMN deficits affecting the sacral spinal cord or nerve roots. In mild or moderate UMN spinal cord lesions (grade 2 or 3), increased urethral tone may prevent the patient from fully emptying the bladder. Initially, in severe UMN lesions (grade 4 or 5), the detrusor muscle is paralysed and urine is retained. It leaks when the bladder is full and intravesicular pressure exceeds sphincter pressure-urinary retention and overflow. After a month or so, reflex emptying of the bladder develops. In LMN lesions, the sphincter tone is decreased and so urine will tend to leak continuously (**Table 38**).

15. POSTOPERATIVE CARE

488 The physiological control of micturition is complex and involves the integration of spinal cord reflexes with the modulating effect of higher centres. Any lesion in the spinal cord is likely to alter either the reflexes, their higher control, or both. This may then alter the ability of the bladder to store urine efficiently and to empty itself completely.

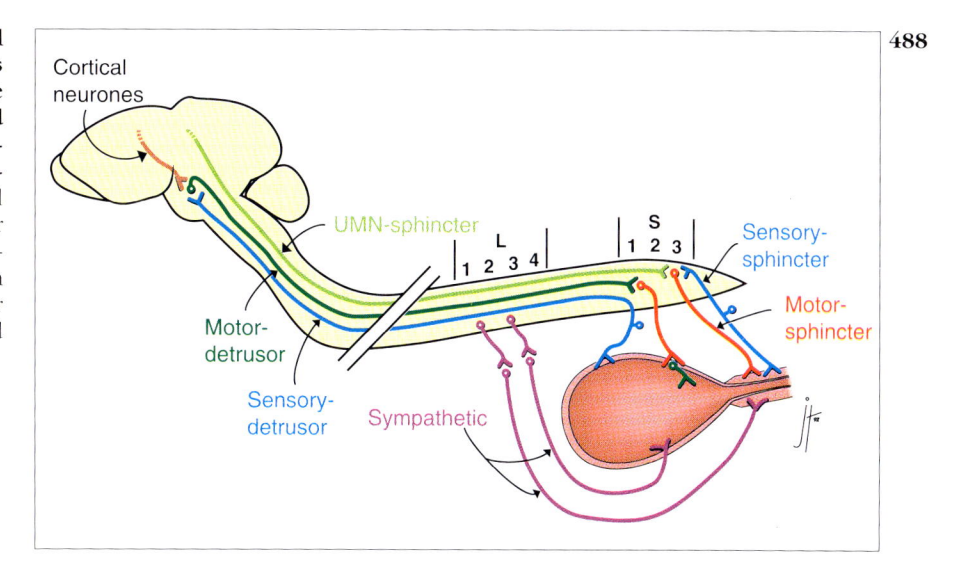

489 Innervation of the bladder and urethra. Parasympathetic fibres run in the pelvic nerves, which originate from S_1–S_3 spinal cord segments, and cause the detrusor muscle of the bladder wall to contract. Sympathetic fibres run in the hypogastric nerves, which originate from L_1–L_4/L_5 spinal cord segments, and cause the urethral smooth muscle to contract. Somatic nerve fibres run in the pudendal nerves, which originate from S_1–S_3 spinal cord segments, and cause the urethral striated muscle to contract.

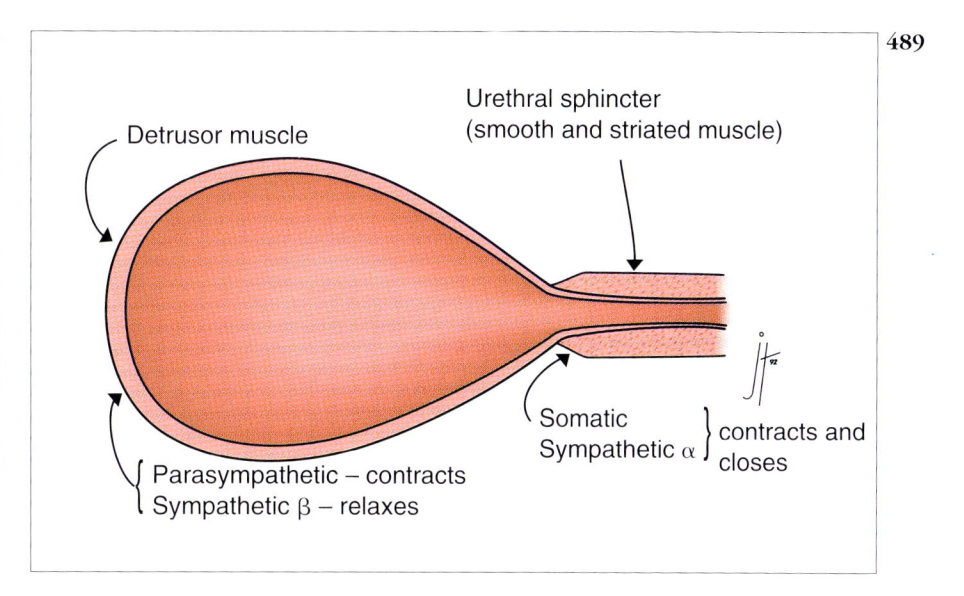

Table 38 Differences in urinary function associated with UMN or LMN lesions

	UMN paraplegic (acute)	UMN paraplegic (chronic)	LMN lesions
Detrusor function	–	+	–
Striated muscle sphincter tone	+ or ++	+ or ++	–
Smooth muscle sphincter tone	+ or ++	+ or ++	+

(+, normal; ++, increased; –, decreased.)

Pharmacological manipulation of micturition

By far the main problem is excessive urethral sphincter tone in UMN bladder dysfunction. The patient's voluntary efforts to void, or attempts at manual expression of the bladder, may be unable to overcome this excessive urethral tone. The result is an increase in the residual volume of urine in the bladder. As it is not usually possible to distinguish smooth from striated muscle effects in any individual patient, the simplest approach is to block the activity of both sphincters (see **489**).

DIAGNOSIS AND SURGERY OF SMALL ANIMAL SPINAL DISORDERS

- Diazepam (2–10 mg q8 hours) reduces striated muscle tone. It may work best given a short time before the bladder is expressed. It is not effective in cats. Dantrolene is an alternative (1–5 mg q8 hours in dogs; 0.5 mg/kg increasing to 2 mg/kg q12 hours in cats).
- Phenoxybenzamine (0.5 mg/kg q12 hours or q8 hours) reduces the smooth muscle tone (sympathetic α antagonist). There is usually a delay of 2–3 days before phenoxybenzamine takes effect.

All patients with UMN lesions that cannot walk unaided should be started on these drugs the day after surgery, or as soon as nonsurgical treatment is embarked upon.

Assisted emptying of the bladder

Assisted voiding has three crucial roles.
- To prevent overflow of urine and urine scald by keeping pressure within the bladder low.
- To empty all urine from the bladder periodically to reduce the risk of retention cystitis.
- To prevent overstretching of 'tight junctions' by maintaining a relatively low bladder volume at all times.

Retention cystitis will develop in any patient where large volumes of urine are allowed to accumulate and the bladder is not emptied. No antibiotic, regardless of its potency or spectrum, can substitute for an empty bladder. Use of antibiotic cover in these circumstances only succeeds in selecting the most resistant organism. Incontinent animals with either UMN or LMN bladder lesions require assisted emptying at least three times daily, with pharmacological assistance recommended for UMN lesions. Repeated cystocentesis is not recommended as a means of keeping the bladder empty.

Manual expression

Probably the best method for assisted voiding is simple manual expression of the bladder (**490, 491**).

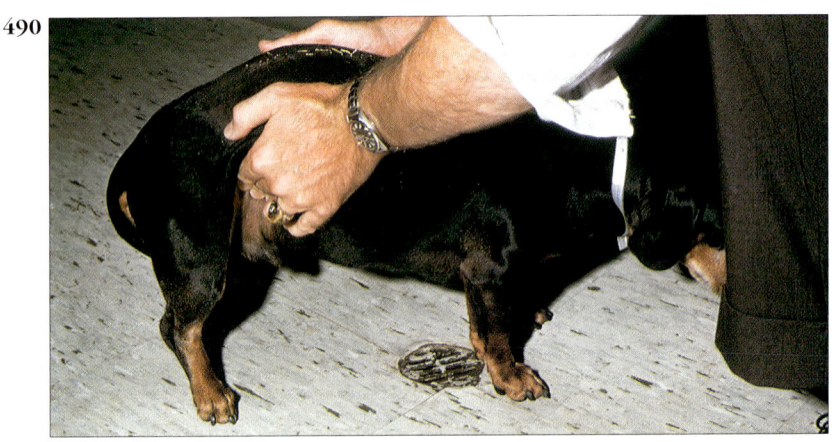

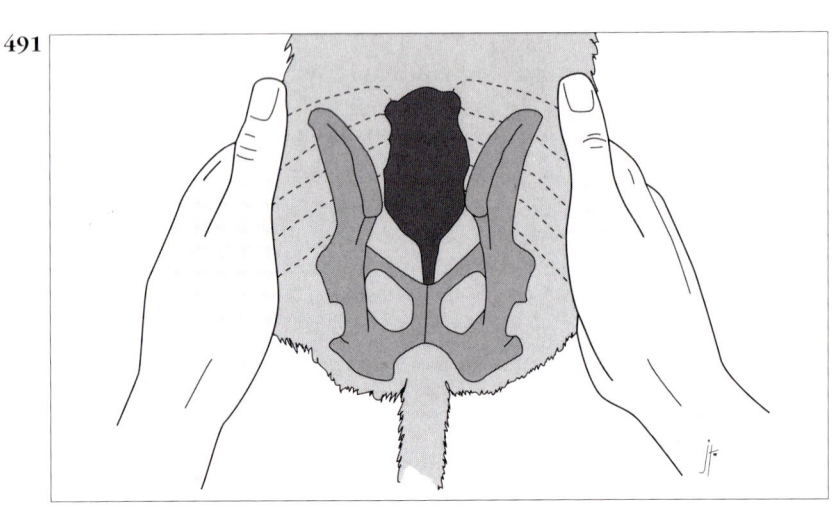

490, 491 Manual expression of the bladder. This relies on gentle, continuous, caudal abdominal pressure to overcome the resistance of the urethral sphincter. The procedure is best performed over a grate or drain. The advantage of manual expression is that, in contrast to catheterization, it avoids the introduction of bacteria into the normally sterile bladder. Even if only performed twice daily, with the third emptying done by catheter, this approach is preferable to catheterization each time. The disadvantages of manual expression are that it can be difficult to perform effectively in some animals, especially those with large or tense abdomens, those with external splints, or before increased urethral tone has been modified by drugs. Care should be taken not to use excessive force to try to overcome high sphincter resistance, as it might result in damage to the bladder wall. It can sometimes be difficult to estimate the completeness of bladder emptying without subsequent catheterization or ultrasound scanning. Occasional use of one of these objective methods for determining bladder volume is useful, but with experience, the effectiveness of manual expression can usually be assessed quite well by palpation.

15. POSTOPERATIVE CARE

Intermittent aseptic catheterization (492–494)

This may prove necessary in some difficult or fractious patients, or in dogs whose sphincter tone has not yet been successfully modified. Strict attention must be paid to aseptic technique. Even with these precautions, bacteria may be introduced into the bladder because the distal urethra has a normal bacterial flora that includes *Staph. intermedius* and *E.coli* (Stone and Barsanti, 1992). Nosocomial organisms may also be introduced by poor technique.

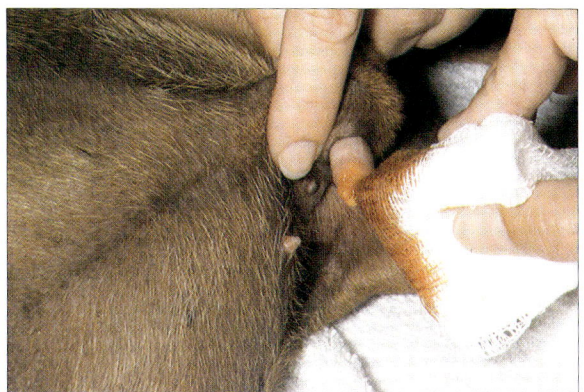

492 Aseptic technique is crucial when catheterizing the bladder. After extruding the penis, the tip can be irrigated with sterile saline and then dilute iodophor or chlorhexidine solution. In female dogs, the vulva should be prepared in a similar fashion and a sterile speculum or a gloved finger should be used to locate the urethral opening.

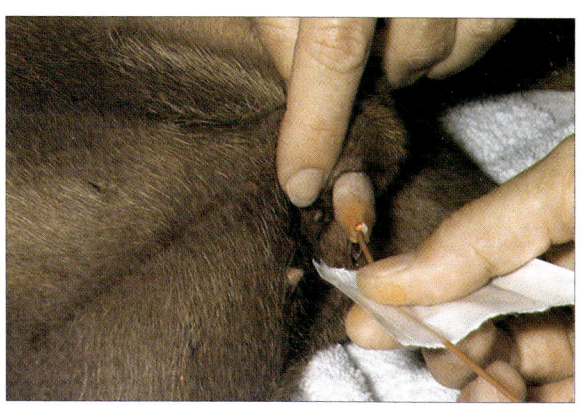

493 A sterile, soft rubber urinary catheter has been introduced into the urethra after first applying sterile lubricating jelly to the tip. The catheter is advanced using a 'no touch' technique, holding it instead by using a short length of the sterile catheter wrapping, which can be slid backwards as required. The remainder of the catheter is kept protected inside its wrapping to prevent contamination until it has been inserted into the urethra.

494 Once the catheter is inside the bladder, a sterile syringe is used to aspirate urine. If large volumes of urine are anticipated, then a sterile three-way tap or stopcock is useful to allow urine to be emptied from the syringe without repeated disconnection and potential contamination.

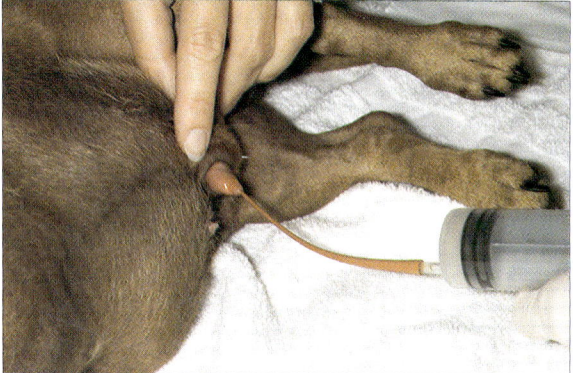

213

DIAGNOSIS AND SURGERY OF SMALL ANIMAL SPINAL DISORDERS

Closed collection system (495–497)

This system is useful in incontinent patients with severe established UTI that require aggressive treatment, and in patients with reduced renal function. Closed collection should preferably be replaced by another means of assisted voiding within 24 hours. After four days of closed urine collection most patients develop UTI even with antibiotic administration.

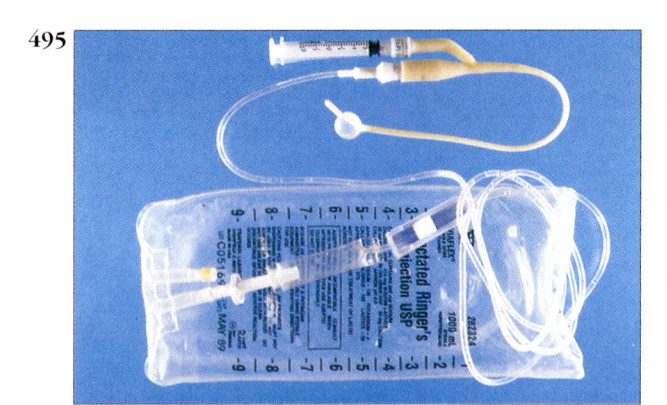

495 Female dogs are usually easy to express, but a Foley catheter can be sutured to the vulva and the bulb inflated as shown. The catheter can then be connected to a closed collection system (see **496** and **497**). Closed drainage has the advantage of allowing diuresis, while keeping the bladder empty. Diuresis is useful if the patient is toxaemic and helps flush debris and bacteria from the bladder. This technique is useful for the short term management of incontinent animals with severe UTIs. It also keeps the animal clean and dry, which reduces the development of urine scald and the chances of direct contamination of a surgical wound. The catheter should preferably be removed after 24 hours, to be replaced by some other means of assisted voiding.

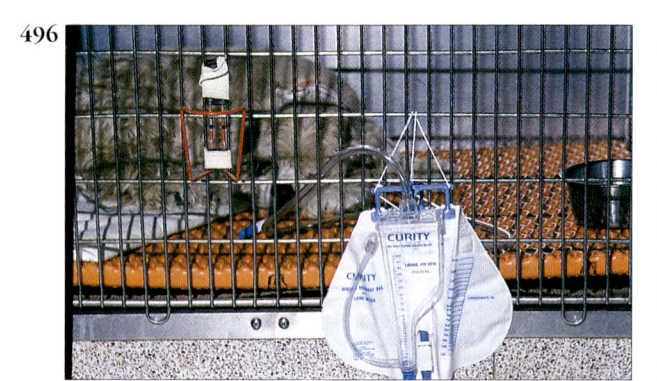

496 A commercially available urine collection container is preferred for the closed technique. This apparatus prevents reflux of urine into the bladder and has a much lower likelihood of introducing bacteria into the urinary tract than IV drip tubing and an empty fluid bag.

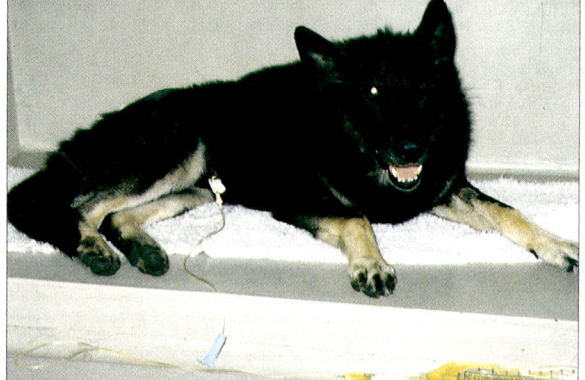

497 Urine output was monitored for 12 hours after surgery in this nine-year-old German shepherd dog with chronic renal failure. Adhesive tape was placed around the catheter, which was then sutured to the prepuce. Drip tubing was used to connect the catheter to an empty IV fluid bag. The collection bag should always be kept lower than the animal so that urine drains passively from the bladder into the bag and never vice versa. If the animal is moved for any reason, reverse flow of urine should be prevented by clamping the drip tubing. This dog tolerated the catheter very well, but some dogs need an Elizabethan collar to prevent catheter removal. These bags are very difficult to empty aseptically, and it is undesirable to lie the collection bag on the floor, as shown here, as this further increases the likelihood of contamination. The preferred collection apparatus is shown in **496**.

POSTOPERATIVE COMPLICATIONS

The most important potential complications are UTI, gastrointestinal disturbances, pancreatitis, urine scald, decubital ulcers, and surgical wound problems.

Urinary tract infections

Stagnant urine remaining in the bladder after voiding will predispose the patient to lower UTI. Animals with Cushing's disease or diabetes mellitus are also predisposed to UTI. An important consequence of UTI is for transient episodes of bacteraemia to occur, which may lead to wound infection. The potential for increased residual urine and an associated UTI should be recognized in all patients with a lesion severe enough to disturb motor function, until proven otherwise by urinalysis or urine culture. Urinalysis should be performed on urine collected by cystocentesis.

Evidence of inflammation on urinalysis, such as the presence of inflammatory cells or bacteria, warrants the following.
- Urine culture.
- Institution of assisted voiding.
- Specific antibiotic therapy.

In an animal with a severe, established UTI, a 12–24 hour period of diuresis combined with continuous evacuation of the bladder via a gravity assisted closed drainage system is useful. Before urine culture results are available, the initial antibiotics of choice are trimethoprim-sulpha (30 mg/kg PO q12 hours) or amoxycillin (22 mg/kg PO q12 hours) given for 14 days (Aronson and Aucoin, 1989). A repeat culture is performed once the animal has been off antibiotics for seven days. Methenamine (10 mg/kg PO q6 hours) is a urinary antiseptic agent that can be helpful in chronic UTI, especially those associated with long-term incontinence. The drug is hydrolysed in the bladder to ammonia and formaldehyde at a pH of less than 6; to achieve this mandelic or hippuric acid supplements are often required.

Gastrointestinal disturbances

Up to 15% of dogs with disc disease will develop gastrointestinal problems and 2% may die. The major risk factor in one study was use of dexamethasone; dose and duration of therapy were not important (Moore and Withrow, 1982). Vomiting can have a variety of causes including corticosteroids, antibiotics, NSAIDs, or pancreatitis. Effective postoperative analgesia should be used to minimize the contributory effects of patient stress. If vomiting occurs, food, water, and unnecessary medications should be withheld for 24 hours, and intravenous fluids given to replace losses. Drugs used to treat gastrointestinal disturbances are listed in **Table 39**. Persistent vomiting warrants antiemetic therapy and suggests an underlying cause such as pancreatitis. Diarrhoea will increase the risk of UTI or wound infection and every attempt should be made to prevent it, or at least to shorten its severity and duration. Opioids are the preferred antidiarrhoeal drugs (Strombeck and Guilford, 1990).

Table 39 Drugs acting on the gastrointestinal system[1]

Use	Drug	Species	Dose	Notes and side-effects
Antiemetic	**Prochlorperazine**	Dog, cat	0.1 mg/kg IM q6 hours	Hypotension, increased risk of seizures
Antiemetic	**Chlorpromazine**	Dog, cat	0.5 mg/kg IM q8 hours	Hypotension, increased risk of seizures
Bleeding	**Ranitidine**	Dog	1–4 mg/kg PO q12 hours	More effective than cimetidine
Bleeding	**Sucralfate**	Dog	15 mg/kg PO q6 hours	Can bind other drugs including cimetidine
Bleeding	**Cimetidine**	Dog, cat	5–10 mg/kg PO q6 hours	
Bleeding	**Misoprostol**	Dog	1–3 µg/kg PO q8 hours	Diarrhoea (usually transient), abortion[2]
Diarrhoea	**Diphenoxylate**	Dog	0.05–0.1 mg/kg PO q8 hours	Narcotic overdose
Diarrhoea	**Loperamide**	Dog, cat	0.08 mg/kg PO q8 hours	Narcotic overdose
Diarrhoea	**Bismuth salicylate**	Dog, cat	0.25 ml/kg PO q6 hours	For enterotoxic diarrhoea

[1]Strombeck & Guilford 1990.
[2]Murtaugh et al., 1993.

Bleeding into the GI tract, presenting as 'coffee ground' vomit or melaena, should be treated aggressively because of the high potential mortality rate. All oral intake and non-essential drugs are stopped and therapy begun. Misoprostol has beneficial effects in both the stomach and intestine (Murtaugh *et al.*, 1993.). This would seem to be the most appropriate therapy for NSAID- or corticosteroid-induced bleeding. If sucralfate is used, certain other oral drugs need to be given after an interval of two hours: consult specific drug data sheets.

Control of defaecation rarely causes a problem, as reflexive emptying will occur periodically even in animals with functional transection of the spinal cord. Stool softeners can be useful.

Pancreatitis

Acute pancreatitis has a high mortality rate, and should be considered in any neurological patient that develops a sudden onset of vomiting, anorexia, and pyrexia postoperatively. It has been estimated that approximately 12% of all cases of pancreatitis are associated with corticosteroid administration, usually at dexamethasone doses over 2 mg/kg (Strombeck and Guilford, 1990).

Diagnosis is based on serum lipase and amylase measurement, lipase being the more sensitive. Treatment entails withholding all oral intake for five days until the clinical signs are in remission. Intravenous fluid therapy must keep up with fluid losses, which can be dramatic.

A minimum initial rate is 6.5 ml/kg/hr, up to 40 ml/kg/hr. It is preferable to measure the animal's central venous pressure during fluid administration. Metabolic acidosis and electrolyte derangements are common and warrant regular blood gas and electrolyte measurements where available. Urine output should also be monitored. Potassium chloride must be added to the fluid if therapy is continued for more than 24 hours. An antiemetic such as chlorpromazine should be used at the lowest possible dose to control vomiting. Metaclopramide is not recommended. Procaine penicillin and an aminoglycoside are the antibiotics of choice (Strombeck and Guilford, 1990).

Wound infection

Many factors play a role in wound infection (see **Table 12**, page 62). A sterile adhesive dressing is recommended to protect the wound after surgery (**498**). This should be kept in place for several days, but the wound must be checked daily for seroma formation, swelling, redness, or discharge. Significant seromas should be drained, paying careful attention to aseptic preparation of the skin.

Wound infection after thoracolumbar laminectomy has been associated with a surgical time over 90 minutes, and use of multifilament absorbable suture material to close the epaxial fascia. In that study, corticosteroid, NSAID, or antibiotic use did not influence the infection rate (Hosgood, 1992).

If infection occurs, a culture should be taken from the depths of the wound after aseptic preparation of the skin. Antibiotic therapy should be instituted, initially directed at staphylococcal involvement (cephazolin 5–15 mg/kg IV, IM q8 hours, or cephadroxil 20 mg/kg PO q12 hours). Depending on the severity of the infection, consideration should be given to surgical debridement and irrigation of the wound.

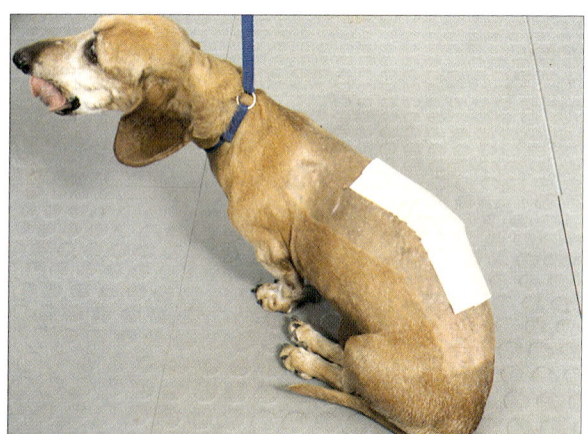

498 A sterile, self adhesive dressing has been applied to the laminectomy wound of this Dachshund. This should be lifted to inspect the wound daily, but can usually then be reapplied several times. The dressing can be removed after two or three days, but should be maintained if the dog has a UTI or diarrhoea, in order to provide additional protection.

15. POSTOPERATIVE CARE

Urine scald
Urine scald is an important cause of dermatitis and also predisposes to decubital ulcer formation (**499**).

Decubital ulcers
Decubital ulcers result mainly from unrelieved compression of tissue between a hard surface and a bony prominence. Even small paraplegic animals sometimes develop decubital ulcers (**501**). The skin should be kept clean and dry at all times, and in recumbent animals, the bony prominences should be examined at least daily for the onset of decubitus. The early appearance is erythema, oedema, and tenderness, followed by serum exudation and alopecia. Skin and subcutaneous tissue loss then develops rapidly. Decubital ulcers may give rise to episodes of bacteraemia, with the potential risk of infecting the surgical wound or implant (**500–503**).

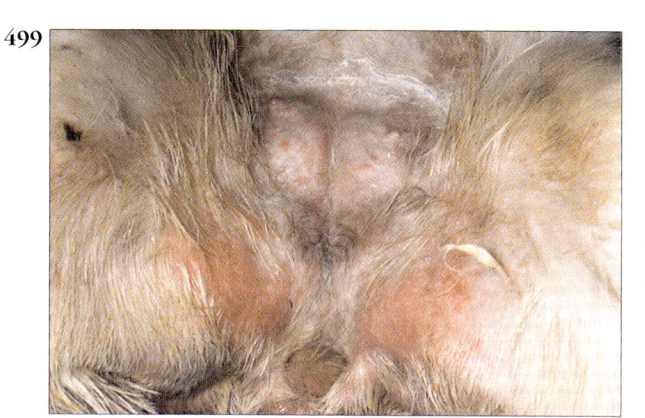

499 Early urine scald around the vulva. This dog was incontinent because of a fracture of the L_6 vertebral body that had been managed using an external splint. Manual expression of the bladder was made difficult by the abdominal straps used to attach the splint to the dog. The problem was successfully overcome by regular replacement of the straps, washing and drying the skin and then by applying an emollient followed by a water repellent ointment.

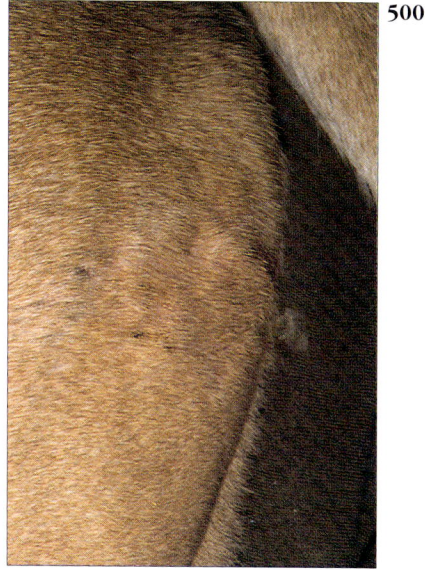

500 The area over the ischiatic tuberosity in the early stages of decubitus formation, to show oedema and the onset of hair loss. Inspection of underlying skin revealed erythema and early serum exudation. At a more advanced stage, areas of decubitus may appear simply as a wet area on the hair coat due to serum exudation. Skin overlying the shoulder, elbow, rib cage, pelvis and hip, and the lateral stifle is most at risk.

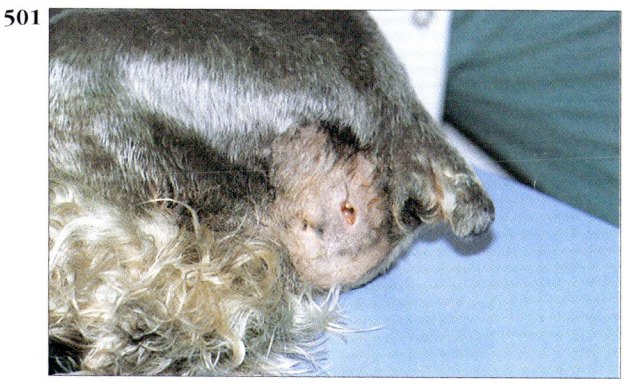

501 Decubital ulcers occasionally occur in small paraplegic animals. For example in this Miniature schnauzer with a disc extrusion that had resulted in an effective spinal cord transection. Most small paraplegic patients will shift their weight frequently enough to avoid decubital ulcers.

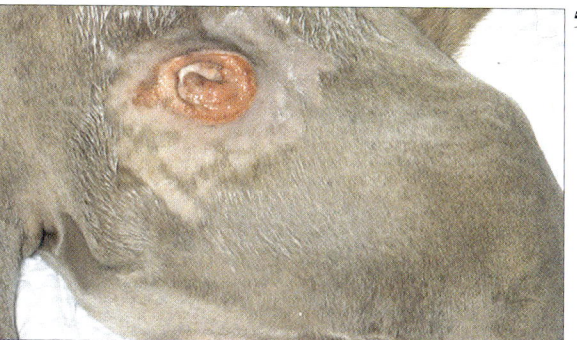

502 An advanced decubital ulcer over the greater trochanter that will require aggressive management.

217

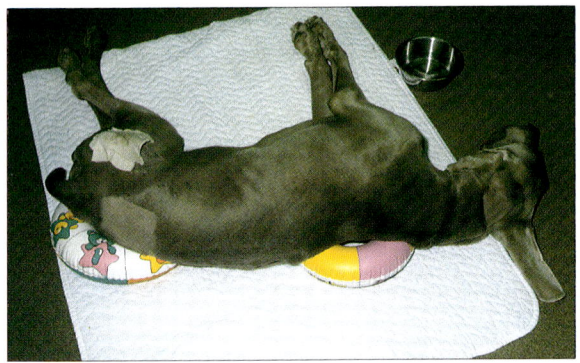

503 The same dog illustrated in 502 is shown here lying on two inflatable rings, one placed under the shoulder and one under the hip. A good alternative would have been to use the plastic bubble packing material discussed in **476**. Note that an ulcer on this dog's opposite hip has been covered by a sterile dressing held in place with Elastoplast. The rings are difficult to keep in place for a long period of time. They were used to allow this tetraparetic dog to be moved temporarily from his waterbed into an area where there was a lot of activity. Such attempts to improve the animal's mental status, by affection from nursing staff, several short physiotherapy sessions rather than one long one, allowing the animal to be in a location where it can see a lot of activity, a regular look at the outside world, and frequent contact with owners, even extending to overnight stays at home, can actually mean the difference between success and failure in some animals.

An appropriate flooring material (see **473–477**) is essential to prevent, or at least retard, the onset of decubitus. Resolution of established decubitus is obviously difficult until the inciting cause is eliminated. Prompt removal of devitalized tissue and regular irrigation with an antiseptic solution (such as 0.4% chlorhexidine) are recommended. Surgical debridement and primary closure, possibly using skin flaps or grafts, may be required to resolve an indolent ulcer, even after neurological function returns.

Miscellaneous

In humans, prolonged recumbency combined with inactivity significantly increases the risk of deep vein thrombosis and pulmonary thromboembolism. These are almost certainly under-recognized as a cause of morbidity and mortality in veterinary neurosurgical patients (Feldman, 1986). Treatment is difficult, and so every effort should be directed toward avoiding circulatory stasis by providing adequate physiotherapy and intake of fluids. Pneumonia and gastric dilation or torsion are additional problems that can occur during the postoperative period, especially in recumbent animals.

REFERENCES

Aronson, A.L. and Aucoin, D.P. (1989) Antimicrobial drugs. In *Textbook of Veterinary Internal Medicine*, 3rd edn, pp 383–412. (Ed. S. J. Ettinger.) W. B. Saunders Co., Philadelphia.

Berry, W.L. and Reyers, L. (1990) Nursing care of the small animal neurological patient. *Journal of the South African Veterinary Association* **61**, 188–193.

Crane S. (1987) Perioperative analgesia: a surgeon's perspective. *Journal of the American Veterinary Medical Association* **191**, 1254–1257.

Dodman, N.H., Clarke, G.H., Court, M.H., Fikes, L.L. and Boudrieau R.J. (1992) Epidural opioid administration for postoperative pain relief in the dog. In *Animal Pain,* pp 274–277. (Eds C. E. Short and A. van Poznan.) Churchill Livingstone, New York.

Donoghue, S. (1989) Nutritional support of hospitalized patients. *Veterinary Clinics of North America, Small Animal Practice* **19**, 475–495.

Feldman, B.F. (1986) Thrombosis–diagnosis and treatment. In *Current Veterinary Therapy IX*, pp 505–509. (Ed. R. W. Kirk.) W.B Saunders Co., Philadelphia.

Haskins, S.C. (1990) Analgesics and sedatives. *Proceedings of 14th KalKan Symposium Emergency and Critical Care*, pp 33–39.

Haskins, S.C. (1992) Advantages and guidelines for using agonist opioid analgesics. *Veterinary Clinics of North America, Small Animal Practice* **22(2)**, 360–361.

Holtsinger, R.H., Parker, R.B., Beale, B.S. and Friedman R.L. (1992) The therapeutic efficacy of carprofen (Rimadyl-VTM) in 209 clinical cases of canine degenerative joint disease. *Veterinary and Comparative Orthopaedics and Traumatology* **5**, 140–144

Hosgood, G. (1992) Wound complications following thoracolumbar laminectomy in the dog: a retrospective study of 264 procedures. *Journal of the American Animal Hospital Association* **28**, 47–52.

McKellar, Q.A., Lees, P., Ludwig, B. and Tiberghien, M.P. (1991) Pharmacokinetics, tolerance and serum thromboxane inhibition of carprofen. *Journal of Small Animal Practice* **31**, 443–448.

Moore, R.W. and Withrow, S.J. (1982) Gastrointestinal hemorrhage and pancreatitis associated with intervertebral disc disease in the dog. *Journal of the American Veterinary Medical Association* **180**, 1443–1447.

Murtaugh, R.J., Matz, M.E., Labato, M.A. and Bourdrieu, R.J. (1993) Use of synthetic prostaglandin E, (misoprostol) for prevention of aspirin-induced gastroduodenal ulceration in arthritic dogs. *Journal of the American Veterinary Medical Association* **180**, 251–256.

Sackman, J.E. (1991) Pain. Part II. Control of pain in animals. *Compendium on Continuing Education for the Small Animal Practitioner* **13**, 181–192.

Stone, E.A. and Barsanti, J.A. (1992) *Urologic Surgery of the Dog and Cat*, pp 20–22 urine culture; pp 86–90 catheter associated infection. Lea and Febiger, Malvern, Pennsylvania.

Swain, S.F., Lee, A.H. and Hughes, K.S. (1989) Heating pads and thermal burns in small animals. *Journal of the American Animal Hospital Association* **25**, 156–162.

Strombeck, D.R. and Guilford, W.G. (1990) *Small Animal Gastroenterology*, 2nd edition, pp 45–46 prostaglandins; pp 200–205 gastritis; pp 286–295 diarrhoea; pp 402–403 colon; pp 431-436 pancreatitis. Stonegate Publishing Company, Davis, California.

Valverde, A., Dyson, D.H., McDonell, W.N. and Pascoe P.J. (1989) Use of epidural morphine in the dog for pain relief. *Veterinary and Comparative Orthopaedics and Traumatology* **2**, 55–58.

GLOSSARY OF ACRONYMS

CCSM	Caudal cervical spondylomyelopathy	LMN	Lower motor neuron
CDV	Canine distemper virus	MRI	Magnetic resonance imaging
CMC	Cerebellomedullary cistern	NSAID	Non-steroidal anti-inflammatory drug
CNS	Central nervous system	PO	Per os
CSF	Cerebrospinal fluid	RBC	Red blood cell
CT	Computer tomography	SQ	Subcutaneous
ECG	Electrocardiogram	UMN	Upper motor neuron
FCE	Fibrocartilaginous embolism	UTI	Urinary tract infection
FeLV	Feline leukaemia virus	VW	Von Willebrand's
FIP	Feline infectious peritonitis	WBC	White blood cell
FIV	Feline immunodeficiency virus		
IM	Intramuscular		
IV	Intravenous		

INDEX

A
Acepromazine, 63, 199
Acetaminophen, 205
Albuminocytological dissociation, 42
Aminocaproic acid, 194
Aminoglycoside, 216
Amoxycillin, 62, 195, 215
Amphotericin B, 198
Ampicillin, 195
Anaesthesia,
    complications, 63–4
    premedication, 63
    procedure, 63
    recovery from, 64
    seizures, 48
Analgesia,
    opioid, 203–4
    post-traumatic, 172
    postoperative, 168, 205, 215
        NSAID, 204–5
        opioid, 203–4
        other drugs, 205
Anti-inflammatory drugs, 88, 89, 111, 127, 196
    see also Corticosteroids, Non-steroidal anti-inflammatory drugs
Antibiotics,
    prophylactic, 62
    vomiting due to, 215
    see also specific drugs
Aortic embolism (iliac thrombosis, ischaemic neuromyopathy), 198–9
Arachnoid cysts, 192
Articulations, synovial, 15, *see also* Intervertebral discs
Aspirin, 61, 199, 205
Astocytoma, 51 fig.
Atlantoaxial fracture (subluxation), 68, 109–21, 193
    anatomical relationship C1/C2, 109
    in cat, 31, 121
    clinical signs, 110
    diagnosis, 35, 110
    differential diagnosis, 110
    nonsurgical treatment, 111
    surgery, 180
        complications, 120–1
        dorsal wiring, 111, 117–20
        indications, 111
        postoperative care, 121
        prognosis, 121
        ventral fusion, 111–17
Atlantoaxial joint, radiography, 44
Atlas (C1),
    anatomy, 13
    myelography, 47 fig.
    radiography, 44 figs., 44 fig.
Atracurium, 63
Atropine, 63, 204 table
Axis (C2), 43 figs., 44 fig., 47 fig.
    anatomy, 13
    fractures, 180
Azotaemia, 61

B
Bacterial meningoencephalomyelitis, 41
Beagle, 50 fig., 68, 197
Bed,
    air, 207
    water, 207
Bedding,
    non-retentive, 207
    waterproof foam mattress, 207
Bence-Jones proteinuria, 34
Bernese mountain dog, 42 fig., 197
Bile duct rupture, 172
Biochemistry, 34
Biopsy, 55
Bismuth salicylate, 215
Bladder,
    emptying, 210 fig., 212–14
        closed collection system, 214
        intermittent aseptic catheterization, 213
        manual expression, 12, 212, 217 fig.
    innervation, 211
    LMN/UMN systems and dysfunction of, 25, 211–12
    sensory tract associated, 11
    traumatic rupture, 172
Blanket,
    electric, 207
    water, 207
Bleeding disorders, 139–40
Bleeding time tests, 139–40
Bleeding times, 35
Blood supply, 18–30
Bone scintigraphy, 54
Bone screws, 178
Boston terrier, 192
Boxer, 156 fig., 201 fig.
Brachial plexus,
    avulsion injury, 26, 54
    tumour, 156, 167
Brain herniation, 35, 36, 38
Brain involvement, 30
Brucella canis, 35, 194, 195
Buccal mucosal bleeding time, 140
Bulldog, 192, 193 fig., 200
Buprenorphine, 204 table
Butorphanol, 204 table

C
C1/C2, 109, *see also* Atlas; Axis
C2/C3, 47 fig., 68
C3/C4, 69 fig., 181
C4/C5, 69 fig.
C5/C6, 50 fig., 69 fig., 137 fig.
C6, 43 fig.
C6/C7, 68, 136 fig., 137 fig.
C7/T1, 50, 68
Cage rest, 70, 88, 111
Calcinosis circumscripta, 192
Canine distemper virus (CDV), 35, 42, 197
Cardiac arrhythmias, 61, 63, 64, 83, 172
Cardiomyopathy, 140
Carprofen, 107
Cart, paraplegic, 210
Castration, 195
Cat,
    atlantoaxial subluxation, 31, 121
    bacterial meningoencephalomyelitis, 41
    cervical spine, 31, 84
    dens, 109
    discospondylitis, 194
    hypervitaminosis A, 196
    ischaemic neuromyopathy, 198–9
    lumbosacral disease, 33
    lymphoma, 156, 158, 159
    Manx, 200
    meningioma, 51 fig.
    neuroaxonal dystrophy, 199
    neurofibroma, 157 fig.
    neurological examination, 23
    osteochondromatosis, 199
    postoperative analgesia, 204 table, 205
    sacrocaudal injuries, 122
    spinal cord infections, 198
    spinal tumours, 168–70
    splinting, 190
    tail avulsion, 181
    thoracolumbar disc disease, 108
    vertebral malformations, 192
Catheterization, intermittent aseptic, 213
Cauda equina, 9, 15, 54, 122, 123
Caudal cervical myelography, 47 fig.
Caudal cervical spondylomyelopathy (CCSM), 31, 32
    aetiology, 135
    clinical signs, 135–6
    concurrent disease, 61
    diagnosis, 52, 136–8
    dynamic/static lesions, 137
    myelopathy, 48
    nonsurgical treatment, 140
    other disorders, 139–40
    presurgical evaluation, 139–40
    prognosis, 154
    surgery,
        algorithm, 141, 142 fig.
        complications, 64, 83, 153–4
        dorsal decompression, 141, 149–52
        general indications, 141
        multiple lesions, 152
        operative considerations, 142
        postoperative deterioration, 153–4
        reported results, 141
        self-induced trauma, 153
        ventral decompression, 139, 141, 142–3
        ventral fenestration, 152
        vertebral distraction/fusion, 141, 143–148, *see also* Lag screw, fixation; Metal implant and bone cement; Screw and washer technique
CDRM (chronic degenerative radiculomyelopathy), 193–4
Cephadroxil, 216
Cephazolin, 62, 145, 188, 216
Cephradine, 195
Cerebellomedullary cistern (CMC) puncture, 35, 36–8, 110
Cerebrospinal fluid (CSF),
    functional anatomy, 10
    see also CSF (cerebrospinal fluid) analysis
Cervical disc disease, 25, 29, 30
    in cat, 84
    clinical signs, 68
    diagnosis, 69–82, 110
    disc herniation, types of, 68
    nonsurgical treatment, 70, 83
    palpation and site of lesion, 68
    predisposing factors, 68
    surgery,
        choice of, 70
        complications, 64, 82–3
        deep anatomy, 73 fig., 75 fig.
        disc identification, 74 fig.
        dorsal laminectomy, 70
        hemilaminectomy, 70, 82
        indications, 70
        postoperative care, 83
        prognosis, 83–4
        ventral approach, 71–6
        ventral decompression, 70, 78–82
        ventral fenestration, 70, 76–7
Cervical intumescence, 29
Cervical myelography, 46–7, 48
Cervical spinal nerves, 8
Cervical spine,
    blood supply, 18
    fractures, 110, 180
    radiography, 43–4
    vertebrae, 9, 13
    see also Cervical disc disease
Chemotherapy, 159, 169
Chihuahua, 68
Chlorhexidine, 209 fig.
Chlorpromazine, 215, 216
Chondrodystrophoid breeds, 15, 68, 85
Chondroid metamorphosis, 16
Choroid plexus tumours, 42
Cimetidine, 215
Client communication, 66
Cloxacillin, 195
Computed tomography, 52–3
Conscious proprioception, 10, 12, 23, 24
Corn starch powder, 183
Corticosteroids, 62, 215
    acute pancreatitis due to, 216
    bleeding into gut, 216
    CDRM, 194
    inflammatory CNS diseases, 197
    thoracolumbar disc disease, 85 fig., 89
    vomiting due to, 215
Cranial nerves, 21, 27
Crossed extensor reflex, 28, 30
CSF (cerebrospinal fluid) analysis,
    abnormal values, 42
    albuminocytological dissociation, 42
    blood contamination, 41, 42
    collection, 36–40
    contraindications, 35
    from cerebromedullary cistern, 35, 36–8
    from lumbar spine, 35, 36, 39–40
    indications, 35
    interpretation, 41
    normal values, 41, 42
    pleocytosis, 42, 46
    sample handling, 40
Curettage, 195

Cushing's disease (syndrome), 61, 215
Cuticle bleeding time, 140
Cystitis, retention, 213

D
Dachshund, 15, 30, 68, 206, 209
Dantrolene, 212
Decubital ulcers, 183, 217–18
Deep pain sensation, 11, 12, 30, 85
   assessment, 29
   following trauma, 172
   spinal fractures, 178–80
Deep vein thrombosis, 218
Defaecation, 216
Degenerative myelopathy, 33, 48, 124–5
Dens,
   congenital absence/hypoplasia, 109
   fracture, 109
   functional anatomy, 13
   ligaments, 17
   radiography, 44
Dermoid (pilonidal) sinus (epidermoid cyst), 200
Desatin ointment, 183
Desmopressin (DDAVP), 139
Dexamethasone, 62, 85 fig., 215
Diabetes mellitus, 61, 215
Diagnosis, differential,
   cervical spine, 31–2
   DAMNIT formula, 31
   lumbosacral spine, 33
   orthopaedic disorders, 21
   sacrocaudal spine, 33
   thoracolumbar spine, 32
Diarrhoea, 215
Diazepam, 48, 63, 70, 83, 153
   bladder muscle tone, 212
   in recovery from anaesthesia, 64
Differential white cell count, 41
Diphenoxylate, 215
Disc herniation,
   diagnosis, 49
   Hansen type, I, II, 16
   see also specific spinal regions ; Intervertebral discs
   traumatic, 171
Discharge information, 203
Discography, 48, 127
Discospondylitis, 33, 34, 68, 156, 194–5, 201
   after cervical disc surgery, 83
   bone scanning, 54
   diagnosis, 35, 110
   lumbosacral, 122, 125 figs., 126, 127
Dobermann,
   bleeding diseases, 139–40
   C5/C6 disease, 50 fig.
   CCSM, 48, 135, 136–7 figs., 152, 153
      UMN signs in, 29
      ventral fenestration, 152
   cervical disc disease, 68
   discospondylitis, 195 fig.
   hepatitis, 140
   hypothyroidsm, 139
   nursing plan, 206
   Von Willebrand's disease/factor, 82, 139
Domino effect, 48, 147, 152, 154
Dorsal decompression, for CCSM, 141, 149–52
Dorsal foramenotomy, 127–34
Dorsal fusion fixation, 134
Dorsal laminectomy,
   in cat, 169
   cervical disc disease, 70
   thoracolumbar, 160–3, 167
Dorsal spinal plate, 173, 184–5
   biomechanics, 177
   with vertebral body plate, 173, 176, 177, 185
Dorsal wiring, 111, 117–20, 121
Dressings, 216
Durotomy, 65, 106–7

E
Electromyography, 54
Electrosurgery, 64
Endocrine disorders, 61
Epidermoid cyst (dermoid (pilonidal) sinus), 200
Epidural, 203
Epidurography, 48, 126

Erythrophagocytes, 42
 Escherichia coli , 194, 213
Extensor postural thrust, 25
External splints, 173, 181–3, 184, 185, 208
   biomechanics, 177
   disadvantages, 181
   technique, 182–3

F
Fat grafts, 65, 97
FCE (fibrocartilaginous embolism), 196
Feline immunodeficiency virus (FIV), 35, 61
Feline infectious peritonitis (FIP), 31, 197
Feline leukaemia virus (FeLV), 61
Fenestration, lateral, 100–6, 107
Fibrocartilaginous embolism (ischaemic myelopathy), 32, 33, 196
Fibroid metamorphosis, 16
Fine needle aspiration, 55
FIP, see Feline infectious peritonitis
Fleas, 61
Flexor (withdrawal) reflex, 28
Fluconazole, spinal cord infections, 198
Foreign bodies, 194
Free radical–induced lipid peroxidation, 62
Frusemide, 38

G
Gastrointestinal disturbances, 215–16
Gentamycin, 195
German shepherd,
   degenerative myelopathy, 193, 194 fig.
   lumbosacral disease, 122, 124 table
   urine output monitoring, 214 fig.
Giant breed dogs, 61, 135, 140, 196, see also Large breed dogs, specific species
Glioma, 51
Glycopyrrolate, 63
GME (granulomatous meningoencephalomyelitis), 197
Golden retriever, 51 fig., 54, 55 figs.
Granulomatous meningoencephalomyelitis (GME, reticulosis), 197
Grate, raised, 206–7
Great Dane, 135, 136

H
Haematology, 34
Haemorrhage, 196
Haemostasis, 61–2
Halothane, 63
Head trauma, 35, 203
Hemilaminectomy, 82
   cervical, 70, 159, 163–7
   spinal fractures, 179, 184
   thoracolumbar disc disease, 89–98, 106
      complications, 106–7
      prognosis, 108
Heparin, 199
Hippuric acid, 215
Hopping, 23, 25
Horner's syndrome, 27, 142, 149 fig.
Hydromyelia, 201
Hyoid, 44 fig.
Hypercalcaemia, 34, 156
Hypergammaglobulinaemia, 34
Hyperparathyroidism, 34
Hypervitaminosis A, 196
Hypocalcaemia, 34
Hypoglycaemia, 34
Hypokalaemic polymyopathy, 34
Hyponatraemia, 34
Hypothermia, 63, 207, 208–9
Hypothyroidism, 61, 139

I
Iliac thrombosis (aortic embolism, ischaemic neuromyopathy), 198–9
Inflammatory CNS disease, 31, 33–4, 46, 68–9, 110, 197–8
Instrumentation, 57–60
Internal fixation devices,
   biomechanics, 177–8
   see also Dorsal spinal plate; Metal implant and bone cement; vertebral spinal plate
Intervertebral discs,
   chondroid metamorphosis, 16
   disc extrusion, 16
   disc protrusion, 16

   fibroid metamorphosis, 16
   functional anatomy, 15–16
   see also Disc herniation
Intervertebral foramen, 12
Intracranial imaging, 53
Intracranial lesions, 35
Intracranial pressure, raised, 35, 36
Iohexol, 46, 48, 63, 64
Ischaemic myelopathy (fibrocartilaginous embolism), 32, 33, 196
Ischaemic neuromyopathy (aortic embolism, iliac thrombosis), 198–9
Isofluorane, 63

J
Jack Russell terrier, 192 fig.

K
Ketoconazole, 198

L
L1/L2, 87 figs.
L5, 47
L6/L7, 181
L7 spinal nerve, 122
L7/S1,
   disc protrusion, 122
   normal relationship, 123 fig.
Lag screw fixation, 148
Laminectomy, 63
   and dorsal foramenotomy,
      complications, 134
      postoperative care, 134
      procedure, 127–34
      prognosis, 134
   healing, 64–5
   membrane, 134
Laminectomy membranes, 152
Large breed dogs,
   cardiac dysfunction, 61
   cardiomyopathy, 140
   CCSM, 135
   congenital abnormality of dens, 109 fig.
   degenerative myelopathy, 193
   discospondylitis, 194
   FCE, 196
   lumbosacral disease, 122
   myelography, 48
   see also specific species
Leukoencephalomalacia, 199
Ligaments,
   dorsal atlantoaxial rupture, 109 fig.
   functional anatomy, 17–18
   tranverse ligament of atlas rupture, 109 fig.
Limb flexion, passive, 208
LMN, see Lower motor neuron system
Longus colli muscle, 82
Loperamide, 215
Lower motor neuron (LMN) system, 11
   bladder, 25
   electromyography, 54
   lesion severity, 30
   lumbosacral disease, 122, 123
   patient examination, 27, 28–9, 30
   thoracolumbar disease, 86
Lumbar intumescence, 29
Lumbar myelography, 47–8
Lumbar spinal puncture, 39–40
Lumbosacral discography, 48
Lumbosacral disease, 122–34
   clinical signs, 123–4
   diagnosis, 124–7
      clinical electrophysiology, 127
      differential, 124–5
      epidurography, 126
      myelography, 126
      other techniques, 127
      survey radiography, 125–6
   discospondylitis, 125 figs., 126, 127
   dorsal fusion fixation, 134
   dorsal laminectomy and foramenotomy, 127–34
   nonsurgical, 127
   spondylosis deformans, 126 figs., 126
   surgery, indications, 127
Lumbosacral intumescence, 48
Lumbosacral joint, 122, 181
Lumbosacral myelography, 47, 48
Lumbosacral plexus tumour, 156, 167

Lumbosacral spine,
   epidurography, 48
   MRI, 53
   radiography, 46
Lumbosacral vertebrae, 9, 14–15
Lymphoma, 34, 42, 158, 159, 168

M
Magnetic resonance imaging (MRI), 53
Mandelic acid, 215
Mannitol, 38
Manx cat, 200
Massage, 208
Melaena, 216
Meninges, 10
Meningiomas, 42, 168
   in cat, 51 fig.
Meningitis,
   aseptic, 42 fig., 197
   breed–specific, 197
   myelography, 48
   steroid-responsive, 197
Meningoencephalomyelitis, 41, 198, 200
   bacterial, 42
   granulomatous, 42
   noninfectious suppurative, 42
Mental attitude, 183, 208 fig., 210
Meperidine (pethidine), 63
Metabolic diseases, 34
Metaclopramide, 216
Metal implant and bone cement, 173, 176, 185
   in CCSM, 144–5
   complications, 154
   implant failure, 153–4
   pin, 187–8, 190
   pin/screw, 178
   screw, 187, 188–90
Methenamine, 215
Methocarbamol, 70, 83, 107, 205
Methoxyfluorane, 63
Methylprednisolone sodium succinate, 38, 62–3, 159, 167, 196
   after trauma, 171, 172, 179
   postoperative, 108, 142, 190
Microbiology, 34
Miniature schanuzer, 196, 217 fig.
Minihemilaminectomy, 98–9, 107
Minocycline, 195
Misoprostol, 215, 216
Morphine, 203, 204 table
Multiple cartilaginous exostoses (osteochondromatosis), 199
Muscle,
   atrophy, 27, 156
   postoperative spasm, 205
   relaxation, 63
   strength, 23
   tone, 28
Myelodysplasia (spinal dysraphism), 200
Myelography,
   cervical, 46–7, 48, 69
   complications, 48
   contrast medium, 46
   indications, 46
   interpretation, 49–51
      column splitting, 50 figs.
      compression patterns, 49
      extradural lesions, 49–50
      'golf tee' pattern, 50 fig.
      intradural extramedullary lesions, 49, 50–1
      intradural intramedullary lesions, 49, 51
   lumbar, 47–8
   prevention of seizures following, 205
   special positions, 48
   stress, 48
   technique, 46–8
Myeloma, 34, 55 fig.
Myelomalacia, 65, 86–7, 179, 192
Myelotomy, 65

N
Naloxone, 204 table
Naltrexone, 204 table
Neck,
   brace, 111, 153
   palpation, 25, 26
Neoplasia, 31, 33, 122, 156–70
   clinical signs, 156
   diagnosis, 42, 55, 156–7
   extradural, 48, 158
   intradural-extramedullary, 158–9
   intramedullary, 159
   nonsurgical treatment, 159
   pathology, 158–9
   surgery,
      complications, 167
      dorsal laminectomy, 159, 160–3, 169
      general principles, 159
      hemilaminectomy, 159, 163–7
      postoperative care, 168
      prognosis, 168
      tumour dissection, 167
Neospora caninum, 35
Nerve root signature, 68
Nerve sheath tumours, 31, 50 fig.
Neuroaxonal dystrophy, 199–200
Neurofibroma, 157 fig.
Neurological examination,
   cranial nerves, 21, 27
   deep pain sensation, 28
   extensor postural thrust, 25
   flexor reflex, 28
   following trauma, 172
   hopping, 23, 25
   in lateral recumbency, 27–9
   locomotor status, 23, 27
   muscle mass, 27
   muscle tone, 28
   panniculus reflex, 25, 26
   patellar reflex, 28
   paw position test, 24, 25
   placing test, 25
   reflex step, 24
   Schiff-Scherington sign, 28, 29 fig.
   spine palpation, 25, 26
   in upright position, 23–7
   wheelbarrowing test, 24
Nitrous oxide, 63
Non-steroidal anti-inflammatory drugs (NSAIDs),
   analgesia, 204, 205 table
   bleeding into gut, 216
   cervical disc disease, 70
   induced platelet dysfunction, 61
   thoracolumbar disc disease, 107
   vomiting due to, 215
Nonchondrodystrophoid breeds, 15
NSAIDs, see Non-steroidal anti-inflammatory drugs

O
Obesity, 61
Opioids, 203–4, 215
Orthopaedic disorders, 21, 124
Osteoarthritis, 61
Osteochondritis, 126
Osteochondromatosis (multiple cartilaginous exostoses), 199
Osteophytes, 136, 148
Osteosarcoma, 54, 156, 157 figs.
Oxymorphone, 204 table

P
Pancreatitis, 203, 215, 216
Panniculus reflex, 25, 26, 86
Patellar reflex, 28, 33
Patient examination,
   aims of, 21
   behavioural response, 28
   history, 21
   lesion localization, 29–30
   lesion severity, 30
   LMN/UMN deficits, 25, 27, 28–9, 30
   neurological, see Neurological examination
   physical, 21
   reflexes, 28–9
Paw position test, 10, 24, 25
Pekingese, 68, 109 fig.
Penicillin, 216
Peripheral neuropathy, 54
Pethidine (meperidine), 63
Phenoxybenzamine, 212
Physiotherapy, 82, 88, 107, 208–10
Pilonidal (dermoid) sinus (epidermoid cyst), 200
Placing test, 25
Pleocytosis, 41, 42, 46

Pneumonia, 61, 153, 203, 206
Pneumothorax, 184
Pomeranian, 109 fig.
Poodle, 109 fig.
Postoperative care,
   flooring for recumbent patients, 206–8
   gastrointestinal disturbances, 215–16
   important clinical signs, 203 table
   nursing,
      cleanliness, 205
      hydration/nutrition, 205
      moving patients, 205
      myelography, 205
      recumbency, 205
      treatment plans, 205, 206
      urinalysis, 205
   pancreatitis, 216
   physiotherapy, 208–10
   urinary tract infections, 215
   urine scald, 216
   wound healing, 216
Prednisolone, 197
Prednisone, 194 table
Preoperative assessment,
   anaesthetic, 63–4
   clinical, 61
   pharmacological, 62
   surgical, 64–6
Pressure sores, 183
Prochlorperazine, 215
Pseudohyperreflexia, 29, 124
Pug, 192, 200
Pulmonary thromboembolism, 218

R
Radial nerve injuries, 26
Radiculomyelopathy, chronic degenerative, 193–4
Radiography,
   atlantoaxial joint, 44
   cervical spine, 43–4, 69
   chest, 61
   general principles, 49–51
   lumbosacral spine, 46
   positioning aids, 43
   stress, spinal fractures, 177
   thoracolumbar spine, 45
Radiotherapy, 149, 168, 169
Ranitidine, 215
Recumbent patients,
   and decubital ulcer, 218
   flooring for, 206–8
Reflex step, 24
Reflexes, 28–9, 30
Reperfusion injury, 62, 159
Reticulosis (granulomatous meningoencephalomyelitis), 197
Rhodesian ridgeback, 192, 200
Rib head disarticulation, 184, 185 fig.
Rottweiler, 52–3, 195 fig., 199
Rub sores, 181, 182

S
Sacrocaudal dysgenesis, 200
Sacrocaudal fracture (luxation), 181
Sacrum, 15, 122
Schiff-Scherrington sign, 12, 28, 29 fig., 30
Sciatic nerve, 29, 54
Scintigraphy, 54
Screw and washer technique, 146–8, 154
Sedation, 172
Segmental fixation, modified, 184, 186
Self-mutilation, 210 fig.
Serology, 34
Seromas, 216
Scrum creatinine kinase, 34
Shih Tzu, 68, 200
Skin disorders, 61
Slings, 208
Spaniel, 68, 157 fig.
Spina bifida, 33, 200
Spinal cord,
   atrophy, 53, 138
   concussion, 171
   functional anatomy, 8–9
   ischaemia, 64
   motor tracts,
      ascending, 13
      descending, 11–12

segments, relationship to vertebrae, 9
sensory tracts, ascending, 10–11
swelling, 51 fig., 65
transverse section, 8
Spinal cord evoked response, 55
Spinal dysraphism (myelodysplasia), 200
Spinal fracture (luxation), 122
    classification,
        anatomical, 173–5
        stability, 175–7
        stress radiography, 177
    treatment,
        cervical, 180
        conservative, 181, see also External splints
        deep pain sensation, 178–80
        hemilaminectomy, 178, 179
        L6/L7 and lumbosacral junction, 181
        sacrocaudal and tail avulsions, 181
        thoracic/lumbar spine, 181
    see also External splints, Internal fixation devices
Spinal nerves, 8
Spinal plates, see Dorsal spinal plate, Vertebral spinal plate
Spinal stapling, 186
Spinal trauma, 33, 54, 173
    analgesia, opioid, 203
    associated injuries, 171
    and atlantoaxial subluxation, 110
    concurrent disease, 61
    CT scan, 173
    initial assessment, 171–2
    neurological examination, 172
    radiography,
        myelography, 173
        survey, 172–3
    treatment, general principles, 171
Spinal tumours, 168, see also Neoplasia
    feline, 168–70
Splints, external, see External splints
Spondylosis deformans, 122, 126, 201
Staphylococcus intermedius, 194, 195, 213
Steptococcus faecalis, 190
Stool softeners, 216
Storage diseases, 201
Streptococcus spp., 194
Streptomycin, 195
Stress leukogram, 35
Sucralfate, 215
Surgical drains, 65–6
Surgical draping, 64
Swimming, 208, 209 fig.
Syringomyelia, 201

T

T12/T13/L1 disc disease, 85
Tail avulsions, 181
Thermal burns, 207, 208 fig.
Thiopentone sodium, 63
Thoracic injuries, 203
Thoracic spinal nerves, 8
Thoracic vertebrae, 9, 14
Thoracolumbar disc disease, 29, 30
    in cat, 108
    chondrodystrophoid/non-chondrodystrophoid, 85
    clinical signs, 85–6
    diagnosis, 85, 87
    dorsolateral hemilaminectomy, 89–98
        compared to dorsal technique, 90
        fat graft, 97
        with fenestration, 90, 97
        indications, 90
        procedure, 90–7
        wound closure, 97
    durotomy, 106–7
    high-dose methylprednisolone, 63
    lateral fenestration, 100–6
    minihemilaminectomy, 98–9
    non-surgical treatment, 88–9
    progressive myelomalacia, 86–7
    surgery,
        complications, 64, 107
        postoperative care, 107
        prognosis, 108
        treatment, results compared, 88–9
        UMN/LMN deficits, 30, 86
Thoracolumbar junction, 15

Thoracolumbar spine,
    blood supply, 19
    fracture/luxation, 171
    palpation, 26
    panniculus reflex, 26
    radiography, 45
    trauma, 181, 203
Thrombocytopenia, 61
Thrombolytic therapy, 199
Towel walking, 208
Toxoplasma gondii (toxoplasmosis), 35, 198
Tracking harness, 208, 209 fig.
Transilial pin techniques, 186–7
Trauma,
    analgesia, 172, 203–4
    associated injuries, 171
    differential diagnosis, 173
    head, 35, 203
    initial assessment, 171–2
    neurological examination, 172
    spinal, see Spinal trauma
Trimethoprim-sulpha, 62, 215

U

Ulcer, decubital, 183, 217–18
UMN, see Upper motor neuron system
Unconscious proprioception, 11
Upper motor neuron (UMN) system, 11
    bladder, 25, 211–12
    deficits, and lesion severity, 30
    electromyography, 54
    lesion severity, 30
    thoracolumbar disease, 86
Urethra, innervation, 211
Urinalysis, 34
Urinary function,
    anatomy/physiology, 210
    micturition,
        disorders, 210–11
        pharmacological approach, 211–12
Urinary incontinence, 25, 30
    closed collection system, 214
    urinalysis, 205
Urinary tract,
    infection, 34, 62, 215
    traumatic damage, 172
Urine culture, 34, 35
Urine retention, 34
Urine scald, 181, 183, 214 fig., 216

V

Ventral decompression (slot),
    for CCSM, 139, 141, 142–3
    complications, 82–3
    indications, 70
    postoperative care, 83
    prognosis, 84
    ventral approach, 71–6
Ventral fenestration,
approach, 71–6
in CCSM, 152
complications, 82–3
indications, 70
postoperative care, 83
procedure, 76–7
prognosis, 83
Ventral fusion, 111–17, 120
Ventral slot, see Ventral decompression
Vertebrae,
    anticlinal, 15
    block, 193
    butterfly, 193
    cervical, 9, 13
    congenital anomalies, 192–3
    functional anatomy, 12–15
    hemi(wedge), 192–13
    intervertebral foramen, 12
    lumbosacral, 14–15
    thoracic, 14
    transverse processes, 13
Vertebral arch, 13
Vertebral body,
    anatomy, 12
    biomechanics, 177
    combined with dorsal spinal plate, 173, 176, 177
    metal and cement fixation, seeMetal implant and bone cement
    tumours, 54, 156

Vertebral body plate, 184
    with dorsal spinal plate, 173, 176, 177, 185
Vertebral canal stenosis, 122, 135, 136 fig., 149
Vertebral distraction/fusion, 141, 143–148, see also Metal implant and bone cement; Screw and washer technique
Vertebral fixation devices,
    biomechanics, 177–8
    see also External splints, Internal fixation devices
Vertebral fracture, 171, 173
Vertebral instability, 83, 122
Vertebral sinuses, see Vertebral venous plexus, internal
Vertebral (sub)luxation, 171, 173 fig.
Vertebral tumours, 49, 52–3, 54, 156
Vertebral venous plexus, internal, 19, 82, 107, 139, 142, 153
Vitamin supplements, 194
Vomiting, 215, 216
Von Willebrand's factor (disease), 35, 61, 66, 82, 139

W

Weimaraner, 192, 200, 201
Wheelbarrowing test, 24
Whirlpool bath, 208, 209 fig.
Withdrawal (flexor) reflex, 28
Wound healing, 61, 216
Wound infection, 35, 62, 66, 190

X

Xanthochromia, 42

Y

Yorkshire terrier, 109 fig.